THE CURSE OF BONGOLO FALLS

Dr. David Thompson

THE CURSE OF BONGOLO FALLS

Published By: Trinity Alps Media, Redding, CA @2025

Printed in the United States of America

DEDICATION

"Not to us, O' Lord, not to us,
but to your name goes all the glory
for your unfailing love and faithfulness."

- Psalm 115:1 (NLT)

PRAISE FOR THE CURSE OF BONGOLO FALLS

We have been friends with Dr. David Thompson and Nurse Becky Thompson over four decades and have worked with them at the Bongolo Mission Hospital many times. As detailed in the compelling stories in this book we have seen so many incredible "coincidences" of events in their ministry, frequently at the "11th hour" to know that God was hovering over the development of this amazing medical mission work.

The Curse of Bongolo Falls is a story that will inspire you and make you want to further your impact on the world around you in the name of your Creator.

This book is a comprehensive look at the trials, stresses, victories, and surprises of providing medical care in a resource limited setting—there is a *MacGyver*-like quality, prayerfully sought out by the author, to save lives of people in the middle of the night without all the equipment, personnel, or medications usually available.

Just as one meaningful story concludes, another scene is set that makes you not want to put the book down.

So many of us who have worked at Bongolo Hospital have been inspired by our lessons learned at this mission hospital to continue medical ministry at many other sites in the low- and middle-income countries. We have done over 100 medical trips teaching in Africa frequently with young medical trainees along because of this inspiration."

Ron Johannsen, Clinical Professor of Medicine/Department of Medicine/ University of Minnesota

Colleen Johannsen, Director of International Cardiology/ Division of Cardiology/Hennepin HealthCare

I love this book! I'm not sure whether to categorize it as an adventure story, an autobiography, a collection of (really interesting!) medical cases, a devotional, or a sequel to *Foxe's Book of Martyrs*. But regardless of its classification, once you start reading, you won't be able to put it down. The stories recorded here are not sentimental piety written by a religious humanitarian. Dave Thompson is a realist who lives in the real world, working with real people, who struggle with real pain. Most importantly, he serves a real Savior who offers a real salvation. *The Curse of Bongolo Falls* will ignite your imagination, engage your mind, warm your heart, and make you want to fall on your knees in prayer. I cannot recommend this book strongly enough.

Stan Key
OneWay Ministries – Minister at Large

What a privilege it was to read this stunning autobiography! It is so much more than just another missionary biography. The book you hold in your hands will take you on a journey spanning several continents and multiple generations. Dr. David Thompson tells you so much more than just his story and the story of his beautiful family. Above all, he tells of the wonders of our Almighty God who has faithfully walked with His children through the deepest challenges and highest joys. This book is a testament to the faithfulness of God! Get ready to laugh out loud and shed lots of tears, and when you are finished, you will want to pick it up again and start over! I know I will!

Cindi Taylor - Bethel Missions Pastor

Reading *The Curse of Bongolo Falls* was like being welcomed into the living room of Dr. David Thompson and hearing the stories that shaped his heart and calling. His words carry both the grit of hardship and the joy of God's faithfulness, drawing us into the moments where Christ's light pierced the darkness. As I turned each page, I was reminded that PAACS was born out of this same obedience and courage—a willingness to trust God completely and follow wherever He leads. This book is a beautiful reminder that the "yes" of one faithful servant can ripple across generations, and I am profoundly grateful for the legacy Dr. Thompson has given us.

Susan Koshy, JD, MPH
Chief Executive Officer
Pan-African Academy
of Christian Surgeons (PAACS)

I'm very grateful to Dr. Thompson for preserving the many fascinating, powerful and God-glorifying stories that have led to the establishment of this ministry which has brought the love of Christ to countless people. You'll be encouraged and inspired as you read.

Rev. John Stumbo
President, Christian &
Missionary Alliance

LETTER FROM THE EDITOR

Dear Reader,

Did you know that writers dream in stories? The author's mind is constantly scrutinizing the undulations of life in hopes of finding the mysteries worth sorting out. Like a miner, the writer pans constantly searching for the glimmers of gold that can be woven to into words capable of making the world a better place. When a good story comes from the recesses of the imagination and the experiences of a life lived, it is simply *everything.* Every writer waits his or her entire life for a story like this, and every editor does the same, hoping for something incredible to land upon her desk. *The Curse of Bongolo Falls* is not only a once-in-a-lifetime, extraordinary story, it is also a *true* story. It is the type of story that one could only hope to dream up and yet it all *really happened.*

I still don't know how I was chosen to edit *The Curse of Bongolo Falls.* It is and will always be one of the greatest honors of my life. Dr. David Thompson has chronicled for us a history of how Christianity and modem medicine came to Gabon, Africa. His stories are uniquely human and center around the lives of the people who made these advancements of light into the darkness possible. A child of missionary patients, Thompson grew up witnessing his patient's work in Cambodia and then experiencing their untimely death as they were martyred in Banmethuot, Vietnam. With a call from God to be a missionary doctor, Thompson depicts the origins of missionary work in Gabon with the story of Donald and Dorothy Fairley. Later, he and his family become the torch bearers, witnessing countless miracles during their extensive time with the Gabonese people. Thompson's message throughout the book is how one is to trust and to fully surrender to God, even in the most bleak and heartbreaking situations. Thompson demonstrates how God, never failingly shows up.

Thompson's stories show the astounding and profound ways in which God reveals His nature in the least likely places, like finding a wheel bearing for an old Dodge dump truck in the midst of the jungle. Gabon is a place of mysterious black magic and curses; a place where the history of human sacrifice permeates the spiritual atmosphere. From battling herds of goats, to building a large outhouse, to navigating and crossing the perilous Loutesi River, Thompson's life is an exciting and wild ride within the pages of this story. He is more than a doctor to the people of Gabon; he is a servant in every sense of the word. You'll never forget the scene where Dr. Thompson digs a grave for his patient with his own two hands.

The Curse of Bongolo Falls demonstrates the intersection of the supernatural with the natural world. The novel is woven throughout with the workings of evil spirits scheming against the goodness of God that always prevails. Thompson writes, "A feeling of apprehension passed over me. There was indeed something terribly evil with us on that porch. I could feel the hair stand up on the back of my neck, and my arms were covered with goosebumps!" This book will have you on the edge of your seat and move your heart. Through the author's incredible characterization, you will feel as though you have traveled to Africa and have gotten to know the Gabonese people. Memorable moments such as the tale of "one-eyed Bernard" killing a deadly black mamba with a machete in the attic of the hospital will stay with you forever.

Jesus saves one soul at a time, working through Dr. David, his wife Becky and their team as they establish a hospital in Gabon. Thompson's dedication to the physical and spiritual health of the people of Gabon is an embodiment of the love that God has for these people. This book reveals how much a talented physician and faith in Christ can do with limited resources. Reader, you will see that modern medicine and medical miracles are *both* blessings from the Lord. The advancements of science and the miraculous workings of God to save lives do not preclude one another but are of one source: the love of Jesus Christ.

I must disclose that if you read this book, you will be changed. A story of this magnitude cannot and will not leave the reader the same. This book cannot sell you anything because it is absent of propaganda: it simply is authentically real. When I once asked Dr.

Thompson how he decided to write his stories, he told me that he did not wish to do so. An extremely humble man, Thompson told me that he never wished to write about himself. However, a close friend guided him towards an irrevocable truth: that Thompson's stories were not his own; that they belonged to God. Thompson directed me to Psalm 77 where the psalmist writes, "I will remember the works of the Lord; / Surely, I will remember Your wonders of old. / I will also meditate on all Your work, / and talk of Your deeds," (NKJV, 1.11-12). Some stories simply demand to be told, and this is one of those stories. I am not the same as I was after reading *The Curse of Bongolo Falls.* I feel in my soul the lovely and mysterious heartbeat of Africa, and as a writer I find myself more intrigued by the writings of God than anything my own mind could dare to dream up.

Warm Wishes & Best Regards,
General Editor
Sarah Elizabeth Bartlett

TABLE OF CONTENTS

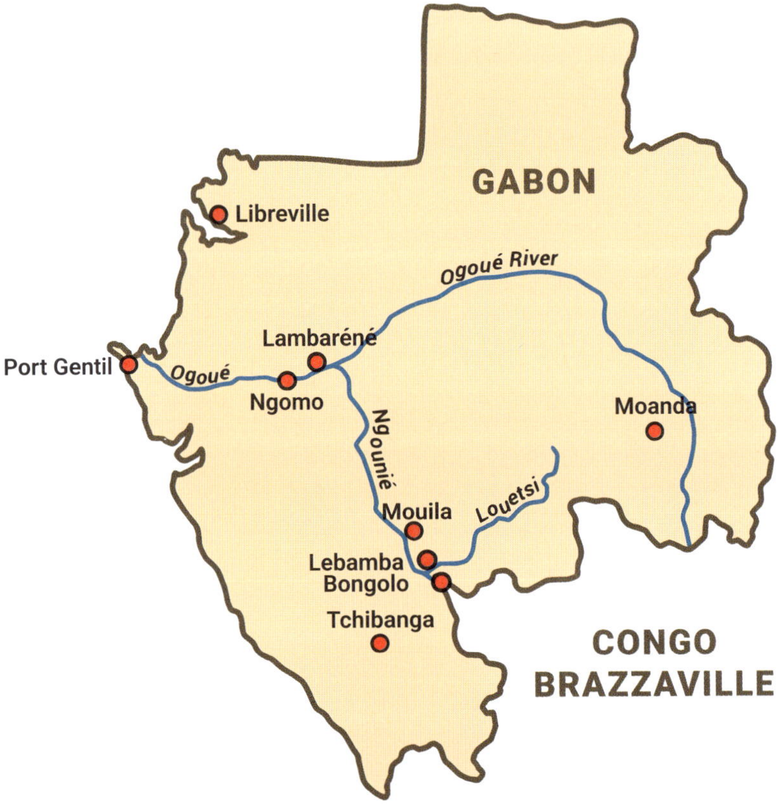

RIVER MAP OF GABON, AFRICA

INTRODUCTION: "WHERE IS THE LORD, THE GOD OF ELIJAH?" (2 KINGS 2:14)

A man's destiny is a curious thing. We often believe that with a good education, a supportive family, and sufficient resources, we can chart a straight course to personal significance. But then God intervenes— and everything changes. He takes over. The path we once imagined for ourselves has become quite different.

In the Old Testament we read where after Elijah the Tishbite was taken up to heaven. Elisha the son of Shaphat picked up Elijah's cloak and struck the waters of the Jordan. The waters parted, and Elisha crossed over. In that moment, Elisha's life and purpose were forever altered. His past was on one side of the Jordan, but his destiny was on the other. His destiny was no longer his own—it belonged to God. Yet the message here is that it wasn't the cloak of Elijah the Tishbite that parted the Jordan, it was Elisha's trust and unconditional dependence on God.

Something similar happened to Dr. David Thompson— "Dr. Dave"—on a remote road from Kratie to Phnom Penh in Cambodia. While still a young man, a harrowing vehicle accident unfolded before his eyes:

"My father knelt beside him and greeted him in Cambodian. As I poured water into a cup for him, my hands were shaking. The man tried to drink, but he was breathing fast and couldn't seem to swallow. My father spoke Cambodian fluently, and he began talking to the man, asking him if he was ready to meet God. But the man shook his head and gasping, said, "Don't—tell me —about— your—God, just help me!"

"In that moment I realized the dying man in front of us was turning away from his only hope for God's forgiveness. My dad prayed for him, and we returned to our car and continued on. But I will never forget the overwhelming sorrow that gripped my heart. In the weeks and months that followed, I thought of the dying man often and grieved for him. I couldn't stop thinking, 'If we could have *helped* him, he might have lived long enough to listen to us, hear the gospel, and believe in Jesus!'"

In that moment, everything changed. Before, Dr. Dave was a gifted young man with ambitions of success and prosperity. Afterward, he was marked by God and filled with purpose and unwavering commitment. A new destiny began—along with a path of hardship and faith.

What can God do with a man whose heart is fully surrendered to him? That is the story that unfolds here. In a larger sense, this is also your story. There is a pattern here of what happens to all who are called and stamped by God. For those who are called, Jesus is our destiny, our only hope, and our sole reward as we listen, observe, and obey Him in the work He has set before us.

Because of Dr. Dave's willingness to allow God to work through him, thousands of people were healed and thousands more turned from demon worship (with all the horrific consequences) to a living and dependent trust in Jesus. The lives of the Gabonese people were changed, the nation of Gabon was changed, and through the organization he founded, the continent of Africa was forever altered for the glory of God. Moreover, other dedicated God-fearing missionaries were also challenged as they serve the poor, the widow, the orphan, and the outcast.

Here is a story that compels.

Once we adjust to the *what* and the *why,* we are drawn into the stories of *how* God worked powerful miracles through David's life. Only about 20% of these are given here. The full picture is much larger.

Yet this is not just a catalog of miracles. It is the gradual unfolding of a man's relationship with the living God—refined through trials, humility, despair, and patience. The outcome is a profoundly humble servant whose steps are guided by the Living God.

Dr. Dave is neither a legend nor a symbolic figure. He is a real person, and he is easily approachable. He lives among us, offering his life generously to others. He repairs the bodies of men, but he also repairs their souls. Moreover, he never shies away from speaking honestly with his patients about the state of their spiritual lives.

After reading this remarkable work, you may find yourself asking, *"What about me? Could God change the world through someone like me? Does He have plans for me that I'm missing? Am I allowing His Spirit to guide me through life?"*

The answer to the first questions is "Yes." God will work through anyone who is willing, obedient, and fully surrendered to Him. The road may be long. The cost may be great. But no matter. God is in charge. He will shape your character to His satisfaction in ways you never expected.

You see, God is in the character business. May these stories give you the courage to take God's hand and walk with Him.

Les Reading

Chapter One:

SPYING OUT THE LAND

Chief Boudiongo's Gift

In 1933 two Americans men trudge wearily into the village of Makombo. Ten African porters and a young man named Ndoba follow them, carrying loads on their heads. The largest thatched house in the village belongs to the village chief. A fence of sticks pounded into the ground around the house gives it a kind of ragged prominence. The rest of the village includes thirty or forty thatched houses with bark walls. Ndoba is a young man from a friendly tribe 4-1/2 days march to the north and serves as their cook and interpreter. The foreigners' khaki clothes and leather boots are soaked with recent rains and stained with grime and mud. For the past several months, they've been searching for a place to establish a base among South Gabon's southern tribes. One tribe refused to welcome them because they had nothing to trade for ivory. Two others showed interest but lacked what the Americans were looking for. The unexpected appearance of the foreigners produces a flurry of barking dogs, squawking chickens, excited children, and elders staring at them from darkened doorways. Eventually, a muscular, bare-chested African in his 30's steps out of his house and approaches the travelers. He is the village chief, and he greets them in French and asks who they are. The older white man introduces himself as Joseph and his younger colleague as Donald. Joseph explains they are Americans, and their porters are from a friendly tribe 10 days away.

The chief introduces himself as Boudiongo and invites the strangers to put down their backpacks and sit on several benches in front of his house.

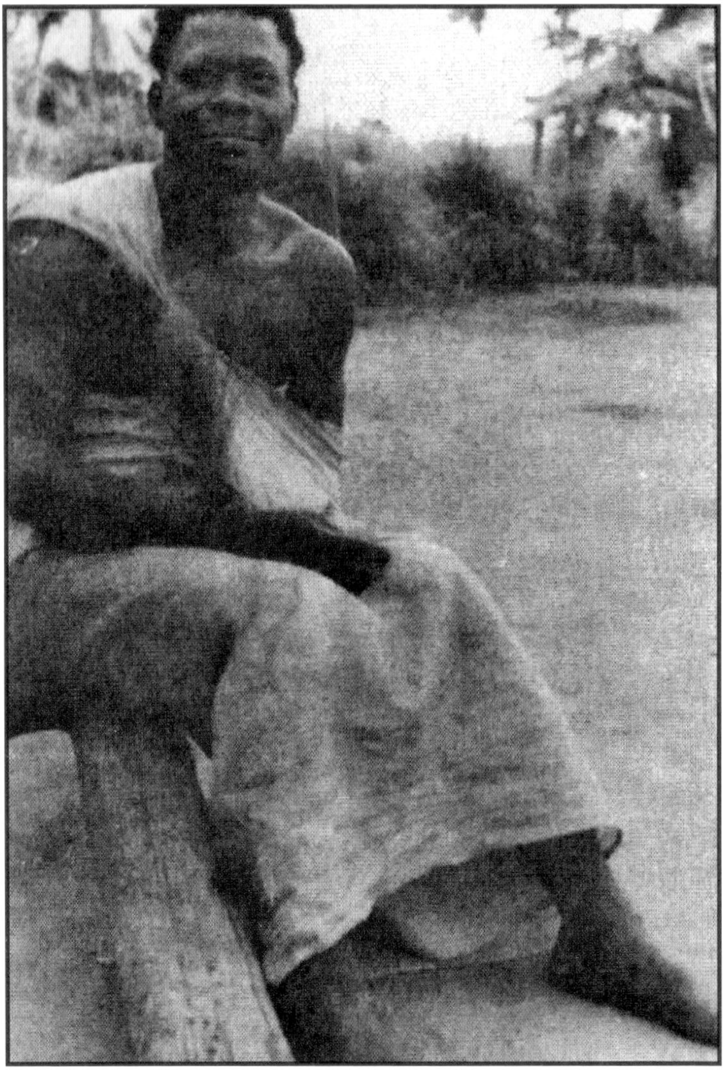

Photo of Chief Boudiongo, 1934

The porters gratefully lower their loads and seat themselves in the shade of a nearby tree. After everyone is seated, Chief Boudiongo asks the strangers why they have come. Joseph explains they are seeking a place that is near a waterfall and has plentiful sand and gravel. They are looking for workers they could hire to help them clear land, build houses, and plant gardens.

By this time the village children are peeking from neighboring houses to get a glimpse of the strangers. White people are rare this far south, and now there are two of them in plain sight, in the middle of their village!

Boudiongo's experience with Gabon's French masters has made him wary, but after hesitating, he acknowledges there is a waterfall upriver about half a mile away, and abundant in both sand and gravel. He also states that his people know everything there is to know about making gardens and growing food in the jungle. When the white men politely request to see the falls, Chief Boudiongo seems reluctant at first, but then gets up and motions for them to follow. A few minutes later they stop at the confluence of two rivers: the Louetsi River on their left that flows from the west and joins the larger Ngounié River that flows from south to north. Boudiongo motions them to a 30-foot dugout canoe tied to a tree on the bank and calls five of his men to row them upriver. The Americans are surprised when the men row them upriver standing completely upright.

After 30 minutes, they round a curve and see a modest waterfall 100 yards upriver. White water from the top of the falls pours roughly 25 feet down to a jumble of massive rocks. The waterfall is about 40 feet wide, and as they approach it, the chief points to clean sand on both banks.

Boudiongo directs his men to row to the left side of the river where there is a sandy bank. The white men take a few minutes to wash the mud off their clothes and boots and wet their faces. Then one of them takes out a strange black box with a glass eye, puts it to his face, and points it at the falls. He tries to explain to Boudiongo that he is taking a photo, but Boudiongo is looking around nervously. Joseph asks him if the falls have a name, and the chief says one word, "Bongolo." Donald asks what it means, and Boudiongo explains that it has no meaning, but is a repetitive sound the river makes during the Dry Season when the flow of water is greatly reduced. During that season the sound it makes is "bong-go-lo."

Boudiongo then leads his visitors upriver along whitewater rapids. As they walk, he stops and points across the river to magnificent, one-hundred-foot-high limestone cliffs. As he leads them downriver toward the falls, Joseph and Donald note that the limestone cliffs on the opposite shore gradually drop in height until they reach the falls.

Boudiongo stops and because of the roar of the whitewater rapids, silently points out the limestone cliff directly above the falls. Then he turns abruptly and leads them back to the canoe. As his men row them back to the village, Donald asks Boudiongo why he pointed to the cliff above the falls. Boudiongo shakes his head and says to them, "later." As they paddle downriver the roar of the falls is gradually replaced with the singing and chirping of myriads of birds and millions of insects that thrive in the dense forests on both sides of the river.

Back in Makombo, the visitors notice a man sitting outside the chief 's house. He is wearing a loincloth and has a collection of parrot feathers in his hair. He seems displeased to see the strangers. Boudiongo introduces him in French as "the Nganga," the tribe's name for a traditional healer. The Americans greet him politely, but the Nganga rudely ignores them, turns, and walks away.

As the sun dips behind the trees, Boudiongo leads them inside a large bark and thatch house at the edge of the village that is furnished inside with beds, a table and chairs, kerosine lanterns for light, and a living area with armchairs. He explains it is the guest house for colonial officials and foreign visitors, then bids them a good night. Young Ndoba builds a fire behind the house and cooks a simple meal for the Americans and their porters. As they enjoy their meal, a thunderstorm announces it coming with wind, lightning, and thunder. The men take shelter in the guest house, and for the next hour, a torrential storm pummels the village.

Early the next morning, Boudiongo invites Joseph and Donald to a guided tour of the land on the other side of the falls. They are surprised that this time the Nganga will accompany them. The chief leads everyone to the river's edge where the oarsmen wait in the dug-out canoe. Before they board, the chief picks up a stick and draws a half-circle in the sand. He then explains that above the falls the river descends in a broad half-circle, until it reaches the falls.

It takes the oarsmen half an hour to row them upriver until they reach the falls. This time Boudiongo has the oarsmen pull to shore on the right side of the river. The Nganga takes the lead, followed by the chief and his rowers. They walk up an overgrown path that leads them through heavily wooded hills. Remarkably, the land shows no sign of human activity or presence. As they climb, the visitors are impressed by massive hardwood trees on every side, many of which would have taken more than 400 years to grow so large. When asked why there are no gardens, the chief explains, "The spirits in this place are angry and evil. It's not safe for anyone to come here without the Nganga."

Thirty minutes later the visitors find themselves on the edge of the 50-foot cliff above the falls that Boudiongo silently pointed out to them the previous day. They step to the edge and peer over the ledge, surveying the breath-taking drop to the whitewater and rocks below. The Americans are surprised that they are the only ones to look over the edge at the falls. During the next hour, the chief leads them away from the falls and upriver to the top of the 100-foot limestone cliffs that they marveled at the day prior. Their amazement and admiration of the property seems to please the chief and irritate the Nganga. A short time later, the Nganga and the chief get into a heated argument that continues until they return to the river and are rowed back to the village.

The next morning, the chief and several of his wives bring a large basket of ripe mangoes for their breakfast. As they eat the luscious fruit, the chief asks what they thought of the property and what their plans are.

Joseph asks him if he, Donald, and Ndoba can go alone to see the land on the other side of the falls and explore. Boudiongo's smile fades and he explains, "It's too dangerous for you to go over there without the Nganga. When we argued today, the Nganga told me he didn't want you over there again."

After a silence, Joseph says, "Thank you for your concern, Chief Boudiongo, but we are not afraid of the evil spirits on the other side. The God who made the world and the stars is protecting us, and he is far more powerful than any spirits!"

The chief shakes his head and walks away, but half an hour later returns and says, "I'll have my men take you up to the falls in the canoe. They'll wait for you at the river's edge until an hour before the sun goes down. May your God guide and protect you."

The next day, Boudiongo's men row Joseph, Donald, and their helper Ndoba to the land below the falls. For the rest of the day, the three men explore the land, going much farther than before. They discover that the river curves around more than half of the site, enclosing more than 30 acres of forested land. Eight hours later when they return to Boudiongo's canoe, his men are waiting for them. When they arrive back in the village, the chief is visibly relieved to see that no harm has come to them.

That night the chief invites them to a feast of antelope meat, pounded and fermented manioc, boiled plantain, roasted giant palm caterpillars, mangoes, and palm wine. It is a magnificent feast, and though the Americans decline the palm wine, they eat everything else.

After the meal, Joseph asks Boudiongo a question that is on the Americans' minds: "What spirits are you and your people afraid of on the other side of the river? Today as we explored, nothing troubled us."

Boudiongo is silent for a minute or two, then says quietly, "That your visit was peaceful is a good sign, a very good sign. If you will come here with your wives and children and build houses and gardens on the land on both sides of the falls, I will give you all the land inside the half-circle of the river that you explored today. I will also give you land on the other side of the falls!"

Joseph and Donald thank Boudiongo for his generous offer, but they are surprised that he has asked nothing from them in return. Joseph finally asks "Chief Boudiongo, you have received us with great kindness, even though we are strangers and have offered you and your people nothing in return." He hesitated, for a moment, then asks, "Why?"

As the chief 's wives collect the leftovers and slip away, Boudiongo is quiet. Then he says to the Americans, "There is something more I need to tell you. There is a terrible secret about Bongolo Falls and the land on both sides of it that you need to know. The land is cursed!" He pauses, as though looking for words. "Everyone who has challenged the curse and has tried to live on that land has disappeared without a trace, usually within days! As long as we have lived in this village, this has been true. Is your God able to protect you from the angry spirits that live there, and from this fearsome curse?"

Donald replies without hesitating, "There is no spirit in the world more powerful than our God Jesus." When Boudiongo shakes his head Donald asks, "How do the people die when they try to live on that side of the river?"

Lowering his voice to almost a whisper and looking around fearfully, Boudiongo says "The spirits that live under the falls are the spirits of the *evil* people the Ngangas have executed."

Stunned by Boudiongo's revelation, Donald inquires further, "How do the Ngangas execute people?"

Boudiongo is silent for several minutes, thinking about his answer. Finally, he says, "The Ngangas and their helpers tie up those who are guilty of killing our people by sorcery. Then we take them up to the cliff above the falls, tie them up, and throw them over!"

Boudiongo's admission has left Joseph and Donald speechless! Finally, Joseph asks, "How do the Ngangas know who is using sorcery to kill your people?"

Boudiongo sighs, then explains, "The Nganga's ask the *good* spirits—Bwiti and Mwiri, to tell them who in the village is killing our people with sorcery."

Struggling to understand such a bizarre concept, Donald asks, "How do people in your village kill their neighbors with sorcery?"

After glancing around again to be sure no one else is listening, Boudiongo says, "Evil spirits kill our people when they're fishing and fall into the river and drown! Others are injured when they chop down a tree and it falls on them! Sometimes when people go to the river to bathe, a giant python drops on them from a tree above, crushes them in its coils, and eats them! Sometimes when a woman is washing clothes at the river a crocodile comes out of the water, drags her into the river and devours her! Others die when evil people use sorcery and call leopards to attack people as they work in their gardens, or when they call on evil spirits to bring fevers that don't go away until the victim goes crazy and dies! Many of our young women die in childbirth. None of these deaths are accidental! No deaths here are accidental, except when really, really old people die, or babies born too soon die. It's always the sorcery of secret enemies that cause my people to die!"

The Americans are genuinely shocked by the chief 's explanation. Joseph finally asks, "Why do the spirits of people who are thrown over the cliff live under the falls? Don't their dead bodies go downriver?"

Boudiongo shakes his head. "I don't know why their spirits live there, but that's why we stay away from Bongolo Falls and the land around it. The bodies of the people the Nganga executes float downriver, but their spirits remain under the falls forever and seek revenge. When anyone enters their forbidden land across the river without the protection of the Nganga, the angry spirits of the dead kill them."

Shaking his head in amazement Joseph asks, "How many have died this way?"

Boudiongo sighs and answers softly, "Too many, too many. In my lifetime, maybe twenty or thirty. I've lost count. But before my time, there were more killings. And every time one of my people dies because of sorcery, we execute the guilty person, and two more of my people are gone from our village."

Joseph asks one final question, "Do the accused ever confess before they are thrown off the cliff?"

Boudiongo shakes his head. "No, they always claim they're innocent, but the good spirits Bwiti and Mwiri who protect us never lie!" After a long silence, Boudiongo sweeps his hand toward the bark huts that make up his village and says, "In my grandfather's day we were a great village, and we had two or three times as many people. But now, we are all who are left. Many who are accused run away and never come back. If I knew how to stop the killings, I would." And that was the end of their conversation.

Their hearts heavy, the two Americans realize that the curse of Bongolo Falls is certainly not from angry human souls that live under the Falls, but from the very gods the people worship. They soon learn that when the Ngangas smear white clay on their faces and induce the men to drink the drug that's made from the root of the Iboga plant, the men will pound their drums and dance for Bwiti and Mwiri all night long, without stopping. The punishment for any woman or child who dares watch is death. Claiming to be "good spirits" and the healers and saviors of the people, Bwiti and Mwiri have in fact become their worst enemies.

God saw it all, and He did not forget them.

Challenging the Curse

No one is alive today who knows when and at whose invitation the dark and evil gods of Mwiri and Bwiti entered the forests of south Gabon. There are few forests in the world today as great in trees and fauna, and as rich in wildlife, grandeur, and beauty as the forests of Gabon. The first people came to the land were the Pygmies, and they did not worship demon Gods but the unknown Creator of their world, though they knew very little about him except from the beauty of his works. When invaders twice their size crushed them in battle, the little people found refuge in the dense forests, and learned to live in tiny, temporary huts, moving frequently. But the little people were not afraid of the forest. Using their silent Basenji dogs and setting traps with nets woven from bark, they herded deer, antelopes, and other small animals into their nets and swiftly clubbed them to death. When Gabon's fierce forest elephants attacked them, the little people's greatest hunters learned to slip under the largest of them, and with a single thrust of a spear, pierce the elephant's heart! Until the bigger tribes showed up, the Pygmies were the only humans who lived in Gabon's southern forests.

But then the "big people" came into south Gabon in successive waves, with tribal names like Bapounou, Banzebi, Mitsogo, Massangou, Eshira, Bateke, and Bavoumbou. Each tribe carved out its own territory, and all of them despised the little people, considering them to be only slightly more intelligent than animals. But the big people soon learned that the "little people:' as they called them, could appear and disappear like ghosts, and when threatened, could shoot lethal, almost invisible poison-tipped arrows from their tiny bows.

The migrating tribes established large villages and brought with them the demon gods that had failed them in the lands they fled. They called their high priests "Ngangas:' which means "healers:' though their natural cures were only occasionally helpful and often made their patients worse. As migrating tribes entered Gabon's forests, they encountered sleeping sickness, a mysterious disease transmitted from the bite of an infected Tsetse fly that caused madness. Not until 1892 would the origin of the disease be discovered by Europeans. Until then, Africans living in Gabon's forests attributed the disease to evil spirits that sent by secret enemies.

In time, another disease appeared, causing people affected to lose feeling in their fingers, feet and toes until they rotted and dropped off. Some even lost their lips and noses. The Ngangas attributed the new disease to evil spirits, never guessing that it was carried by anteaters and other small animals that the people frequently trapped, butchered, and ate. Regardless of the cause, every tragedy served to increase the Nganga's power and the people's fear of "evil spirits."

In time, Bwiti and Mwiri did what all demons do: they enlisted hosts of other demons for the people to worship or fear, making the Ngangas more powerful than the village chiefs. But there was one far more powerful than the Ngangas, and He was grieved by the suffering of the people.

Donald and Dorothy Fairley[1]

On November 26, 1905, a boy was born to Archibald and Emma Fairley, in the town of Zion, Illinois. His parents named him Donald. His father was a Presbyterian pastor who had emigrated from Scotland. By the time Donald was a teenager, he demonstrated unusual intelligence and an almost uncanny ability to do anything he put his mind to. By the age of 15, he could cook delicious meals, fix anything mechanical or electrical, build and repair houses, raise bees, grow all kinds of garden foods, graft fruit trees, hunt, and drive trucks! But his greatest fascination was animals, especially wild animals. But though his father preached the gospel from his pulpit, and his mother entreated young Donald to follow Jesus, he had different plans for his life.

In 1920 when he was 15, his father accepted a call to pastor a church in Oregon. Leaving his family in Illinois, he traveled ahead to find a house. When the house was ready, Donald drove his mother, brother and two sisters and all their belongings from Illinois to Oregon in a rented truck.

The following year he surprised his parents by announcing his plans to travel by ship to Alaska for the summer so he could earn big money at a Salmon canning factory. Against his parents' wishes, he purchased a train ticket to Seattle. During the night as he slept, he

1 The stories of Don Fairley come from his book, *Hunting Pygmy Hunters,* 1929

was robbed of everything he owned. Though he knew no one and had lost all his money, when he arrived in Seattle he went to the docks and finagled his way onto a boatload of Filipino workers headed for a Salmon canning factory in Alaska! The only non-Filipino on the boat, Don volunteered to help in the kitchen. His cooking skills surprised and delighted the passengers and crew and soon won their admiration. When the ship arrived in Ketchikan, Alaska, he found work at a Salmon packing plant. He was the only Caucasian worker in the factory, and his hard work, mechanical skills, and leadership abilities caught the attention of the plant manager. A month later and at the age of 16, Donald was promoted to the job of foreman!

During his time in Alaska, Donald thought little about God. He had heard the plan of salvation so many times that it had ceased to mean anything. One night he got into a violent argument with a Filipino worker about religion. Don became so angry that their discussion escalated into a shouting match. Don was ready to kill him and headed to his room to get a pistol he carried in his bag. But as he pulled the gun out of the bag, he heard God say to him, "*Donald Fairley, you are at a crossroads in your life. What you do now will decide if you will go up or go down.*" Sobered and surprised, Don put the gun away and instead opened a New Testament he had packed in his bag. As he read God's word, he realized that if he continued to live for himself, he would end up in hell. Closing his eyes, he asked God to forgive him and save him. Later that same night he made peace with the Filipino man he had contemplated murdering. When the Summer ended, Don returned to Seattle and his family with a changed heart.

Over the next two years Don became a leader among the youth in his church, even leading other young men and women to faith. On July 4, 1924, something unexpected happened that changed his life. A large group of high school students and recent graduates decided to spend the day swimming in the Willamette River near Springfield, Oregon. Don took his two younger sisters with him and joined them. As he stood on the shore keeping an eye on his sisters, he noticed four young women playing in the river, including a sixteen-year-old who was not the least bit timid in her knee-length bathing suit! As the young people played, a log drifted serenely down the river. The four girls pulled the log closer to shore and climbed onto it. As it drifted into deeper water, some boys nearby slipped underneath the log and playfully tipped the girls off. Three of them squealed and laughed as they fell, but the fourth girl was totally surprised and fell backward into the water.

Don watched for her to reappear, but as seconds passed, she didn't resurface. The other girls were swimming back to shore, oblivious to what was happening to their friend. As the seconds ticked on, Don shouted, "There's a girl missing! There's a girl drowning!" Nobody seemed to hear him, so he dove into the water and swam to where she had disappeared. Seeing no sign of her under the water, he surfaced and yelled for help. By now over a minute had elapsed, and he realized the current was probably carrying her downstream. In a panic, he swam back to shallower water, ran downriver 30 yards, and dove under water to look for her. Almost immediately he bumped into her! She was struggling weakly, but when she felt Don brush against her, she wrapped her arms and legs around him. Remembering his training as a lifeguard, Don brought his knees up into her stomach as hard as he could. Stunned, she let go. Circling behind her, he grabbed her hair and headed for the surface.

By then the current was pushing them both downstream, and Don was tiring in water over his head. Just then a fisherman saw what was happening and waded out into the river as far as he could. As the current swept Don and the now unconscious girl downstream, Don grabbed the fisherman's outstretched hand, and the two of them pulled the unconscious girl to shore. Don immediately began CPR, and an anxious crowd gathered. After several minutes the girl coughed and began to breathe. As she recovered, her friends told Don that her name was Dorothy Knowles.

A few days later Don tried to visit Dorothy at her home, but her mother, though grateful to the young man who had saved her daughter's life, told him he couldn't see her and asked him not to come back! Dorothy was only 16, and her mother wanted her to get a college education before getting into a serious relationship with a young man. Don was only a year older, but when he continued to persist, Dorothy's mother went to see Don's mother. They both agreed that their children were too young to be dating. Two years later Don's family moved to southern California.

Within a few months of moving to Los Angeles, Don found a job at the Featherhill Ranch Zoo. His love for animals and his willingness to work hard made him an instant favorite with the zoo's owner, his animal caretaker, and his animal trainer. One of the animals Don took care of was a large male elephant. Later that year there was a minor earthquake in Los Angeles, and the elephant broke the chain on his foot and ran out of the zoo in a panic. Don followed him on foot, calling for the elephant to stop. In a rage, the elephant turned on Don. Without thinking, Don laid down on the road in front of the panicked animal. The move confused the elephant and saved Don's life. Eventually, Don was able to calm the animal and lead him back to his cage. For the rest of the night, he slept next elephant. In the days that followed, the grateful owner of the Zoo promoted Don and invited him to join in the animal shows. Don had an uncanny ability to win the trust of animals, and soon included in shows involving chimpanzees, lions, and even tigers!

In the Spring of 1926, Dorothy Knowles and her mother came to Santa Barbara to visit the Fairley family. Dorothy had never forgotten Don's courage in rescuing her from drowning and still cared deeply for him. At the same time, she felt God was calling her to become a missionary. As they talked, Don described his work at the zoo and explained that he saw no reason to leave it and become a missionary. A few days later Dorothy and her mother returned to Seattle.

Several months later as Don was walking home from work, he passed the open door of a church. A missionary was showing a black and white film with scenes of the jungle. Thinking he might see pictures of wild animals, Don quietly entered and sat in the back of. But instead seeing animals, Don saw pictures of tribal people in the mountains of Vietnam and Laos, living under the most primitive conditions imaginable. As he sat transfixed, God's spirit said to him, "*What is more important, Don, animals that live for a time and then die, or these people whose souls live forever?*" It was the first time Don had considered that people should be more important to him than animals, and that God might hold him personally responsible for the fate of people who lived and died without ever hearing the gospel!

Within days, Don realized that God was calling him to preach the gospel to people who had never heard of Jesus and were living in darkness. At first, he was reluctant to tell Dorothy about the movie that had so affected him, but he finally called her and shared what happened. Surprised, she told him that she had already made plans to enter Bible school at BIOLA. Now it was Don's turn to be surprised! Not one to hesitate when he saw an opportunity, soon after her mother brought her to Los Angeles to start school, Don asked her to marry him. She smiled, took his hand, and without hesitating said, "Yes, I will marry you!"

The next day Don asked Dorothy's parents for permission to marry her, but Mrs. Knowles again said "no!" She wanted her daughter to complete her education before marrying and was not willing to consider anything else! But a month later, Don and Dorothy were no longer willing to wait. On September 1, 1926, they slipped over to the Alliance Chapel in Santa Barbara where a sympathetic pastor married them, without either set of parents in attendance. Don's two sisters served as witnesses.

The news came as a shock to both sets of parents. Not surprisingly, Dorothy's mother tracked the newlyweds down and surprised them on their honeymoon! After a long and awkward conversation, she made peace with her daughter and new son-in-law and blessed them. Soon after, Don quit his job at the zoo, and for the next two years he and Dorothy studied the Bible at BIOLA. Two years later, they transferred to the Alliance's Missionary Training Institute in Nyack, New York.

Midway through their last year at the Missionary Training Institute in Nyack, the Foreign Secretary of the Alliance and his wife invited the Fairleys to their house for dinner. His name was Dr. Snead, and he and his wife were retired Alliance missionaries. After the meal Dr. Snead laid out on the living room floor a huge map of Africa and pointed out places where no missionary had ever gone. The couple explored the map on their knees and were stunned to see vast areas in Equatorial Africa where countless tribes were still living in spiritual darkness. After they stood up, Dr. Snead pointed out that the indentations on the map from their knees were over the southern half of the country of Gabon, an area that France had kept closed to all missionaries for 50 years!

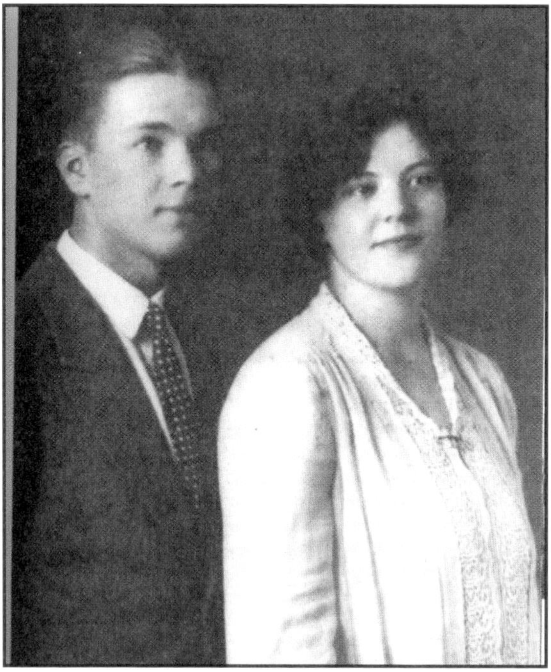

Donald and Dorothy Fairley

Midway through their last year at the Missionary Training Institute in Nyack, the Foreign Secretary of the Alliance and his wife invited the Fairleys to their house for dinner. His name was Dr. Snead, and he and his wife were retired Alliance missionaries. After the meal Dr. Snead laid out on the living room floor a huge map of Africa and pointed out places where no missionary had ever gone. The couple explored map on their knees and were stunned to see vast areas in Equatorial Africa where countless tribes were still living in spiritual darkness. After they stood up, Dr. Snead pointed out that the in- dentations on the map from their knees were over the southern half of the country of Gabon, an area that France had kept closed to all missionaries for 50 years!

At the end of their training at the Missionary Institute, the Alliance appointed the Fairleys to the western side of Belgian Congo, now known as the Democratic Republic of Congo. The Fairleys were assigned to the Alliance's Congolese team that by then included 20 missionaries.

In 1933, the French colonial government ended an economic agreement that it had signed in 1894 with the Society of the Upper Ogooué (S.H.O). The agreement gave the S.H.O. vast land concessions for the purpose of resource exploitation. It would seem that an economic agreement would not preclude the entrance of Christian missionaries into the S.H.O. concession, but the S.H.O. saw it differently, since their greatest profits would require free labor, and the concessionary system often involved forced labor where local people were compelled to work for the companies in lieu of paying taxes. Since missionaries might interfere in their freedom, the S.H.O. refused to allow any evangelistic work south of the Ogooué River, an area that included roughly 50,000 square miles and half a million people.

American and French Protestants had been preaching the gospel and planting churches north of the Ogooué River for more than 100 years, so when France ended its agreement with the S.H.O., the French Protestant mission contacted the Alliance in the Congo and invited their missionaries to move personnel into the territory.

The news was received with great joy by the Alliance, and the Congo field made plans to send a survey team to south Gabon to "spy out the land." They chose veteran missionary Joseph Nicholson and young Don Fairley, and in February two men traveled by ship up the West African coast to Gabon's port city of Port Gentil. The next day Nicholson and Fairley boarded a steamboat that over the next two days, took them up the Ogooué River to the mission at Ngoma.

After several days at the French Protestant mission at Ngoma, Nicholson and Fairley met a young African Christian named Ndoba. He had come to the school from the Yishira tribe that lived two hours south on the Ogooué River. Ndoba volunteered to go with the Americans as their cook, and the missionaries were glad to have him. Ndoba helped them hire ten porters to accompany them, and the next day they started their journey south. Over the next two months the missionaries visited more than ten villages and multiple potential sites for a permanent mission station, but none had all the things they were looking for, until the day they walked into the village of Makombo, and met Chief Boudiongo.

Desperate Giving for the Desperate

Six months later, Don and his family were back in the U.S. speaking in Alliance churches. Don didn't seem troubled that he and Dorothy would have to raise the equivalent today of $115,000 from Alliance churches in America during one of the worst days of the Great Depression! Whatever the odds, God's hand had so clearly directed them to Makombo, to Chief Boudiongo, and to Bongolo Falls that as far as Don was concerned, it was only a matter of time before God would come through with everything that they would need to win the tribes of South Gabon to faith in Christ, even if it took decades!

When the Fairleys arrived back in California in 1934, America's economy was just beginning to climb up from its lowest point. Unemployment had soared to 25%, and there were so many bank failures that President Franklin D. Roosevelt declared a "bank holiday," and temporarily closed all banks to stabilize the financial system and implement reforms. The Alliance mission board was forced to cut missionary allowances by 40%, and churches struggled to support their pastors. Despite these challenges, Alliance leaders were keenly interested in Nicolson and Fairley's positive report of their survey into South Gabon. France's recent reopening of the region gave the Alliance a golden opportunity to proclaim the Good News to multiple unreached tribes—if they could afford it! The Alliance decided that if the Fairley's succeeded in raising $5,000 in advance, it would be enough to pay their transportation expenses, build a mission station with four or five homes, and have enough money to support the Piersons and the Fairleys for the next few years.

Undaunted by the challenge and brimming with optimism, Don and Dorothy began telling their story in Alliance churches across America. The economy might be on its knees, but God wasn't, and didn't He own the cattle on a thousand hills? What was $5,000 to the Creator of the Universe?!

Over the next twelve months, Don spoke in more than 30 churches in Nebraska, Iowa, Wisconsin, Colorado, Washington State, Oregon, and Southern California, each time telling the stories of what he saw and experienced and how God led them. But despite his zeal and story-telling gifts, his efforts produced little excitement. Don and Dorothy were still in their twenties; they had spent a mere two years in Africa. Next to the legendary missionaries who spent their lives reaching "the dark continent," the Fairleys were kids who had yet to plant a single church!

But Don and Dorothy's stories were not the only weapons in God's quiver! The most notable who championed the dream of reaching Gabon's southern tribes, was the treasurer of the Alliance, Dr. William Christie. He was known for his years of service as a pioneer missionary in Northeast Tibet and China. In several of the churches where Don preached and appealed for support, Dr. Christie followed him. Little by little, funds began to trickle in. But by the end of the year, only 40% of the amount needed had come in.

The last church Don Fairley was to speak in was the Gospel Tabernacle, in Omaha, Nebraska. Weighing in at around 100 pounds and just five feet six inches tall, Don looked like a teenager behind the pulpit. But Don's message was passionate: he had filmed black and white movies during his survey trip to Gabon that showed how the people lived and worshipped demon gods. His movies showed half-naked people dancing like zombies, and young men with teeth who despite agonizing pain had filed their teeth to points! Reaching them with the gospel was an amazing challenge, but God's people faced an equal challenge. The Depression had wiped out many of their nest eggs, bank accounts, businesses and jobs. As Don ended his messages, he pleaded with congregations to send them back so Gabon's tribes could be saved from the demons they worshipped and reborn with the love and forgiveness of Christ. When the elders of the Omaha Tabernacle finished passing the offering plates, the amount collected was far short of what they would need to return.

Just then Dr. Christie arrived at the back of the church, having just traveled for two days by train from New York City! He walked directly to the front, climbed onto the platform, and stood at the podium. Over the next forty-five minutes the old missionary preached with such passion that God's people began to weep, not for themselves, but for the lost people of south Gabon! He ended by announcing that another offering would be taken. As the plates went down the pews, women in the congregation removed their wedding and engagement rings, and the jewelry they were wearing, and dropped them into the offering plate. Men took out their prized pocket watches and their wedding rings and put them in the plate. When everything was counted and valued, the total came to over $5,000! The congregation erupted with shouts of joy and weeping! Dr. Christie turned to Don on the platform and said, "Young man, you are on your way back to Gabon!"

The goal of raising $5,000 had been reached, but God's people continued to give for the Gabon project. By the time the Fairleys boarded a freighter to Gabon, a total of $8,000 had come in, enough to pay for the construction of five mission residences in Bongolo and financially support two missionary couples for the next five years.

On November 19, 1934, the Fairleys arrived in Gabon's southern port of Port Gentil with their four children. After unloading their crates and barrels onto a barge, they reloaded them onto a paddle wheel steamboat and chugged up the wide Ogoué River. Two days later they arrived at Ngoma where the students and French missionaries welcomed them warmly.

The Fairleys stayed at Ngoma for six weeks, waiting for Harold and Ozzie Pierson. There could hardly have been two more different people in the world than Harold Pierson and Donald Fairley. Harold was tall, balding, slow-moving, and methodical. He strongly believed that God was leading their mission into South Gabon, but unlike the ever-optimistic Don Fairley, Harold believed that poor planning would inevitably result in failure. When decisions were needed, Harold could not be rushed. His answers to questions were long in coming and reflected an innate caution.

In sharp contrast, Don Fairley had the unshakable belief that if God was with them, no problem was too great to overcome! Don was short, had plenty of hair, and moved like a nervous gazelle. He was fluent in French and learned tribal languages with ease. He also overflowed with energy, optimism, enthusiasm, and untried ideas. Innately adventurous, he believed that failure to try was the worst failure of all. He seemed to believe that God could overcome any blunder, as long as it sprang from a rightly motivated idea! He was so accustomed to looking at the bright side of disaster that discouragement slid off him like water off a duck's back.

While they waited, Don commissioned the French mission's skilled carpenters to build a 20-foot-long by seven-foot- wide roofed boat that he painted it white. To power it, he brought in his crates one of the first outboard motors manufactured in America. While they waiting at Ngoma Don encountered Paul Ndoba again, the Yishira Christian who had accompanied him and Joseph Nicholson during their survey trip to south Gabon the previous year. When Don invited him to join them in Bongolo, he said "Yes, but I can't come right away."

An important perspective that Harold Pierson and Don Fairley agreed on was the importance of recruiting a small number of discipled African Christians from the northern Protestant Church of Gabon. Protestant missionaries had made many disciples and had planted churches, established schools, and had trained many teachers and pastors.

Six weeks after the Fairleys arrived in Ngoma, Harold and Ozzie Peterson and their 10-year-old son finally joined them. During their six weeks at the Ngoma mission, Don had talked the French missionaries into "loaning" him and Harold Pierson five high school-educated Gabonese Christian men to help them establish the Bongolo mission and disciple new believers. Paul Ndoba was one of the five, and all five of them were fluent in French, in addition to their tribal languages.

A week after the Pierson family arrived, Don, Harold, and the five Gabonese men recruited from Ngoma boarded the new 20-foot launch and sped upriver, marveling at the speed and power the new motor provided. The women and children would remain in Ngoma until the men had built temporary housing and had cleared enough land to plant gardens. It was the Rainy Season, but that day the river was relatively calm, making the portages around the waterfalls easier. The outboard motor was a great success, and their first voyage between the Ngoma and Bongolo took only three days.

The launch's arrival at Makombo took the village by surprise, but Chief Boudiongo welcomed them with evident pleasure. Once again, he invited his guests to stay in the large thatch and bark guest house.

The next day Boudiongo took the visitors in his 30-foot canoe to the Bongolo Falls and showed them the land he had promised Don and Joseph Nicholson during their initial visit. Harold wanted to see every inch of the property Chief Boudiongo had given them, so their survey took the entire day. The next morning Harold announced that he, Don, and Ndoba would spend the day on the Bongolo property fasting and praying for confirmation from the Lord that Bongolo was God's choice. At the end of a day of prayer and fasting, Harold and Donald were satisfied that Bongolo was indeed God's choice for the new mission station. The next day when Chief Boudiongo heard the news, he shouted his approval! Better yet, from that day forward there were no more executions at Bongolo Falls!

That night the team ate with Chief Boudiongo, and Harold asked how many of his people might be willing to work for pay to clear the land and help them build temporary houses. Chief Boudiongo promised 20 men from his village, and up to 100 in another few weeks, once he sent word to the regional governor and the surrounding villages. The chief 's only condition was that the missionaries and their helpers work alongside the Africans, since they were still fearful of angry spirits and the curse of Bongolo Falls.

Once Harold and Don and their five colleagues were settled in the village guest house, they began planning what they would need to do in the coming weeks and months, and in what order. First, they agreed to work alongside the villagers as they cleared the land. Second, they would build temporary housing and move their families to Bongolo. Third, they would begin learning the local language.

Other priorities that would come later would be to hire as many workers as possible to clear the underbrush from as many acres as possible and cut down trees only where they were planning to build houses and roads. The first houses they built would have to be made entirely of forest materials, since they had not had room in the launch to bring nails, carpentry tools, heavy axes, or the two-person saws required to saw boards. The construction of permanent houses out of burned bricks and hardwood would come later and would be required by the French government before granting the missionaries a deed to the land. Soon after their arrival they sent a letter with a runner to the provincial governor 75 mile2s1away, inviting him to visit them as soon as possible.

Don and Harold agreed that the first house not made of bark would be made of mud-wattle, which the Africans had never seen. The missionaries showed them how by first pounding wooden posts into the ground every 2 feet to frame the walls. The posts were then linked together horizontally with split palm branches that were tied to the posts every four inches from top to bottom, with small, tough vines. Once the framework of the walls was finished, the workers packed moist clay inside the framework from both sides of the walls. When the mud dried, the result would be sturdy, 6-inch-thick walls. The roof was then framed with 8-inch tree trunks and thick, palm branch shingles. In dry climates, a mud wattle house could be completed in a month, but in Gabon's 90% humidity, the walls took so long to dry that eventually the workers had to light small fires in each room and keep them burning for weeks!

Harold and Don also agreed on a long-term plan to share the gospel with their workers. At the beginning of every workday, they would provide a meal and a one-hour chapel service where the missionaries and their African helpers from Ngoma would preach the gospel, beginning with the Creation story and ending with the return of Christ. Before being baptized, workers who repented and believed in Jesus would be asked to burn their fetishes as evidence of their sincerity. Pierson and Fairley also agreed to a long-term plan to establish churches in as many villages as possible and train both men and women evangelists who would return to their own villages with the gospel.

Among their other pivotal decisions, Harold and Don decided that as soon as their families were housed and they had learned the tribal languages, they would begin work on translating the gospel of Luke into the local languages. They would then use the translated scriptures to teach literacy classes for men, women, and children. As God called more missionaries to join them, they would establish additional mission centers and churches among other tribes until all the tribes south of the Ogoué River had heard the gospel message and were being discipled. They would not insist on Western church and worship forms but would establish a self-supporting African church led by Africans. Finally, as soon as God enabled, they would establish a Bible school to begin training pastors for all the southern tribes.

The first problem Harold and Don encountered in carrying out their plan surfaced when Boudiongo's men refused to set foot on the Bongolo property. The chief did his best to convince them to work, but because of their fear of the curse, only a few showed up. All of that changed a week later when a representative of the French governor arrived, threatening punitive consequences for any village in the region that did not immediately send all of its able men to work at Bongolo for two weeks, without pay! In anticipation of the arrival of the governor, Boudiongo built several small bark houses on the Bongolo land for the Americans to live in temporarily, freeing the Makombo guest house for the governor's visit.

The next evening the Americans met with a sullen group of chiefs from the surrounding villages who had come only because of the governor's threats. They all feared the curse of Bongolo Falls, and like the people of Makombo were devout worshippers of Bwiti and Mwiri. But as Boudiongo explained to the chiefs that Jesus, the American missionaries' God, had sent them to live among them, they listened quietly. With Boudiongo translating, Harold explained they had been sent to Bongolo by the great God who had created the world, the sun, the moon and the stars, and that he had power over all other spirits. He offered as proof the fact that the missionaries and their helpers from Ngoma had already worked on the land for two weeks, and not a single accident or injury had occurred! Finally, the two Americans promised that if any of the workers stayed after their two-week obligation was over, they would pay them good wages!

The next day the conscripted men showed up to work, though at first, they were sullen and fearful. But as Harold and Donald worked alongside them to clear the land, their attitude began to change. By the second week, more than 150 conscripts had arrived. As Harold and Donald worked with them, felling trees and cutting the underbrush, the tension faded and turned to respect. Soon after, the French governor arrived and warmly welcomed Harold and Donald. He congratulated them on what they had already accomplished and were planning, assuring them that he would do everything in his power to help them succeed. In the months that followed, he was as good as his word.

Harold Pierson worked with several crews to cut down five of the massive hardwood trees on the property with a two-man saw the governor donated. Harold had the men saw the hardwood tree trunks into 10-foot sections, then cut the sections into boards. To the amazement of the conscripts and the people of Makombo, despite weeks of clearing the land, not a single worker was seriously injured. By this time five more African Christians from the French

Protestant Mission in Ngoma had joined the missionaries, bringing their total to eight.

Four months after the missionaries and their African colleagues from Ngoma arrived, Harold asked Donald to return to Lambaréné in the launch and bring their wives and children to Bongolo. But when Don arrived at Ngoma, he learned that Harold and Ozzie Pierson's son LeRoy had come down with tuberculosis! Dr. Schweitzer made the diagnosis after hearing his symptoms, listening to the boy's chest, and taking an X-ray. But Dr. Schweitzer did not have the medications required to treat tuberculosis. LeRoy would have to return to American as soon as possible. Don sent a runner to take the news to Harold in Bongolo, and as soon as he received Don's letter, he hired a canoe and six rowers and made the 200-mile trip to Ngoma in two days. Two weeks later the Pierson's were on a freighter to the U.S.

Before returning to Bongolo with Dorothy and their children, Don asked the missionaries at Ngoma to loan the Alliance mission three more educated and gifted African men. The French mission was very reluctant to release these key disciples, but because they knew the work the Fairleys and Pierson's were pioneering was critical to establishing a foothold for the gospel in the south, they agreed to release them for the work in Bongolo. The men who agreed to go with Don were Paul Ndoba, who had accompanied him and Joseph Nicholson on their survey trip to the south two years before; John Mbadinga, an African high school teacher and pastor; and Mark Divingou, a skilled carpenter. Little did they know that in future years, all three men would become pastors, and two of them would serve as presidents of the Alliance church of the south! The three men would follow the Fairleys to Bongolo several weeks later.

Battling the Demon Gods

In preparation for their trip back to Bongolo, Don loaded the launch with carpentry tools, hammers, boxes of nails, heavy axes, and several barrels. The next morning Don, Dorothy, and their two children boarded the launch and began their journey upriver. After three hours of motoring east on the Ogoue River they turned south at the junction of the Ngounie and Ogoue Rivers (see map). Soon after they approached the fearsome Digaba Falls. The river was unusually high, making the waterfall twice its normal size. Don hired twenty men at a nearby village to help him carry and drag the launch around the falls. It took them half a day.

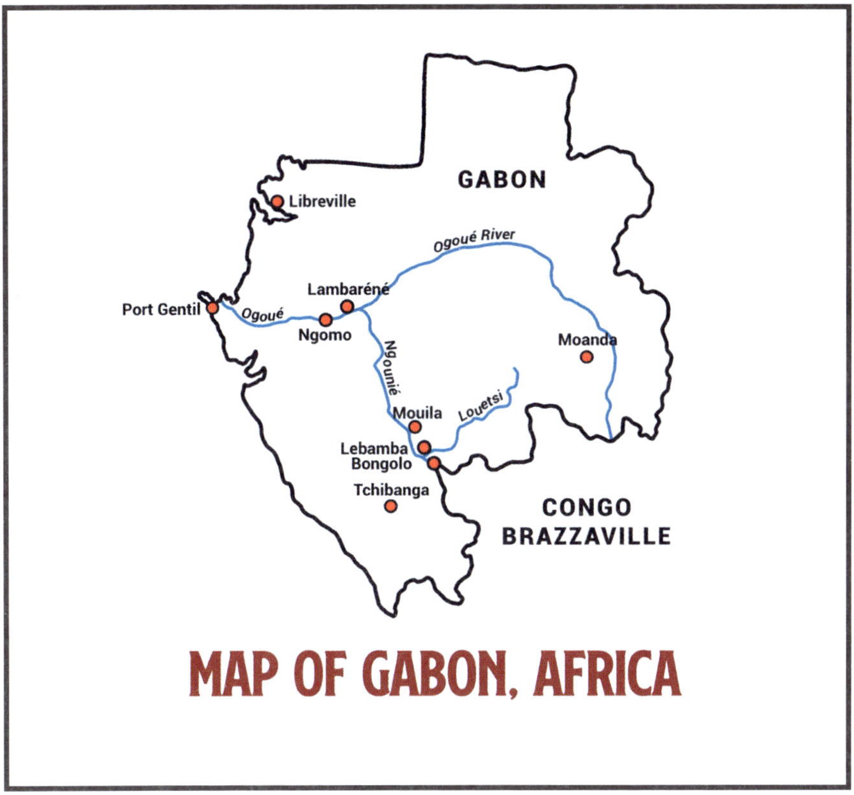

Gabon's Rivers

The next morning Donald hired a guide to help them navigate the miles of treacherous whitewater above Digaba falls. At first, they advanced 25 without problems, but the current was so swift that an hour later they had only advanced about 500 yards. As they continued upriver, they entered an area of wild whitewater. Suddenly, a hidden whirlpool spun them around, turning the launch horizontal to the current. Don forced the boat to face upstream, but then another whirlpool spun them off course and into shallow water. Seconds later the propeller slammed into a partially submerged rock, breaking the cotter pin that secured it to the driveshaft. Without the cotter pin the driveshaft spun uselessly. Don quickly shut off the motor, and as the current dragged them downriver, he and the guide grabbed desperately at rocks and dead tree trunks but weren't able to hold on. As the boat drifted downriver, Dorothy clutched the children and cried out to God to help them! A singular thought and realization occupied their minds: in just minutes they would be at the top of the falls!

Suddenly the launch slammed into a submerged boulder and stopped sideways to the current. The middle of the launch was hung up on the rock, and the useless propeller was in the air. At the same time, the prow was threatening to go underwater. Seeing the danger, the guide leaped into the water and standing chest-deep in the water, held the prow from going under and sliding back into the current. Dorothy looked to her right and saw the large rock they were hung up on. For a moment, she forgot her terror and put her foot over the side into the water to further stabilize the launch.

Don quickly shut the screaming motor off, found another cotter pin in his toolbox, and replaced it. But when he lifted up the motor end of the motor up, the propeller was still above the water. To reengage the propeller, they would have to push the launch off the rock and back into the swift current.

When Don gave the signal, Dorothy pulled her leg back into the launch, the guide pushed the prow up and away from the rock, and the boat spun back into the current. When Don pulled the starter cord motor roared to life, enabling Don to steer the launch into the deeper water in the center of the river and head upstream. During the few seconds it had taken them to free the boat and redirect, the current had swept them to within 100 yards of the falls, but at least now they were moving upstream and knew where not to go!

Hours later as the sun set, they motored into calm water near a village, and they spent the night. The next morning the weather was lovely. As the launch hummed up the winding river, Dorothy and the children gazed in wonder at the beauty of the virgin forest. Troupes of monkeys screamed and chattered in the trees above them, and brilliant blue kingfishers flashed back and forth across the river, catching small fish in their orange beaks.

Around noon, dark clouds began to gather, and soon a strong wind swayed the tops of the trees. Dorothy and the guide lowered the canvas sides to protect them from the coming rain. When the storm hit, a curtain of water roared down upon them. The wind blew so violently that after 45 minutes it tore the canvas off one side of the boat! Half an hour later the storm passed, but soon after a second storm hit, this time tearing the canvas off the other side of the boat and drenching everything in the launch! Eventually the storm passed, and the sun warmed them. But less than an hour later, a third storm poured down on them. The repeated storms and strong winds were causing the motor to consume more and more fuel, each time forcing Don to pull over to the side and refill the tank. As the shadows began to lengthen, Don drained the last of their fuel into the tank. For the first time, he feared they might run out of fuel, out of daylight, or both!

Then incredibly, a fourth storm crashed onto them. This time it seemed as if the demons of hell had been loosed! The wind blew with such force and intensity that the rain came down horizontally, soaking them and flooding into the launch. When it seemed that the storm couldn't get worse, hail began to fall, clattering down on the hapless family and rattling angrily against the roof! By now the children were exhausted and crying, their lips blue with cold. Even Don trembled so violently that he considered pulling over to the shore until the storm passed.

Night was coming, and as it grew darker, they wondered how they could continue. Then suddenly, Don heard shouts and saw people standing on the bank ahead in the pounding rain! Their guide began to shout, waving Don to pull over to the left bank. As the last rays of light disappeared, they reached the village of Makombo and their friends. Don saw Boudiongo and their workers standing in the rain and cheering their arrival. Climbing onboard to help, they gazed in astonishment at the blue-lipped, shivering children, lifted them out of the boat, and ran with them to shelter. Others helped Don and Dorothy step onshore, along with their weary guide. The downpour precluded formal greetings and conversation, so their friends grabbed the water-logged supplies from the launch and half dragged, half-carried the weary travelers into the village and to the guest house. Murmuring in sympathy, they led them inside, seated them, and brought them freshly roasted sweet potatoes to eat. After a few bites, the exhausted travelers laid down fully clothed and fell asleep, oblivious to the amazed stares of the people peeking through the shuttered windows.

It was 1934, and after a wild battle the demon gods had failed to stop God's sent ones!

Fighting Leopards

Don Fairley had hoped that by the time he returned to Bongolo, the workers would have finished the mud-wattle house they were building. The 10-foot-high walls had finally dried, but the house was far from finished. While they waited, Fairley and his family moved into a traditional bark house on the new station. The flimsy walls were made of quarter inch-thick tree bark tied by thin vines to framing posts pounded into the ground, and the roof was made of thatch.

By this time there were more than 100 converts, so Don and his team built a three-sided church out of bamboo and thatch that had room for 200 people. During their first two years at Bongolo, Don and Dorothy worked ten-hour days, and in the evenings before they fell into bed studied the Yinzebi language. As their language skills improved, they learned just how fearful the people —even those who had believed—were of their demon gods Bwiti and Mwiri. To counter their fear, Don and Dorothy and their helpers from Ngoma chose a simple strategy. Every morning at the beginning of the workday, they systematically taught from the gospels and answered the people's questions. The difference between the worship of the demon gods the people had grown up, and the worship of Jesus was worlds apart. The demon gods threatened and bullied their followers and demanded to be worshipped by the men with drums and shouting in terrifying, all-night dances. The demon gods ruled by fear and violence, while Jesus ruled with love, forgiveness, kindness toward others, and joyful songs of worship. The demon gods could not be prayed to by just anyone and anytime, but the people could pray to Jesus whenever they wished. Most surprising of all was to hear that Jesus loved them and asked those who followed him to forgive their enemies and love them!

By the end of the second year, more than 200 former Bwiti and Mwiri worshippers had renounced their demon gods and had believed in Jesus. Before they could be baptized, they had to burn the fetishes the Ngangas had given them for protection against—incredibly—*evil* spirits! Chief Boudiongo was the first to believe and burn his fetishes. Paul Ndoba—who by then had known Don Fairley for almost three years, asked to be baptized. The next Sunday the entire community stood on both sides of the river below Bongolo falls and to watch this strange new ceremony in the middle of the Louetsi river. When Don Fairley asked Paul if he was ready to follow and obey Jesus, he replied in a loud voice that he was ready to follow Jesus for the rest of his life! Don and their helpers had already explained to the somewhat fearful Christians watching what baptism signified. So, when he completely immersed Ndoba and then stood him back up, the people on the shore shouted in relief and began signing! After that, there were many baptisms. Added to the importance and significance of the event was the closeness of Ndoba's baptism to the previously feared Bongolo Falls. The Christians had long since lost the fear that there might be angry souls under the falls, and they no longer trembled at the lies of the Ngangas.

By this time, the Fairleys had moved out of the village of Makombo and had moved into a bark house on the mission property. One night their dog began to bark. Thinking it might be a wild animal, Don grabbed his gun, lit a lantern, and carefully opened the front door. In the dark he saw nothing, but in the morning, he found the tracks of a large leopard all around their house.

A week later while Don was paying his workmen, his dog was sitting on the grass ten feet from him. Suddenly a huge leopard jumped out of the bushes, grabbed the dog, and dragged it into the forest. It happened in just seconds, and a minute later the dog's yelping stopped. That was the beginning of a fierce battle for supremacy over Bongolo. Hunting in packs of two or three, the leopards began killing and devouring the chickens, goats, and pigs of the growing Christian community that was now living in Bongolo. Almost every night they pawed the flimsy bark walls of the houses, looking for weak spots. They were so bold that they even began stalking the villagers during daylight hours!

By this time the mud wattle house made entirely of forest materials was nearing completion. The house was forty-feet long, twenty-feet wide, and featured a large living room, a dining room, two bedrooms, a shower room, a kitchen, and a storeroom. It was five times larger than the temporary bark house they were living in. Unfortunately, the project was months behind schedule because the thick clay walls were taking so long to dry! It was the beginning of the rainy season, so Don finally had the workers build fires in all the rooms and keep them burning until the walls dried. After that the workers framed the roof and using vines, tied on three layers of thatch.

For the floors, Don had the workers lay down two inches of crushed termite mound dirt mixed with water and pound it with the heavy end of palm branches until it was smooth. The result was a durable and easy-to-sweep floor throughout the house. To make whitewash, Don piled up limestone rocks and kept a fire burning on top of them for 24 hours. The result was limestone powder, which when water is added becomes whitewash. The workers whitewashed the inside and outside of the house, giving it a charming appearance!

Next Don made beds by tying a wooden frame together using small vines. For mattresses, Dorothy hand sewed canvas mattress covers, stuffed them with dried grass, and called them "jungle mattresses!" Don used the crates they had shipped from the States a year earlier to make their dining room and living room furniture. When their house was finally finished, the Fairleys invited all their African friends to come for a tour. Amazed and enthralled, the Africans dubbed the Fairley's mud-wattle house a "glorious palace!"

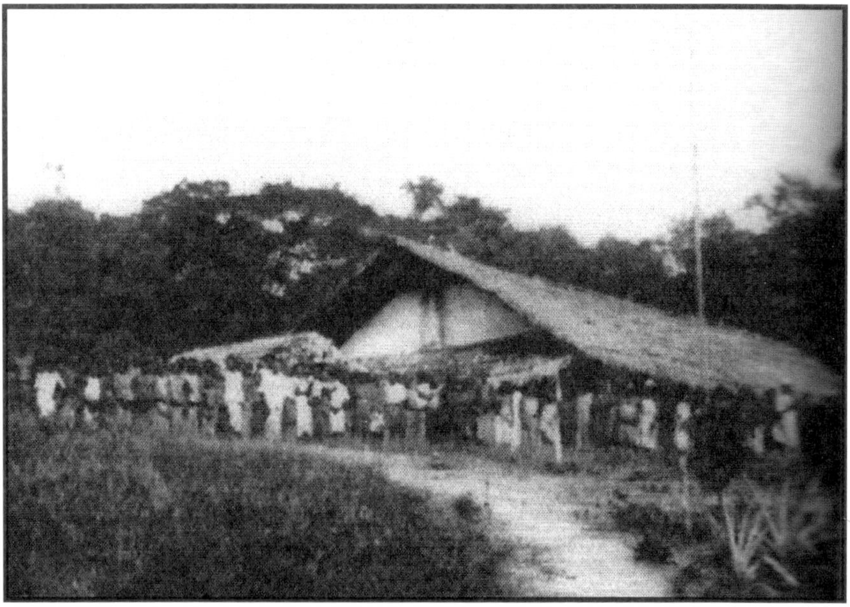

Fairley's lived in for five years!

One evening as Don returned from checking on a work crew, he spotted the spoor of an antelope not more than 100 yards from their new house. Concealed by brush and the roots of a tree, Don imitated the call of an antelope three or four times. Just as he was about to call again, he heard Dorothy banging on a pot from the house, her way of calling him to supper. He treasured the evening meal as the one time of the day when their family could be together without company. Don handed his shotgun to his friend Mbadinga, and giving one more antelope call stepped back onto the path home. He had not gone 100 yards when he heard the roar of the gun. Looking up to the darkening skies and smiling, he thanked the Lord for providing them once again with antelope meat. But it was not an antelope!

Fifteen minutes later, the Fairleys were well into their meal when they heard the workers chanting the way hunters chanted when they had successfully hunted a large antelope or a buffalo. Because they were chanting louder than usual for a mere antelope, Don and his family stepped outside and were astounded to see an enormous leopard lying dead on the ground! Don's antelope call had not attracted another antelope, but a hungry leopard! It was the largest leopard any of them had ever seen, measuring 9 feet from the tip of its nose to the end of its tail! It was also the beginning of what would become a battle for supremacy!

In the ensuing months the leopard attacks that followed so terrorized the people living in Bongolo that they stopped going to their gardens to harvest their manioc, taro, plantains, bananas, sweet potatoes, and peanuts. Night after night the Christians lay awake, listening as growling beasts prowled around their thinly walled bark houses and scratched the walls for weaknesses. Any chicken, goat, or pig that was not inside a hut would be devoured. Over the following months, Don's cleverest attempts to trap the leopards or shoot them proved fruitless. He and John Mbadinga even searched the Bongolo property carefully, their guns loaded, hoping to find how the deadly predators disappeared quickly and like smoke if they pursued them with guns.

The leopards became so bold that Don tried another tactic. He and Mbadinga tied a goat just 20 yards from his mud-wattle house, then climbed onto the thatched roof with their rifles. Don guessed the leopards weren't just hunting because of hunger but were directly challenging the community for control of the land.

There was a full moon that night, and around 2 am the goat suddenly began bleating and pulling on its rope. Less than a minute later, one of the largest leopards Don had ever seen boldly approached. Both men took aim and fired. The leopard leaped six feet into the air and fell to the ground, apparently dead. The two men jumped down off the roof and cautiously approached, then poked the huge animal with the muzzles of their guns. The leopard didn't move. Strangely, there was just one bullet wound, and it went right to the heart! Since the men had identical guns and identical ammo, they couldn't tell whose bullet had killed it, but since John Mbadinga was certain of his aim, Don graciously agreed that he must have missed. When they measured the length of the leopard, they discovered it was just one inch shorter than the huge leopard John had killed a month earlier close the Fairley's house.

But the death of the two huge leopards did not end the battle. A few nights later the leopards again stalked the houses in the village and devoured some of the villager's chickens and pigs. The people living in Bongolo were so afraid that some wondered if the curse of Bongolo falls had returned! In desperation, the Christians and missionaries decided to fast and pray for a week, asking that God would send the leopards away forever. The Christians and the missionaries fasted and prayed for a week, and to everyone's joy, the leopards disappeared and never returned!

Sixteen years later, when my wife and our two sons had made our way to Gabon, Joshua and Jeremy were exploring the 100-foot limestone cliffs behind our house. They found a network of caves near the top of the cliffs. The caves were part of the land Boudiongo had given the missionaries and were only visible when the boys climbed down seven or eight feet from the top of the cliffs. The caves looked as though wild animals had lived in them for years, and on one visit to the caves, Joshua and a visiting pastor encountered a huge python! In any case, it would have been easy for the leopards to kill their prey at night and disappear like ghosts into the caves during the day, especially since some of the caves were less than 50 feet from our house! Leopard cubs hidden in the caves would never be heard, even from our house, and when hunted, they could disappear in minutes! Up until the day our boys discovered them, no one even knew there was a network of caves in the cliffs behind our house.

Looking back to the history of Bongolo before the first missionaries came, anyone who set foot on Bongolo's land—either to clear land for gardens, hunt for antelope, or clear land for a garden or to build a bark house to live there—would have been easy pray for Bongolo's fearsome leopards. What the Ngangas claimed was a deadly curse over Bongolo caused by the wicked souls of those the Ngangas executed might instead have been the unusually large population of leopards that for centuries, ruled over Bongolo with impunity.

We will never know for certain if the leopards were the nidus of what the Ngangas eventually elevated into murderous zeal but knowing how aggressive and fearless the leopards became makes the idea more than plausible!

Power and Light

In 1939, the Fairleys returned to the U.S. for a one-year furlough. That same year, the Alliance sent two new missionary couples to Gabon to join them—the Cooks and the Shindler's. That year Harold and Ozzie Pierson also returned, with their now-healthy son. The Cooks and the Shindler families would build two more of Bongolo's brick and mortar houses, both of which are still housing missionaries to- day. The Piersons would eventually move west and east to take the gospel to other southern tribes, learn their languages, and establish churches among them.

During the 12 months that the Fairley's were in the U.S., Don spoke in countless churches, telling the amazing stories of God's work in opening the door for the tribes of south Gabon to hear the Gospel and believe. The Fairley's stories were so incredible and Don's delivery so breathtaking that people flocked to hear them!

On one of his speaking trips, Don met a wealthy Christian businessman named R.G. LeTourneau. Don shared with him his dream to build a hydroelectric plant at Bongolo Falls. LeTourneau was an American inventor of technologies related to earthmoving machinery, an engineering genius, and the founder of LeTourneau University. He was also an amazingly generous individual. After hearing Donald's story of entering south Gabon with the gospel, LeTourneau agreed to provide him with everything he would need to build a modest hydroelectric plant at the Bongolo Falls and then purchased everything Don would need to build it. He also agreed to send one of his engineers, Furman Lentz, to Bongolo for 10 months to help Don complete project. Before the Fairey's returned to Gabon, Don went to LeTourneau's factory where he learned to weld and better understand the final assembly.

Furman was a gruff and muscular American engineer who loved the challenge of building in the middle of the jungle! Because they would need other resources to complete the project, LeTourneau financed the purchase of a portable sawmill, a gasoline-powered generator, an electric welder, two brick presses, and a Chevrolet Carryall station wagon. Excluding the car, the total weight of the materials and machinery for the project totaled nineteen tons!

When the Fairleys returned to Bongolo they were met by the Piersons, whose son LeRoy had fully recovered from tuberculosis. The Shindlers and Cooks were already supervising teams that were making bricks and burning them for the homes that they were building. During the Fairley's absence, the French colonial government in French Congo, south of Gabon had just completed a gravel road from the Port city of Pointe Noire to the southern border of Gabon, just three miles from Bongolo. It turned out to be a huge and unexpected blessing!

Soon after Furman arrived in Bongolo, he and Don on set about recruiting 50 workers to help them cut a 3-mile road through the jungle to the Congolese border and the new road the French had built. Because they had to construct a number of log bridges, the project took them more than a month to complete. The two men then drove to Pointe Noir in French Congo and hired three heavy trucks to transport all 19 tons of LeTourneau's hydroelectric plant and heavy equipment to Bongolo. As that was happening, Don and Furman made 15 trips between Pointe Noire and Bongolo in the Chevrolet Carryall to ferry 27 tons of cement to Bongolo.

It was 1939, and a year later WW2 would explode across Europe. Hitler's army would conquer France, and General Charles de Gaulle would flee the survivors of France's defeated army to Gabon.

Their presence would ensure that Gabon would remain a jungled haven of peace.

The next step was for the workers to cut down and remove 30 trees from the project site and cut them into boards for the concrete forms needed to make the reservoir and the generator hut. Once that was done, they had to break apart 20 tons of massive boulders at the foot of the falls that were in the way. The boulders were so large that they couldn't be moved. As the African workers watched in amazement, Furman built fires over the huge boulders and kept the fires burning for 24 hours. He then doused the boulders with cold water, which split them into one or two-foot boulders. Furman then took only 2,000 men, but when they saw a sledgehammer and smashed the boulders into rocks small enough for the workmen to carry away. The supposed home of the souls the Ngangas had murdered at Bongolo Falls over a century was now a pile of rubble, and by now, even the African workers were no longer afraid.

When the Dry Season came the river dropped by half, enabling Furman to pour a 40 x 10 x 10-foot reservoir out of steel-reinforced concrete. He also directed the workers to build two-foot-high walls of stone and concrete above the reservoir to channel water from the river into the reservoir. Simple wooden gates controlled and regulated the flow of water into the reservoir that could be closed when too much sand accumulated at the bottom and needed to be cleared.

The most arduous task for Don and Furman was bending the 8'x 8' half inch-thick steel plates, each of which weighed 300 pounds. Once bent into shape and held by chains, Don and Furman welded them together, both inside and outside, creating a 70-foot tube that ran from the reservoir down to the turbine. When they finished welding and let water from the reservoir fill the steel tube with water, there wasn't a single leak! The two men and their helpers then bolted the turbine in place underneath the floor of the generator at the lower outlet of the tube. They then connected the spinning turbine to a 500 KVA generator in the cement hut above. At this point in the project, Furman had to return to the U.S. and resume his job with his boss, Mr. LeTourneau. Don would have to complete the project on his own!

Prior to Furman's departure, Don had managed to purchase 30 steel train rails in French Congo to use as electrical pylons. After they were delivered to Bongolo, Don had his workers clear a path from the cliff above the falls to the four sites where permanent mission houses were in the process of being built. The electrical pole up on top of the cliff was at the very spot from which countless victims had been thrown by the Ngangas to the falls below, before the arrival of the gospel! Now it would be used to bring light to all of Bongolo!

But before that, Don had to cement his train-rail electrical poles into the ground at 100-foot intervals and string three quarter-inch thick aluminum wires from a circuit breaker inside the hydroelectric hut to the pole on the cliff. From there the wires were strung to the mission house construction sites. When the electrical poles and wires were in place, Don began the complicated job of wiring the generator to the fuse box and circuit breakers. To his consternation, the wiring instructions for the generator were missing! It would take months for LeTourneau to send him another manual!

Don had previously purchased a small booklet on the principles of three-phase, 220-volt electricity. During the next few days, he studied them until he had the booklet memorized. But the next morning when he hooked up the generator, nothing made sense! Locking himself in the turbine hut he prayed for several hours, claiming for himself James 1:5: *"If any of you lacks wisdom, he should ask God who gives generously and without finding fault, and it will be given to him."*[2] After praying most of the morning, Don attached the wires in a way that seemed to make sense, then opened the water gates to the turbine. As water rushed down the tube, the turbine began to rotate, spinning the shaft to the generator in the hut above. But the generator seemed to be laboring, so Don shut everything down. Eventually he discovered that the fuses that came in the new control panel were the wrong amperage. After he had corrected the problem, he tried again. Again, the generator continued to labor! Somewhere in the system there was a dead short! Don followed the aluminum wires from the generator to the first pole just outside the hut. It looked fine! But the wires to a second pole at the edge of the river looked odd. Then he saw it: the workman who had helped him earlier hadn't attached each wire to the glass insulators on the light pole, but to the steel arms that held the insulators, creating a dead short to the pole and into the ground!

---

2 All quotes from scripture in this work are derived from the *New Living Translation Bible* (NLT).

After Don corrected the mistake he tried again, and to his joy the entire system ran quietly with the precision of a clock! The Africans working with him had never seen electrical light, so when the glass bulbs in the hut glowed brightly at the flip of a switch, they shouted with surprise and joy! For the first time, twenty-four-hour electricity had come to Bongolo! No longer would it be known for its curse, but for its light!

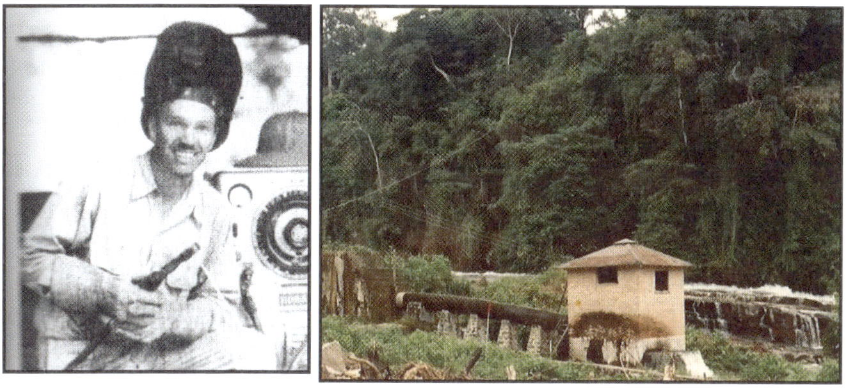

Don Fairley with his welder Reservoir (left), water tube, and "Hydro Hut"

The significance of the transformation of the Bongolo Falls from a fearsome curse that produced death to thousands to a blessing that produced light, peace with God and joy was not lost on anyone who heard of the mysterious power source the missionaries had brought to Bongolo. Even those who had not yet heard the gospel of Jesus understood that their demon gods had experienced yet another crushing defeat.

Chapter Two:

FROM ASIA TO AFRICA

Rebels

In 1945 a lone American drove a black Citroen sedan on the narrow, thinly paved road in northern Cambodia on his way north, to Laos. As the sun set, he stopped in a small Cambodian village for the night. A collection of 30 or so houses perched defiantly on stilts just 30 feet from the often-flooded Mekong River. Behind the houses, golden fields of rice stretched for miles. Though the American knew no one in the village, he stopped in front of the chief 's house, a prominent structure on 8-foot-high Mahogany stilts. A small crowd of villagers soon gathered around the car and the white stranger. Hearing the noise, the village chief stepped out his open front door and onto his front porch to see what was going on. The white stranger below introduced himself in French as "Monsieur Gordon Smith." He asked if he might be allowed to sleep in his car in front of the chief 's house. Intrigued that a French-speaking American had stopped in his village, the chief invited him up to his porch.

As the two men talked, the chief learned the stranger was on his way to Laos. A small group of the chief 's neighbors joined them, including a young Cambodian named PouLop. The American told his listeners the strangest story they had ever heard. It was the story of Adam and Eve, and how after God had created the world, filled it with plants and animals, and put them in charge of a beautiful gar- den. The only tree they couldn't eat from was called "the tree of the knowledge of good and evil." Soon after, God's enemy Sa- tan convinced the woman to disobeyed God and eat the forbidden fruit. She then gave it to Adam, and he ate it too. Their disobedience brought death, sorrow and evil into the world and separated them from God. As Gordon Smith continued his story, the small group on the chief 's porch grew larger. They listened as he explained that because they disobeyed God, evil entered their hearts, and God's curse of death eventually caused them to die. God's curse was passed down to their children and their children, and to everyone in the world. As centuries passed, the world was filled with violence and evil. Then God sent his son to earth in the body of a man. His name was Jesus, and because he was God's son he never sinned. He healed thousands of people by touching them, even people who were lame, blind, and deaf. He even raised people from the dead! But when he told them he was God's son, the religious leaders of that time killed him by beating him and nailing him to a cross. But three days later, God raised Jesus from the dead, and all his followers saw him alive! He told them to tell his story and his teachings to all of the tribes and nations of the world, and then he rose into the sky and returned to heaven.

When the sun began to set, the chief 's wife lit several kerosine lamps and brought them onto the porch. As simply as possible, Gordon shared the gospel to those gathered. When he finished, the people began to murmur: *How could someone who was dead come out of their grave alive? Didn't Lord Buddha teach that when a person dies, he returns as another person, as an animal, or as an insect, depending on how good or bad he was in his previous life?* One by one the people drifted away, talking among themselves. But one young man stayed.

The chief did not believe the white man's story, though he was too polite to say so. The young man, however, was fascinated. He introduced himself to the American in French as "PouLop." As the chief stood silent, PouLop invited Gordon to his bamboo and thatched home by the river so he could hear more. The American thanked the chief for his hospitality and followed PouLop to his house. Late into the night, the two men talked. Hours later, PouLop prayed and asked Jesus to forgive his sins and come into his heart. Gordon spent the night in his car.

The next morning after a breakfast of rice and fish, the American thanked his hosts and prayed that God would soon send someone to teach them and the rest of the villagers more about Jesus. The last question PouLop asked Gordon was when he would come back. With a heavy heart, Gordon shrugged, pointed to heaven, and replied that he didn't know. But he promised to stop and look for him if he passed through the village again.

After the American left, PouLop asked his wife if she would follow Jesus with him. She didn't answer, and he could see she was afraid. His American friend had told him he could talk to Jesus anytime he wanted, and his last words were, "You must pray to Jesus every day and ask Him to help you. He will hear you, and He will show you what to do! And you must do one more thing—you must ask Jesus every day to send someone to teach you and your people about him." Pou Lop looked down at his calloused hands. He would follow this Jesus, this Son of the Creator, but he was afraid. He would have to turn away from Buddhism and for that, he would suffer.

When their rice fields were ripe for harvest, PouLop and his wife harvested more than they had ever harvested before. For the first time, PouLop didn't thank Buddha by participating in the temple worship. Instead, he thanked Jesus. He no longer attended the Buddhist festivals with his friends and neighbors. PouLop's rebellion against Budda angered the village, and the priests no longer stopped at his house for their daily contribution of cooked rice. One night, someone attacked him with a club and beat him up. PouLop's wife became too frightened to stay with him and returned to her father and mother's home, taking their children with her. Years passed, and though PouLop was alone in his faith, he refused to stop praying to Jesus. Eventually, his elderly parents joined the rest of the village and condemned him. Nevertheless, night after night he prayed to Jesus, asking him to protect him and send someone to teach him more.

Nine thousand miles away, a five-year-old boy in Pennsylvania lost his father. The boy's name was Carl, and his father was a coal miner and an alcoholic. One afternoon after a long day of working in the coal mines, Carl's father drank too much beer at a local bar and walked unsteadily to his car. As he drove home that night, he accidently ran over a little girl and killed her. The police put him in jail, and that night he hanged himself.

Times were hard, and Carl's mother had no income to feed her two young sons. She remarried hastily, but within weeks realized she had made a serious mistake. Her new husband took a particular dislike to Carl. When Carl was disobedient or did not obey quickly enough, his stepfather punched him or beat him with his belt, sometimes so brutally that his face and back were bloodied. Some mornings his mother had to use hot water to pull the sheets off his back. As Carl grew older, his beatings turned into lopsided fights. Sometimes his mother intervened with a kitchen skillet, but whenever that happened, her husband beat them both.

One day when Carl was 16, his mother went to the nearby town of New Kensington to shop. As she walked to the bus stop, she heard singing from the open doors of a Christian and Missionary Alliance church. The songs brought back sweet memories from her childhood in Sweden. Battered in soul and body, she entered and sat quietly in a back row. That day she heard for the first time that Jesus loved her, and that he died for her sins. Before she left, she went to the altar and prayed a prayer of confession and faith.

The change in her life surprised the entire family. When her husband got drunk and mocked her faith, instead of arguing she answered him quietly. When he slapped her or punched her, she didn't fight back.

Carl was amazed. When he asked his mother what happened to change her so drastically, she told him about her new faith in Jesus. The following Sunday she took Carl to church with her. Carl's stepfather was not pleased, but he allowed them to go. That day in church, Carl heard that Jesus loved him and had died for his sins. He learned that if he put his faith and trust in Jesus, God would forgive him as many times as he asked. That day Carl believed and asked God to forgive him for hating his stepfather.

When Carl and his mother returned home, their happiness was short-lived. Carl's stepfather called the pastor a "money-grubbing leech" and forbade Carl to return to the church. When Carl argued with him, his stepfather snatched his loaded shotgun from over the fireplace, pointed it at Carl, and threatened to kill him if he didn't leave. Carl threw his few clothes into a bag and walked out the door of his home. He would never live in his stepfather's house again.

When Carl showed up at the church with little more than the clothes on his back, the people welcomed him. A few days later, a widow in the church offered to let him stay in her attic. Church members provided him with food, shoes, and warm clothes. In time, they became his new family. His mother would see him on Sundays, as often as she could get away.

One day a missionary came to the church and talked about the people of Asia who were still waiting to hear about Jesus. Remembering what his life was like before he met Jesus, Carl was deeply moved. Soon after, he announced his intention to become a missionary. After graduating from high school, he applied to the Missionary Training Institute in Nyack, New York. The church bought him a train ticket and took up a collection to pay his school fees for the first semester. Unfortunately, as he slept on the train to New York someone robbed him of all his money for school. Carl immediately notified the church, and as he prayed, God encouraged him not to give up, but to trust him. He was next in line to register and was praying that God would help him when the cashier received a telephone call from his church, informing her that a businessman in the church had wired all the money Carl would need for his first year!

While a student, Carl met a young woman named Ruth. She was a missionary kid who grew up in Vietnam and was a model of decorum and faith but knew little about American culture. Like Carl, she had heard God's call to return to Southeast Asia as a missionary. One day, she and Carl got into a serious conversation. Because Carl had not even heard the gospel until he was 16, he was something of a misfit. But he had a white-hot passion to take the gospel to people who were living and dying without ever hearing of Jesus. Ruth was drawn to Carl by his passion for Christ and Christ's clear command to His disciples to take the gospel to the world.

Ruth's friends and teachers warned her that Carl was wild and unpredictable. Ruth listened for a while, but by their second year at the missionary training school, Ruth and Carl were head over heels in love. After they graduated from the missionary training school in 1946, they married and pastored a small church in Western Pennsylvania. The church paid them $20 a month, so Carl took whatever jobs he could find to pay for his family's needs. The church owned a small parsonage that was furnished with a single bed, a table with two chairs, and a kitchen with a wood-burning stove. One Sunday after the head elder's wife criticized Ruth for wearing the same dress every Sunday, Ruth invited them to come for dinner. Carl had to borrow two chairs from the church so they could all sit at the table.

None of the dishes, silverware, or glasses matched, and Ruth had only an iron skillet to cook on. The elder and his wife were shocked, and soon after, they provided a set of dishes, silverware, pots and pans, and several pieces of furniture. Over the next two years, Carl and Ruth were blessed with two children. In time, the congregation fell in love with them and would be their faithful supporters for decades.

In 1945, Japan surrendered to the United States, ending WWII. Japan withdrew its armies from Cambodia, Laos, and Vietnam, which it had conquered in 1945. France promptly re-invaded all three countries to restore French colonial rule. Within months, rebel movements sprang up. A favorite tactic of the rebels was to bury land mines on the main roads and set ambushes in the jungle on both sides of the road. When either civilian or military vehicles set off a land mine, they were immediately ambushed by armed rebels and killed.

In 1949, the Christian & Missionary Alliance appointed Carl and Ruth to serve as missionaries to Cambodia. In June they traveled to New York City, boarded a freighter with their children, and sailed to Vietnam.

During their first year in Vietnam, Carl and Ruth purchased a used Jeep. To distinguish it from a French Army Jeep, Carl painted it bright yellow with red hubcaps!

After passing their French language exams, Carl and Ruth loaded their Jeep and a trailer with all their worldly belongings and drove from Vietnam to Phnom Penh, Cambodia.

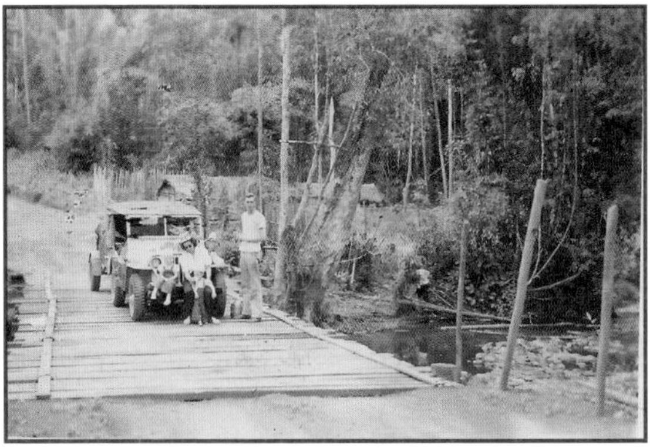

The Thompsons on the road to Kratie, 1950

The mission assigned them to the eastern city of Kratie (pronounced KRA-CHEH), a provincial capital situated on the Mekong River, 150 miles from the capital.

Soon after they arrived in Phnom Penh, Carl asked the French military for permission to travel to Kratie. The French officials strongly advised him not to travel with his family alone, but to wait for a military convoy, and the next convoy wouldn't make the trip for another month. But traveling with the French military would also endanger them, since most Cambodians would conclude they were French colonialists and not Americans. Putting their faith and trust in God, Carl and Ruth decided to make the trip alone. When the French officer they had consulted heard what they were planning, he threw up his hands and said, "You're crazy! But if you're determined to do this, drive as fast as you can and don't stop for anything!"

Carl and Ruth's favorite Bible verse was Proverbs 3:5-6: *"Trust in the Lord with all your heart. In all your ways submit to Him, and He will direct your paths."* In June of 1950, they loaded up their Jeep and trailer and headed for Kratie. But when they were about halfway there, they had a flat tire and were forced to stop to put on their spare tire. As Carl was changing the tire as quickly as he could and Ruth was clutching her children and praying fervently for God's protection, an army truck carrying French soldiers came barreling down the road behind them. Carl and Ruth waved and praised God for sending help when they needed it the most. But to their surprise, the truck drove by them in a cloud of dust! Then fifty yards down the road it set off a landmine! The explosion lifted the truck into the air and rolled it onto its side. Rebels emerged from the jungle on both sides and fired on the French soldiers, killing them all. While that was happening, Carl finished changing the tire and turned their Jeep around. They drove back to the nearest town and spent the night there. The next day they prayed again, asking God to protect them, and resumed their journey. This time they arrived safely in the town of Kratie without further incidents.

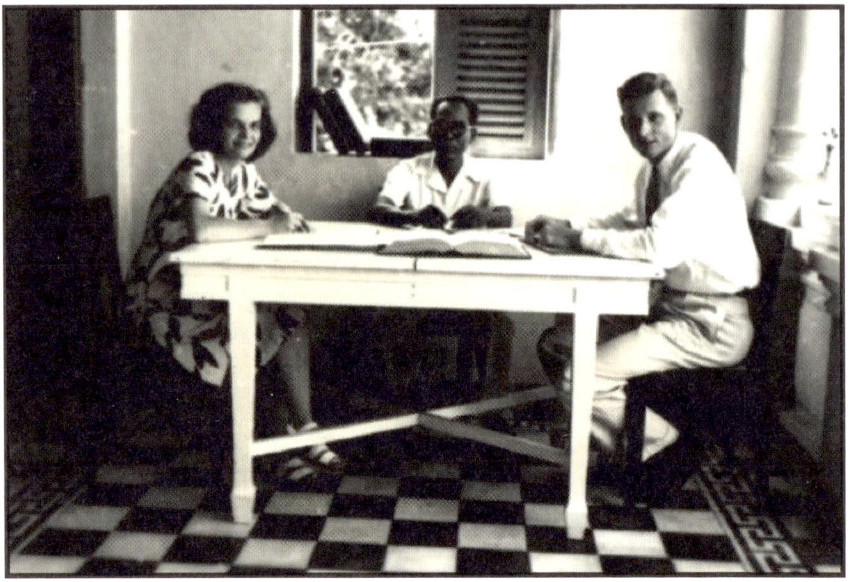

1950 - Carl & Ruth Thompson learn the Khmer language

During their first year in Kratie, Carl and Ruth spent six hours a day studying the Khmer language with a Cambodian tutor, until they could speak, read, and write Khmer. Kratie was a provincial capital, so several thousand French troops were garrisoned in the city to protect it from rebel attacks. One day the French commander received secret information that a large force of Cambodian rebels was planning to attack a French rubber plantation in the town of Snoul, 80 kilometers away. Confident that his information was correct, the commander loaded nearly all of his troops onto trucks and raced to Snoul, hoping to surprise the rebels. But the attack never materialized.

The message the French general had received was a rebel trick. Their actual plan was to trick the French commander into taking all of his troops out of Kratie so they could overrun the town! As the sun set, a French soldier knocked on Carl & Ruth's door and asked if they would like to take refuge in the hotel where the few remaining French soldiers were planning to fight to the finish. They had learned that a force of up to 2,000 rebel fighters would attack their base after dark. Carl and Ruth thanked the French soldier but preferred to stay in their home and pray— not just for themselves, but also for the town and the remaining French soldiers. That night they put their children under their bed, knelt beside it, and begin crying out to God for help!

Around two a.m., a white flare lighted up the sky above the French base. The soldiers had barricaded themselves in with all the weapons they could load. The flare was the sign for the attack to begin.

Soon after, bullets were flying in every direction, some hitting the house. Then exploding hand grenades shook Carl and Ruth's home. Suddenly, a red flare appeared in the night sky, and the shooting stopped. The rest of the night was quiet. In the morning, Carl and Ruth, the Cambodians who lived in the town, and the few French soldiers left behind walked the streets in wonder. There was no sign of the rebels, and no one understood why they had abandoned their attack. Later that day, the French commander returned to Kratie and was surprised that the town had not been overrun.

A year or two later, France agreed to grant independence to Cambodia and return power to Cambodia's king. It was 1953, and the king promised amnesty to all rebels who turned in their weapons on a given day and pledged allegiance to him. On the appointed day, thousands of rebels marched into the town of Kratie and stacked their weapons in a great pile. There were speeches and ceremonies all day long. Towards the end of the day, the retiring French commander asked Carl to translate for him so he could talk to the rebel commander. After introductions, the French commander asked the rebel leader, "On the night I transported nearly all of my soldiers to the rubber plantation 80 kilometers away, there was no attack. You tricked us into moving all of our forces to the rubber plantation, leaving Kratie defenseless. But just minutes after you started your attack on Kratie, you retreated and left! Why didn't you take over the town?"

The rebel commander seemed surprised by the question. He remembered the night well and suggested that the French commander was mistaken. On the night the rebels attacked Kratie, he shot a white flare above the city, and they began their attack. But as they approached the base, they saw thousands and thousands of French soldiers. They were everywhere—behind walls, up on the roofs, in trees, behind bushes. He couldn't believe what he saw! There were more French soldiers defending the town than they had ever seen before! His force numbered thousands of soldiers waiting for them to attack, he realized he had been fooled and withdrew.

With Carl interpreting, the French commander and the rebel leader argued about what happened that night, but Carl understood and could barely contain himself! As he and Ruth prayed that night, *God heard and sent His army to save them, their children, and the town of Kratie!*

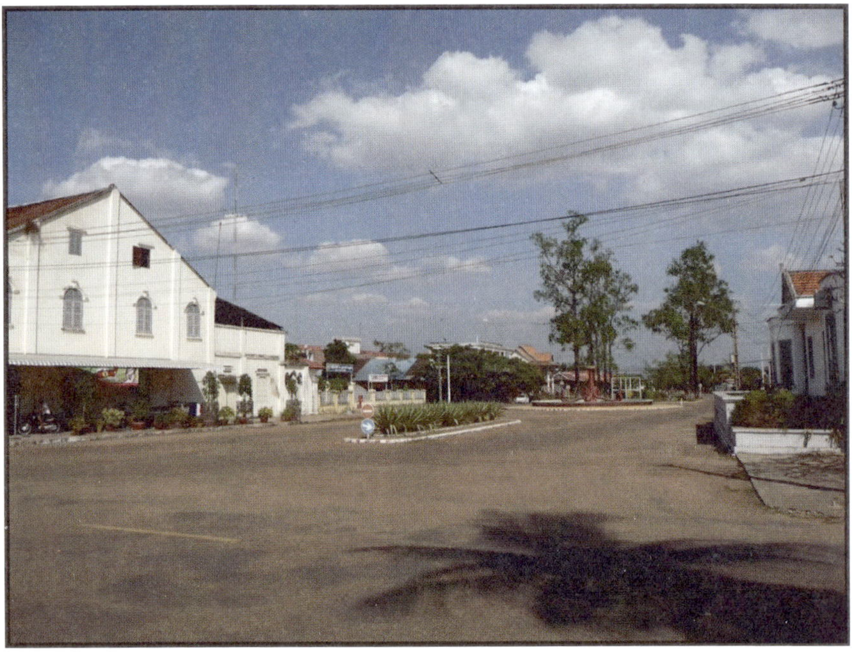

The site of the rebel attack in Kratie, circa 1952. The Thompson apartment was on the second floor of the white house on the left. The window of the bedroom they prayed in as the attack started was the third window from the right. Across the plaza and to the right was the entrance to the French military base where the rebels started their attack at 2 a.m. This photo was taken in 2009.

Church Planting in Kabal Chua

After Cambodia's war for independence from France was over, Carl and Ruth continued to study the Khmer language. Once they had learned to read, write, and speak it, they set their sights on planting a church in Kratie. The governor was a strong Buddhist, however, and when they met with him and asked where in town they could meet, he adamantly refused—unless the church was at least 15 kilometers from the outskirts of the town!

They were disappointed, but trusting God's leading, they complied and began visiting villages outside of the governor's 15-kilometer limit. One day they drove into the small village of Kabal Chua. A crowd quickly gathered, not just to see the white strangers, but also the couple's two small children. They had unbelievably fair skin, and blue eyes! The little girl had light blonde hair, something no one in the village had ever seen or even heard of! Ruth set up a flannel-covered board on the hood of the Jeep, and after introducing his family, Carl began telling them the story of Jesus. The villagers were amused at his strange accent and funny mistakes. The crowd quickly grew to more than twenty people.

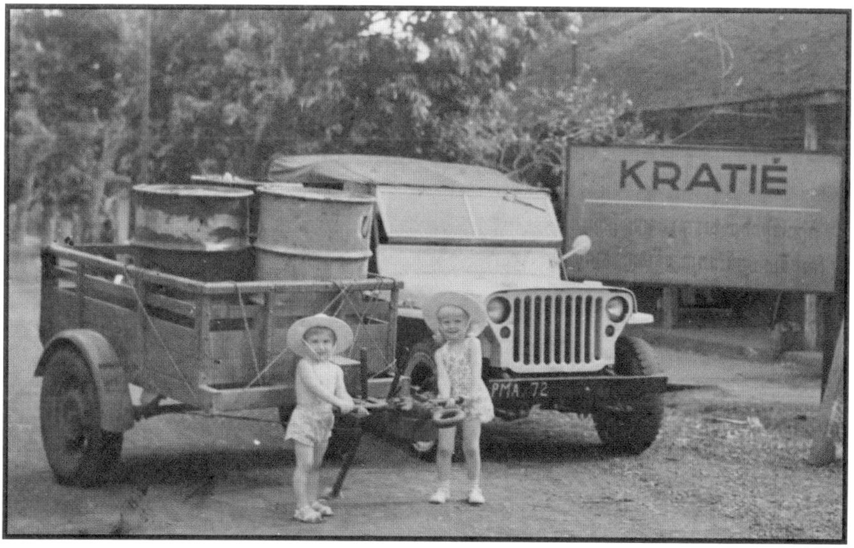

The author and his sister Judy in Kratié in 1952

By this time, it had been eight years since the American in a black Citroen had stopped in the village of Kabal Chua and had led PouLop to faith in Jesus. He had suffered greatly for his faith, and though he knew only what he remembered from the American who had spent the night in his home, he had stubbornly refused to worship Budda. His decision had made him a rebel and a pariah. The growing crowd and excitement in front of the chief 's house attracted his attention, but he was only mildly curious. It wasn't until he saw a tall white man standing near a battered yellow Jeep with red hubcaps that suddenly, his heart started to pound. He tried to move closer. Could this be...? He was afraid to finish the thought! So many times, he had prayed and asked God to send someone to come and teach him, but no one had come. He had almost given up. It was probably just another French- man, but why would a white man stop in a village as small as theirs?

As PouLop elbowed his way towards the front of the crowd and the yellow Jeep, he was surprised to hear the white man and his wife speaking Khmer. He listened with mounting excitement. Then he heard the name of Jesus, and it felt like his heart was going to burst! Could it really be? The white man's woman was putting a picture of a baby on the board, and there were strangely dressed people kneeling in a circle and bowing to him, with cows looking over their shoulders. Then the white man said the baby's name was Jesus!! In an instant, PouLop began shouting, "You've come for me! I'm here! I follow Jesus too! He sent you here for me!" There were tears in his eyes as the white man and his wife turned to him in surprise, but PouLop didn't care. Jesus had not forgotten him, and finally, after so many years, he had sent someone who knew him too!

I marvel at this wonderful story of God's love and grace! He saved an abused rebel from a violence-filled home in Western Pennsylvania and sent him halfway around the world to PouLop's very doorstep. You can't make up stories like this, but God can! That's why Psalms 34:18-20 says, *"The Lord is close to the brokenhearted; He rescues those whose spirits are crushed. The righteous person faces many troubles, but the Lord comes to the rescue each time!"*

PouLop was one of Christ's rebels, and the first Christian in the village of Kabal Chua. Eventually, he became an elder in the church that Carl and Ruth established in Kabal Chua. He served in that role until 1975, when the Khmer Rouge swept over the land, killing all who were known to be Christians. That included PouLop.

I write this story as I heard it from Carl's lips. Carl Edward Thompson was my father, and I was one of the two white children who arrived in Kabal Chua in a yellow Jeep with red hubcaps. In the years that followed, I came to know PouLop and his story. Carl's wife Ruth was my mother, the daughter of Alliance missionaries who went to Hanoi, Vietnam in 1918 and brought the gospel to the people of Vietnam. Between 1918 and their retirement in 1959, God used them to plant more than 20 churches in Vietnam. Today the Alliance church in Vietnam is numbered in the millions.

My father's full name was Carl Edward Thompson, but he preferred to be called "Ed."

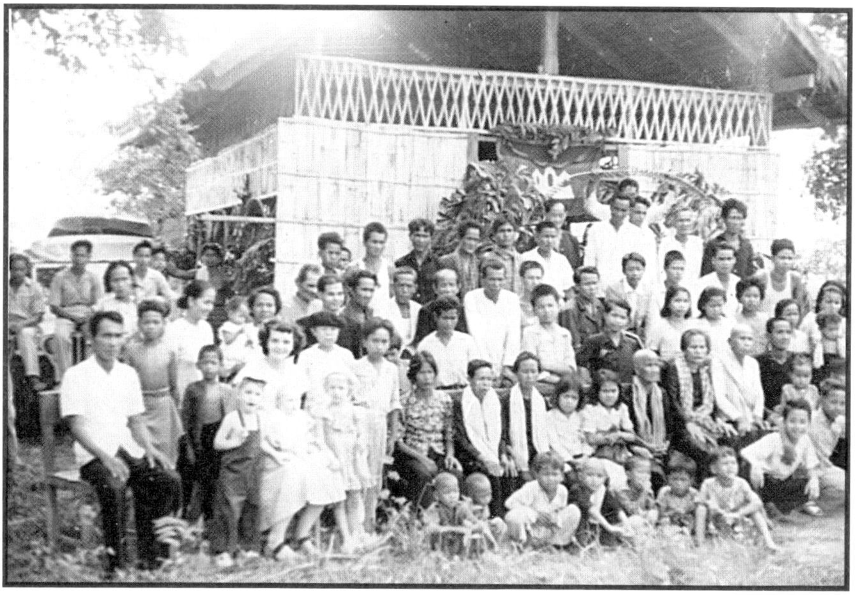

The Khmer church in Kabal Chua, circa 1951.

A Roadside Call

In June of 1959, the Thompson family traveled on a freighter from America to Cambodia for their third four-year term.

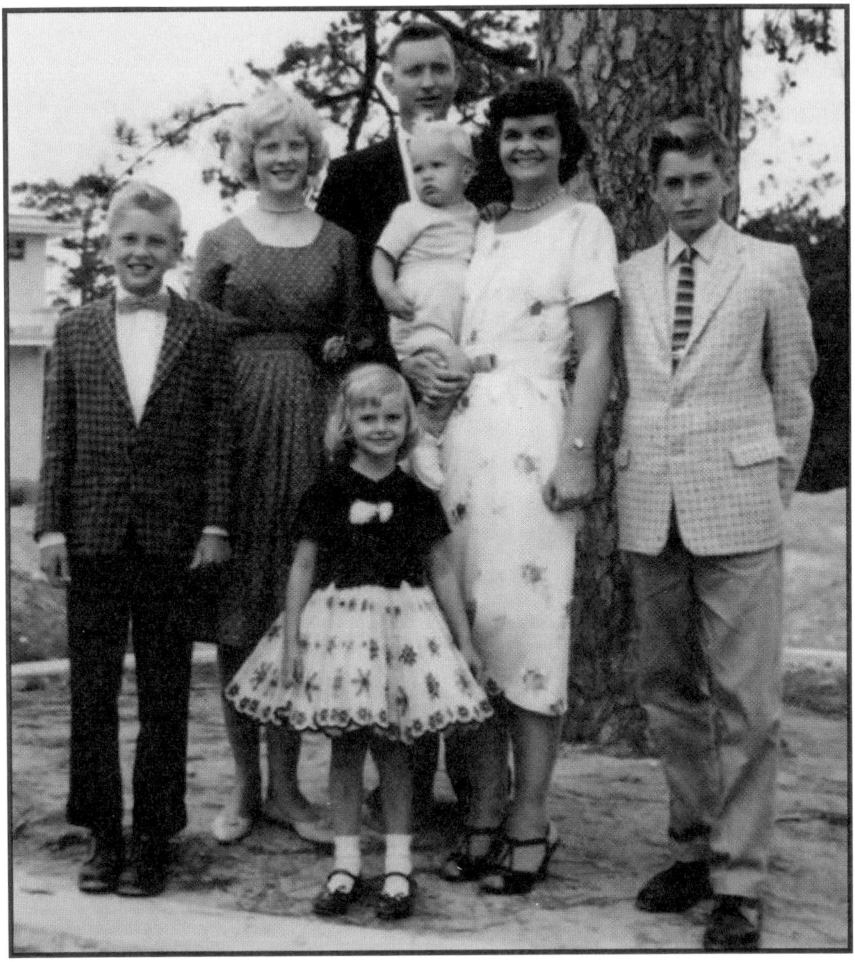

The author's family in 1960, when he was 12.

The trip took two, long months, and by the time we arrived at the school we were half a semester behind in all our classes. I had never had trouble with either math or reading, but halfway through 7th grade my grades plummeted. When my teachers considered holding me back a year, I began praying that God would zap me with a brain upgrade! Sadly, God's zap upgrade never happened, but what did happen was that he sent an extraordinary male teacher to our mission school who taught my class!

The teacher's name was Ralph Bressler, and we called him "Mr. B." From the first day he began teaching he took a worrisome interest in me. One day he said in exasperation, "David, God has given you a perfectly good mind, but you have to *study!*" This was the highest compliment any teacher had given me for a long time, and it was a surprising revelation. With Mr. B's help and encouragement, I began to study.

Towards the end of that first semester Mr. B invited our entire class of eight students to a bonfire outside his house. It was a Friday evening, and someone had previously given us New Testaments to read, but I hadn't bothered to open mine. Our assignment was to bring our New Testaments and pick out a favorite verse to read and comment. I brought my New Testament, but at the last minute I remembered I was supposed to have chosen a verse to comment on! Just then, Mr. B said, "OK, let's go around the circle and read the verses we picked out." I froze, suddenly remembering that we were supposed to have picked out a verse! Mr. B pointed to the classmate on my left and said, "Jim, why don't you start."

As Jim opened his Bible and started reading the verse he had picked ahead of time, I somewhat frantically opened my New Testament randomly. The light of the fi re wasn't good enough to re ad without a flashlight, so when Mr. B turned to me and said, "David? What's your verse?" I grabbed Jim's flashlight and looked where my finger had landed. It was on Matthew 9:12, and I read *"When Jesus heard this, he said, "Healthy people don't need a doctor—sick people do.* "Surprised, I looked up and blurted, 'I think God is calling me to become a medical missionary!'"

Mr. Bressler beamed and said, "That's wonderful, David! Praise the Lord!" A murmur of surprise and admiration went around the circle. Fortunately, nobody could see me blushing in the firelight, because it was entirely fake! Nevertheless, in that moment, something strange had occurred. Beginning that night, I began wondering what it would take to become a missionary doctor. I was such a terrible student it seemed ridiculous. My first thought was to ask God to do a miracle on my brain so I could get all A's, but God didn't seem interested in my solution, and neither was Mr. Bressler. I can laugh at my foolishness now, but at the time hearing that all I needed to do was study was a significant word from Mr. Bressler, because it meant he believed I was not stupid and might actually have the intelligence to become an A student. His encouragement turned my apathy into determination. By the end of that year and with Mr. B's help, my F's turned to D's. When the next school year came around, my D's disappeared. By the end of 9th grade, I had no more C's. By 10th or 11th grade, even my parents agreed that a miracle had taken place: I had become a straight A student. I realized then that God had answered my prayers—not by improving my brain, but by sending Mr. Bressler to be my teacher and mentor. During those years, a missionary doctor came to our school and spoke in chapel. His stories were fascinating, and at the end of his talk he looked at our small group of junior and senior high students and said, "I hope and pray that some of you here today will become missionary doctors." It still seemed impossible, but I felt a strange stirring in my heart to go for it.

That same year, I saw a Cambodian man die from trauma. Our family was traveling in our Land Rover from Kratie to Phnom Penh, Cambodia's capital. Suddenly, we came on the scene of a terrible accident between a truck and a bus. The most seriously injured person was the driver of the truck. The two vehicles had collided on a blind curve in the road at high speed. There were people on both sides of the road with bloody noses and broken arms, but the most severely injured person was the driver of the truck. There were no seat belts in those days, and when the two vehicles collided head on, he was violently thrown against the steering wheel, crushing his chest. People from the bus had dragged him to a nearby tree and had propped him up to help him breathe. He was gasping for air and spitting out blood. Ten or fifteen men were standing around him grimly watching him die.

My dad stopped our car and said, "David, get the thermos of water and come with me." I shakily followed him over to the injured man and was shocked to see his deformed chest. He was gasping for air and spitting up blood, and nobody knew what to do. We were six hours from the nearest hospital, and in those days, there were no cellphones. Nobody knew what to do to help him as he gasped for air fought to breathe. My father knelt beside him and greeted him in

Cambodian. As I poured water into a cup for him, my hands were shaking. The man tried to drink, but he was breathing so frantically he couldn't seem to swallow. My father spoke Cambodian fluently, and he began talking to the man, asking him if he was ready to meet God, and if he had heard of God's Son, Jesus. But as my father spoke, the man shook his head and gasping, said, "Don't—tell me —about— your— God! just help me!"

In that moment I realized the dying man in front of us was turning away from his only hope for God's forgiveness. My dad prayed for him, and we returned to our car and continued on. But I will never forget the overwhelming sorrow that gripped my heart. In the weeks and months that followed, I thought of the dying man often and grieved for him. I couldn't stop thinking, "If we could have *helped* him, he might have lived long enough to listen to us, hear the gospel, and believe in Jesus!"

The rest of the trip I said very little, reliving the experience over and over. The more I thought about it, the more I knew what I wanted to do with my life. I wanted to help the sick and dying people of the world who had no one to help them so that, unlike this man, they could live to hear about Christ's love, believe in Him, and live forever! By the time we reached Phnom Penh I had solemnly promised God that if He would help me, I would devote my life to that task.

The B'nong Chief's Invitation

In 1958, a delegation of chiefs from the largest tribal group in eastern Cambodia appeared at our front door in Kratie. They had walked more than 100 miles from their villages, some of which were only a few miles from Cambodia's border with South Vietnam. The chiefs wore loincloths and loose turbans, carried homemade crossbows, knives and spears, and called themselves the "B'nong." They came because they had heard my mother and father were teaching the story of God to Cambodia's predominant people group, the Khmer.

Somewhere in their distant past the ancestors of the B'nong people had heard about the God who made the world, the animals, and the first man and woman. Then a great flood came that drowned everyone but a single family that built a huge boat to save themselves and many animals. For centuries, the B'nong had passed the story down to their children and grandchildren, who then passed it on to theirs. But over time, they had-lest the rest of the story. When the B'nong chiefs heard that my parents were teaching it to the Khmer people, they wanted to hear it too! They had walked more than 100 miles to invite my dad and mom to come to their villages and tell their people the rest of the story! There were three major problems: first, the only roads into eastern Cambodia from Kratie were logging roads. Second, they were only passable during Cambodia's five-month dry season, from November to April. Third, their villages were scattered across Cambodia's eastern forests in an area the size of Maine!

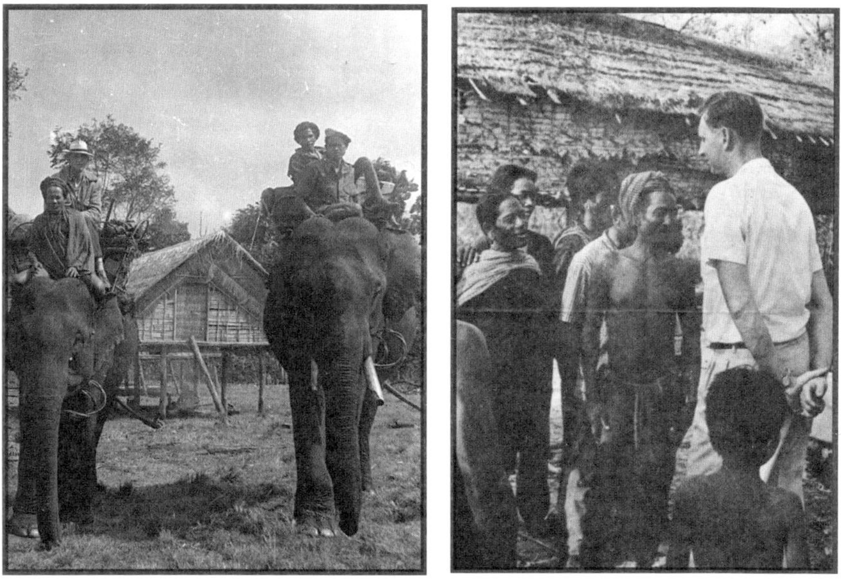

David's dad, Carl, rides an elephant to visit a B'nong village.

Nevertheless, mom and dad were thrilled about the B'nong's invitation. Once again, they turned to God for guidance and help. They would need someone to teach them the B'nong language, they would need something bigger and sturdier than their tired Jeep, and they would need financial support for the project!

The following year our family returned to the U.S. for a year. Dad and mom spoke in churches all across Pennsylvania, Ohio, West Virginia, and New York, telling the story of their first church plant among the Khmer people and the amazing invitation of the B'nong chiefs. Generous friends helped them purchase a new Chevy pickup with a camper on the back, travel money for the next four years, and funds to establish a base camp in in eastern Cambodia.

Our yearly visits to the B'nong villages in Cambodia's Dry Season were unforgettable and would change our lives forever. Over the next ten years, dad became semi-fluent in the B'nong language, and he and mom visited many of the B'nong villages. When there was no road, the village chief would send elephants to carry them.

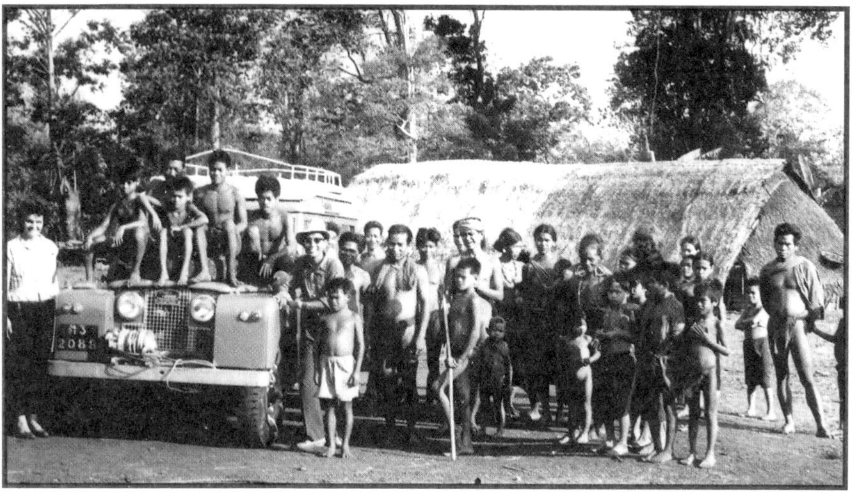

Ruth Thompson during a preaching visit to a B'nong village in Cambodia

In the evenings the chiefs would call the people together around a bonfire, and over three or four nights, my dad would tell the story of God from creation to the crucifixion, the resurrection of Jesus, and his command to take the gospel to all the tribes and nations of the world. In every village the people were fascinated by the story of God, and they believed that "The Great Book" Dad read from was true. But as they heard the story of Jesus, God's Son and learned heard that he was tortured and then hung on a cross by his enemies until he died, they hesitated. If God's enemies could kill his own son, Jesus, how could God and his son be more powerful than the spirits they worshipped? Even if God raised him from the dead, if the enemies of God had the power to torture and kill Jesus, what would stop them from killing and torturing those who followed him? For centuries they had worshipped the spirits and had sacrificed their buffaloes to them. But if they abandoned the spirits to follow Jesus, who would defend them from the evil spirits? Even my father and mother's impassioned preaching and growing friendship with them was not enough to convince them.

Kidnapped!

About that same time and less than a hundred miles to the east, Viet Cong soldiers kidnaped three American missionaries from a leprosy hospital on the outskirts of the city of Banmethuot. The captured missionaries were serving at a hospital that cared for Montagnards who suffered from Leprosy (Hansen's Disease). Their names were Rev. Archie Mitchell, who was the new Director, the hospital's only doctor Ardel Vietti, and Dan Gerber, a Mennonite missionary.

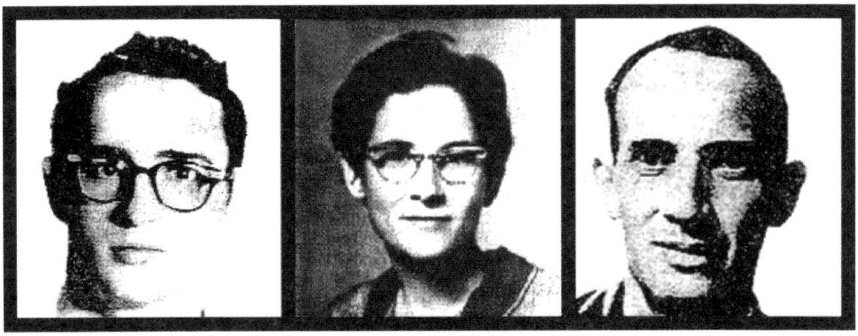

From right to left: Archie Mitchell, Dr. Ardell Vietti, and Dan Gerger

When in 1954 at the tender age of six I arrived at the mission school in the town of Dalat, Vietnam, Archie Mitchell and his wife Betty were in charge of the boys' dormitory. They were like the best aunt or uncle a child could ever have! Mrs. Mitchell was kind, firm, and at first awesome, but she seemed to know a great deal about what went on in the hearts and minds of little boys. She was also a great reader of stories to lonely hearts and a determined scrubber of grime, even if you were the 15th kid in the bathtub lineup! Mr. Mitchell was 6'2," tall and muscular, towered over us, and had scary scars on his hands. But he was also gentle and kind.

The Mitchells had four children, the oldest being Becki who was my age. She was a tomboy, and to our shame she could run faster, jump and climb higher, and play softball, basketball and just about every other game as well or better than we boys! Our main problem with her was that she delighted in proving that in everything athletic, she was better than us! The fact that her parents were the Mitchells made the situation quite difficult, especially when she informed us that if we so much as touched her, her dad would "squish you like a bug!" It seemed plausible and did not endear her to us.

When I was eleven, the Mitchells returned to the United States for a year of furlough, speaking in churches to maintain their support. But when the year was over and Vietnam denied their visas, they ended staying in the U.S. for a second year. When they returned, the Mission assigned them to direct a hospital for Montagnard leprosy patients near the city of Banmethuot, in Vietnam's central highlands.

Just eight days after the Mitchells arrived at the hospital, Viet Cong soldiers destroyed several small bridges on the half-mile access road through the jungle. They also left a threatening note warning them not to repair the ten-foot bridges. Since up until then the Viet Cong had never harmed either missionaries or leprosy patients, the U.S. and the Vietnamese military forces were alarmed and urged the missionaries to close the hospital and leave. After discussing and praying about their advice, the missionaries decided they couldn't abandon their patients and would trust God to protect them.

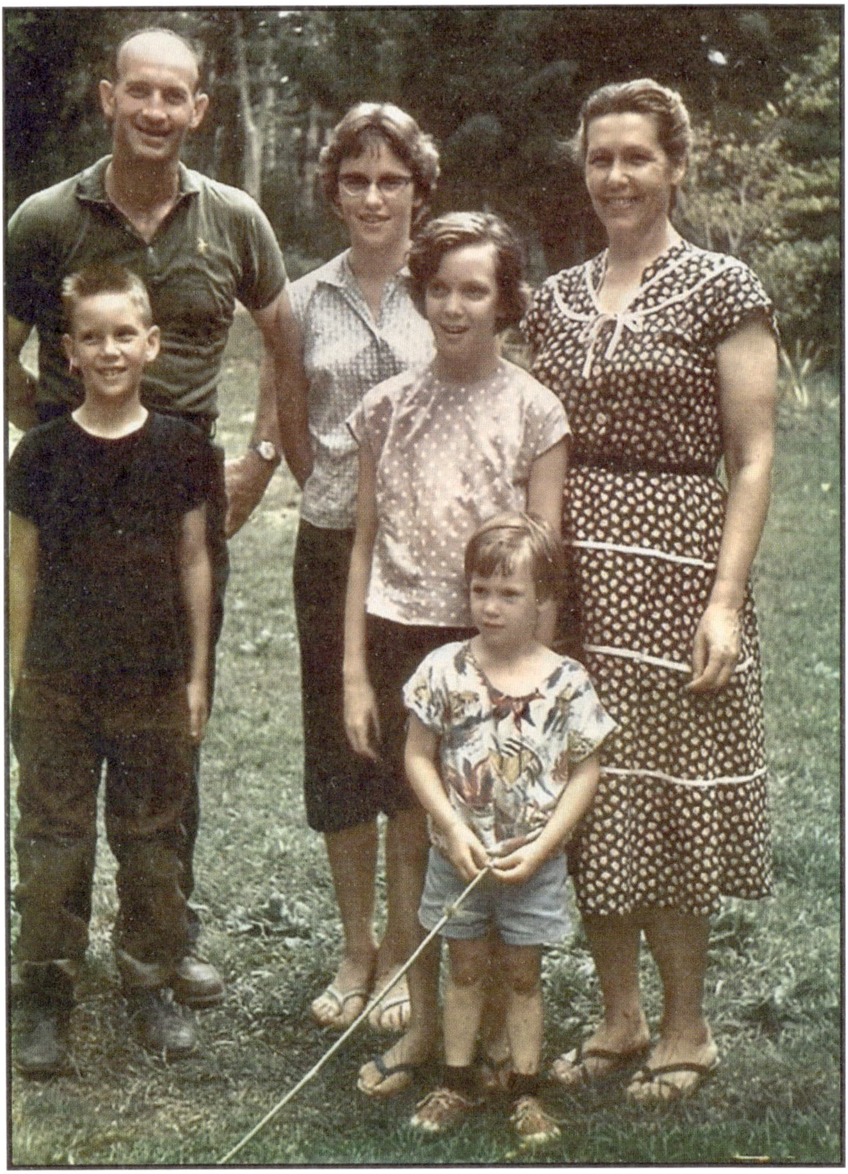

The Mitchell Family, just days before Archie Mitchell and two other missionaries were kidnapped.

On the evening of May 30, 1962, the Mitchells were having devotions in their living room when they heard shouting outside and boots on the stairs. Seconds later a Viet Cong soldier slit the screen door to their porch with his bayonet and burst in. Mr. Mitchell jumped to his feet to protect his family, but the soldier ordered them all outside and tied Mr. Mitchell's hands behind his back. When they started to tie his wife Betty's hands, Archie asked them in Vietnamese to leave her so she could care for their children. For some reason, they listened. Minutes later, Mrs. Mitchell and her children wept in shock as the soldiers marched Archie around the corner of their house and into the darkness of the jungle.

A few minutes later other soldiers brought Dr. Ardel Vietti and three missionary nurses from their houses and Dan Gerber, a Mennonite missionary. Then they tied Dr. Vietti and Dan Gerber's hands behind them and led them away to join Archie.

After that the soldiers forced the remaining missionaries and the Mitchell children to sit on the ground and listen to them lecture about Communist doctrine. While this was happening, other Viet Cong went into the hospital and carried out armloads of medical supplies. They also ransacked the missionaries' homes and loaded the loot into one of the mission Land Rovers until it was full. But then they couldn't figure out how to drive it! Eventually they forced one of the nurses to show them how to start it and drive it away. Before the last of the Viet Cong disappeared into the night, they warned the missionaries that they would kill anyone who left the hospital before daylight.

For Betty Mitchell and her four children that would be the longest night of their lives. As soon as the soldiers left, she and her children ran to their house to check on four-year-old Geraldine. The soldiers had forced them outside without her, and for hours, Betty had been quietly praying for her daughter's safety. When the rest of the family reached Geri's bedroom, they found her sitting on her bed quietly waiting. As they hugged her, she said, "Those were really bad men!"

When daylight finally came the Mitchells and the nurses drove into Banmethuot and reported to the authorities what happened. U.S. Special forces immediately began a search with helicopter gunships and ground forces, but though they continued looking for them for months and even years, they never found a trace of them. To this day, God alone knows what happened to them.

Archie's kidnapping was not the first tragedy to befall him. During World War II, the Japanese army floated more than 9,000 balloon bombs across the Pacific on the Northern Polar Jet Stream that flows from Japan to north America. They hoped that the silent balloons would land on America's forests and explode, resulting in massive forest fires and panic. On May 5, 1945, Archie Mitchell was a young pastor in Bly, Oregon. On a sunny Saturday morning, he and his wife Elsie drove five children on a Sunday school picnic to a favorite spot on Gearhart Mountain, 15 miles from Bly and 50 miles east of Klamath Falls. As Archie unloaded the food from the back of the car, the children and his pregnant wife ran ahead through the trees to find a good picnic site. Instead, they discovered a deflated balloon bomb. When Archie heard their excited voices and sensed danger, he shouted a warning to them to not touch it! He and others in Oregon's mountains had heard rumors of the Japanese balloons. But even as he shouted, the bomb exploded in a tremendous ball of fire. Archie ran toward the explosion and was horrified to see all the children and his wife Elsie lying motionless, surrounded by flames. Elsie's clothes were on fire, and as he desperately tried to stop her clothes from burning with his bare hands he wept. It was no use; he alone had survived, and Elsie and the children were gone.

The exploding bomb created a hole a foot deep and 3-foot-wide, and the trees around it were peppered with shrapnel. It was so powerful that fragments were found 400 feet away. Elsie was 26 and five months pregnant, and the children were 11 to 14 years old.

Today the site is known as "The Mitchell Monument" and is still visited by tourists, though most don't know the details. Archie's wife and the children who died were the only American civilians killed during WWII by enemy action on the U.S. mainland. The Japanese government never learned until after the war that only 300 of the bombs reached the U.S. mainland, and that because most of them arrived in the Spring only the few exploded and caused little damage. It was such a well-kept secret that before the war ended, the Japanese inventor and project director concluded he had failed and committed suicide.

Two years later, Reverend Archie Mitchell married Betty Patzke, the older sister of two of the children who were killed on that fateful day. In 1947, Archie and Betty were appointed by the Christian & Missionary Alliance to serve in Vietnam as missionaries. During their first two years they learned French and Vietnamese in Dalat, a city Vietnam's central highlands. In 1948 their first was child was born, and they named her Rebecca. After completing language study their first assignment was to serve as dorm parents for the boys attending the Dalat School for missionary children. It was the only school for missionary kids in southeast Asia, so in June 1954, my parents brought me there to begin first grade.

Mr. Mitchell had big, hard hands that were scarred but gentle, and unforgettable when tweaking an ear for ignoring clear and well-understood warnings! From the time I came to school until I was ten, I lived with the Mitchells eight months of the year. They provided love and a stability to dorm life that eased the pain of being away from our parents. Before there was a mission school at Dalat or home-schooling, missionaries who wanted to educate their children had only two choices: send them to boarding schools in America for four years at a time or keep them with them and forego formally educating them. Homeschooling was not universally accepted in America until 1992, so mission boarding schools with certified American teachers were an enormous blessing for missionary families, most of whom lived only a few days drive from where their parents were serving.

The news that Mr. Mitchell and two other missionaries had been kidnapped in Banmethuot, spread through the mission school and missionary communities in Vietnam, Cambodia, Laos, and Thailand like wildfire. After all, kidnapping and taking hostages could happen to anyone, including the more than 100 children in the Dalat School, which was just 130 miles away from Banmethuot. We who were at the school watched the Mitchell kids with a mixture of awe, fear, and sorrow. They didn't talk much about their ordeal and I never saw them crying, but we knew they were grieving and praying for their father.

I couldn't help wondering if the kidnapped prisoners would be locked up in bamboo cages like our captured GI's, would be chained in underground caves, or marched every night through the jungle until they arrived in Hanoi. The questions left us shaken and fearful for our own parents. It seemed to me that in an indefinable way, sorrow and faith had made the Mitchells stronger than the rest of us. Their lives went on as before, except that now Becki was subdued and no longer an adversary.

Faith, Hope, and Sorrow

Two years after the kidnapping at the leprosy hospital, my parent's dry season visits to the B'nong villages in Cambodia came to an abrupt halt. The North Vietnamese army had flooded down through Laos and into eastern Cambodia and was threatening a major attack on American and South Vietnamese forces on the other side of Cambodia's eastern border. To stop them, President Nixon sent B-52's to bomb the North Vietnamese army, without the permission of Cambodia's king! The King angrily broke diplomatic relations with America and ordered all Americans out of his country. That included us! Despite all the arduous trips to B'nong villages they had made to win them to faith in Jesus, not a single member of the tribe had believed their message. As we left Cambodia in June of 1965 and returned to the U.S., my parents wept.

In the Fall, I enrolled in a public school in New York State and started my senior year of high school.

My older sister Judy was attending school at Nyack College, so my parents rented a house nearby. That year my parents spoke in Alliance churches all over the country, reporting on what God had done through their ministry in Cambodia and especially their efforts to win the B'nong people to faith in Jesus. If they spoke in churches near us, our whole family went along. At the end of my dad's sermons, he would always ask the people to pray that the B'nong would have another chance to hear the gospel, turn from worshipping spirits, and follow Jesus. It became my earnest prayer, too.

Not long after that we learned that thousands of B'nong people were living in villages on the Vietnam side of the border near the city of Banmethuot. Mom and dad began praying about moving to Vietnam, learning Vietnamese, and joining the Alliance missionary team in Banmethuot and resume their ministry to the B'nong. In the Spring of 1965, they began the long process of packing 55-gallon drums with the things they would need to make a new home in Vietnam.

About that time some dear friends who had supported us generously over the years came for a visit. At the beginning the conversation was light and there was much laughter. But when the subject of Vietnam came up, things grew tense. A few minutes later, my parents led their friends down to our basement to see the barrels they were packing for life in Vietnam. Minutes later, we heard crying, and later we learned that their friends had started pulling things out of our barrels and throwing them to the floor! They were weeping and saying, *"You must not do this, you must not do this! here's a war going on over there, and if you go back the Communists are going to kill you! Please, please, please don't go!"* My mother was crying too, and she replied, "Whether we live or we die, we must go! God has told us to return to the B'nong, and we will obey Him!" Then my father said, "This may be our last chance to win them to faith in Jesus!" When the weeping finally ended, they hugged each other and sorrowfully left. I realized then that the only person who could stop my parents from going to Vietnam and the B'nong people was God himself.

In June of 1966, I graduated from high school and prepared to move to Geneva College, in Beaver Falls, Pennsylvania. By this time Mom and dad had shipped a used Jeep they had purchased and their barrels to a freighter in New York, and the mission had purchased airplane tickets to Saigon for them and my younger sister and two younger brothers.

A friend of mine had spoken so enthusiastically about the pre-med course at Geneva College that I decided to apply. Soon after, I was accepted to start as a freshman in early September of 1966. I was Incredibly naïve and thought that to qualify for a scholarship I had to have straight As in my senior year of high school. Since I had several B's on my report card, I decided to simply trust God and go!

My parent's mission had promised me a monthly stipend of $100 for the next two years, which at the time seemed like a princely sum. Remembering my mother's unshakable confidence that if God wanted me to become a missionary doctor He would provide, I showed up at Geneva College to register for the first semester in early September with just $50 in my pocket. I knew God would supply, but I didn't have the faintest clue how! What I did remember were the last words my mother had said to me the week before we parted. Once again, I had asked her where the money would come from to pay for four years of pre-med, followed by four more years of medical school.

In reply, she put her hand on my arm, looked up at me with a smile, and said "David, if God has called you to become a doctor, *He will provide!"*

Since that day I have learned many times over that God looks for men and women who are willing to trust and obey Him, no matter how great the challenge. Of course, that does not mean we must forgo scholarships and grants to educate and prepare ourselves for God's service! What I got right at the time was the clear understanding that if God could give young David, Israel's second and greatest king, the faith, confidence and courage to kill a bear and a lion with only a club to defend the sheep he guarded day and night, and later challenge a giant with only a sling and a stone, I could start school the money I had. For the rest, I would have to trust God. When I look back, I'm astonished by my ignorance and naiveté, but deeply grateful for the faith that my mother and God gave me as I began my journey to become a missionary doctor.

I had already been told by some of my non-Christian friends that unless I was brilliant or rich, I would never achieve my dream of becoming a doctor. One thing I had learned reading the Bible was that Satan is a liar, behind the lie that God is expects us to plan ahead exhaustively, be self-reliant, and trust only in ourselves. The Bible was full of wonderful examples of how God looked out for those who were willing to trust and obey him, no matter how great or how impossible the challenges they faced!

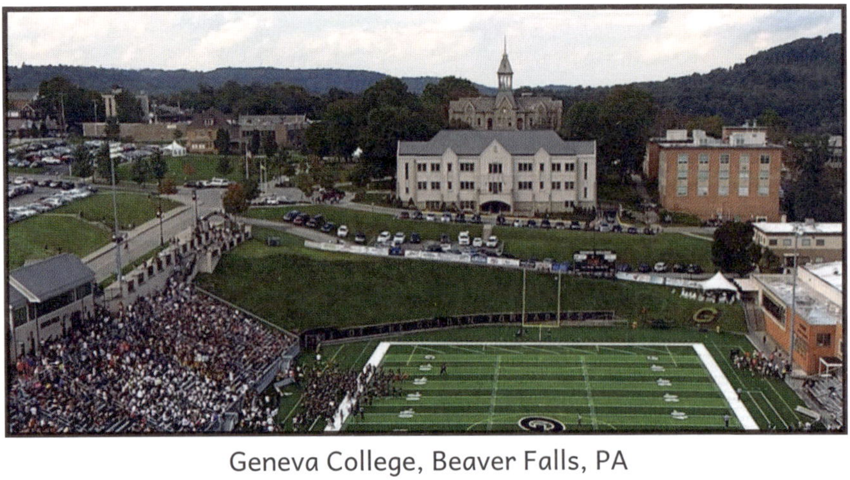

Geneva College, Beaver Falls, PA

On the day I arrived on the campus of Geneva College, there were prominent signs pointing applicants to the gymnasium. There I found tables set up for the different departments. I went to a table that said, "Pre-Med" and found what classes I would need to take during my first semester. Then I paid for some of the books I would need and headed to the cashier. She took a look at my registration card, rang up the cost of the courses I had signed up for, and added the cost of my room and board. My total bill for the first semester would be several thousand dollars! I was somewhat prepared for this and handed her my $50, explaining that my money hadn't come yet, which was certainly true! The cashier looked up at me in surprise, then asked if I had applied for loans, grants, or scholarships. When I said "no," she sighed, handed me my bill, and directed me to a serious looking man in a black suit standing nearby who I later learned was the Dean of Finance.

The Dean greeted me kindly and asked what my problem was. When I explained that my money hadn't come yet he asked when and from where it would be coming. With some hesitation, I explained that I was trusting God to provide for my needs. With that, his eyebrows went up. I hastened to add that I was also planning to work and pay my way through college, but his eyebrows still remained up. After a pause, he suggested I come to his office later in the week so we could talk about "taking out some loans." My heart sank at the thought of borrowing money during my first week of college. How could I pay back eight years of school loans and still devote the majority of my life as a missionary? That would take an even greater miracle, and I would be an old man by then!

Classes started the next day, and I began looking for work. I didn't know anyone in downtown Beaver Falls, or where to start looking for a part-time job. I didn't have a car either, so a job in town wasn't really an option. On the positive side, I had learned to work hard. My first job in America had been helping a neighbor build a retaining wall behind his house. After the homeowner explained that he wanted me to dig out his collapsing bank and then build a wall with railroad ties he had already purchased, I got to work.

For the first two weeks I dug the dirt from the collapsed bank and hauled it in a wheelbarrow to a pile 20 feet away. During the second week it began to rain. In Cambodia, workers were expected to keep working unless it rained hard, and this was a North American all-day drizzle. The homeowner hadn't told me what to do if it drizzled, so I kept working, never considering that I should stop. Later that day when he returned and saw me working drenched to my socks, he was horrified! He asked, "Don't you know not to come to work on a rainy day?" I didn't know, but was immediately grateful that in America, workers could stay home when it drizzled! A month later the rail- road ties were in place, and the bank was handsomely terraced. The homeowner congratulated me for a job well done and paid me $400, more money than I had ever seen! But that money was long gone.

I soon learned there was an opening to daily clean the bathrooms in the men's dormitory. The pay was a dollar an hour, and since there were no other jobs, I signed up. Within a few days I was expert in cleaning sinks, toilets and mopping bathroom floors. Unfortunately, I never managed to stretch the job to more than an hour and a half a day, which meant I was earning only $1.50 a day. Though I persevered, it didn't take a college degree to realize I was never going to pay my way through college cleaning toilets!

During the second week of school, the director of the college's sixty-voice acapella choir announced there would be tryouts. My roommate was a pastor's son from Seattle named David MacMillan. He had a rich baritone voice, so when he tried out, the choir director signed him up right away. He urged me to join the choir too, and since I had enjoyed singing in a choir at the mission school, I decided to try. My tenor voice was a bit reedy, but I could read music and harmonize. Tryouts would resume the following Monday, but just to be sure, I began praying that God would put it on the choir director's heart to accept me.

That Sunday I came down with a cold. By Monday morning I could hardly talk. I was troubled that the Lord had failed to keep me from getting a cold at such an important time in my life. Perhaps, I suggested to him in a brief prayer, he might help the choir director understand? Supremely confident that God would smooth the way, on Monday morning I got in line and waited my turn.

It was a long line, and by the time it was my turn to sing, the di- rector was tired. When he asked me what part I sang, I said hoarsely, "Tenor," and tried to explain that I had laryngitis and could really sing. The director cut me off, handed me a hymnal, and as he began playing said, "Sing! C'mon, sing!" After I horribly sang a few bars, he stopped playing and called for the next student! I was disappointed at my performance, but since I had prayed and trusted God to help me, I remained hopeful.

The following day when my name did not appear on the list of those chosen, I was shocked! Hadn't I prayed and asked God to give the choir director an understanding heart? Instead, he had brushed me off like a fly! Of course, I knew that as a Christian I shouldn't think that way, so I sadly asked the Lord to forgive me and moved on.

A few days later I noticed that my dormmates were wearing very wrinkled shirts to class. There were no "stay-press" shirts back then, so that was the day the "Thompson Ironing Service" was born. I had never ironed a shirt in my life, but I borrowed my roommate's iron and ironing board and began ironing shirts for 25 cents apiece. It was more profitable than the toilet job but still wasn't nearly enough. My typing skills were better than average and I had a good typewriter, so I offered the guys in my dorm typing services for 15 cents a page. Major edits were an extra 10 cents. Soon my every spare minute was taken up ironing shirts, typing papers, and cleaning toilets. When those jobs were done, I got down to studying, often hitting the sack by one or two in the morning.

By this time two weeks had gone by, and the Dean of Finance hadn't contacted me about coming to his office. Whenever I saw him on campus I would slow down and drift behind a tree. I wondered how long I could hold out before he called me in.

Ten days into the semester the school announced there would be a freshman talent show the following Friday. I had recovered fully from laryngitis, and my roommate was vocally gifted, so when he came up with an idea for a humorous musical skit, we signed up. My roommate had a night job cleaning the classrooms in a nearby elementary school, so as he mopped the floors, we practiced our skit. By the day of the freshman talent show we had it down to perfection.

There were many good presentations that day, but when it was our turn, we got so much applause that we won a prize. At the end of the program as everyone was filing out of the gymnasium, the choir director approached me and said, "David, that was a great musical skit you two put on!" I was surprised that he remembered me, so I smiled and thanked him.

"You know, "he said with a laugh, "you can really sing!" Now he had my attention. He continued, "I need more first tenors in the choir, so if you want, you're welcome to join. How about it?" I sighed and glumly explained that though I wanted very much to accept his invitation, I was working three jobs to earn money for school, though of course I didn't tell him what they were! The choir director seemed genuinely disappointed, but not nearly as much as I was.

That afternoon I found a note in my mailbox from the Dean of Finance, asking me to come to his office the next morning at 8 a.m. My heart sank. My earnings by then amounted to less than $150, which I knew were not even close to what I owed. The next morning, I entered the finance office with a sense of impending doom. The Dean greeted me kindly and had me sit down.

After we were both seated, he said, "David, has the Lord provided you with the funds you need for your first semester at school?"

"Not entirely, sir," I said, and placed my $150 on his desk. I was surprised that he only looked at it briefly and didn't even count it. Then he asked, "Have you considered a school loan? We can offer you a loan that you could pay back at very low interest."

I sighed and said, "Several years ago God called me to be a missionary doctor, and I know it's going to take at least eight years for me to do that. If I start taking out loans now it will take me so many years to pay back the loans that I'll never be a missionary!" The Dean nodded and leaned back in his chair.

Then he said, "Mr. Greig, the choir director talked to me yesterday. He told me that he really wants you to sing in the school choir, but that your jobs are making it impossible."

Surprised by the change in direction, I said, "Yes sir, he asked me this morning to join, but I had to refuse because I'm working to earn money to pay for my schooling. I don't have time to work, sing in the choir three afternoons a week, and have time to study." The Dean nodded agreeably, putting his hands together in a steeple.

Then he asked, "What if we were to find some grants and scholarships to pay for your first semester? If we did that, would you consider quitting your jobs and accept Mr. Greg's invitation to sing in the choir?" I stared at him, my mouth ajar.

"Do you mean not work and sing in the choir?" I finally asked.

"That's right. Your professors tell me you seem to be a serious student. If you keep your grades up, we might be able to find additional grants and scholarships for you next semester."

I wanted to hug the guy, but I settled for a handshake and a happy smile! As I walked out the door, my feet barely touching the ground, I realized I had seriously misjudged the Lord. If I had not developed laryngitis when I did, the choir director would never have heard my story and would not have advocated for me! In fact, I realized so many things that day that it took weeks to sort it all out in my heart and mind. Part of that process was remembering the promise my mother had taught me from my childhood: "*Trust in the Lord with all your heart; do not depend on your own understanding. Seek his will in all you do, and He will show you which path to take.*" That night I asked God to forgive me for doubting him and his ways. I also thanked him for teaching me how to trust in Him and for so wonderfully answering my prayers! It was the beginning of understanding that God had every right to allow me to suffer, and that when suffering happened, I had no right doubt him. But how soon, how very soon I would forget!

The Unimaginable

A year and a half later, I was sitting down to breakfast in the college cafeteria when a friend of mine hurried up to me with a message from the Dean of Students. He said, "The Dean wants to see you in his office right now!" Wondering what it might be, I left my tray and hurried to the Dean's' office. A chill of fear shook me as I opened the door to his office and saw five or six faculty and staff members sitting in the Dean's office. Had I done something wrong? Even my pastor from the local Alliance church was there! After they greeted me, my favorite professor cleared his throat and said, "David, we've just received news from the Christian & Missionary Alliance headquarters that your parents have been killed in Vietnam." In the breathless silence that followed, the world stopped turning. A thousand images of my mother and father flashed through my mind, stopping finally at the last day I saw them alive.

It was a warm, summer morning in Nyack, New York. I had to leave for my summer job, and my parents were loading their bags into the back of a car that would take them to La Guardia airport in New York City. Then they would board a plane to Saigon, Vietnam. I was in a hurry to get to work, and I didn't want to be late. As I sat stunned in the Dean's office, that d ay and this moment in the Dean's office were somehow connected. Mom and dad had just finished Vietnamese language study a month before, and now they were in Banmethuot, with eight other missionaries. So how…? How could they have…?

Then my mind switched to the last day I saw them. There were tears in our eyes as we hugged each other goodbye. They promised to pray for me, and I promised to do the same for them. Then I said briskly, like I had urgent business, "Goodbye, Mom, Dad. I'll be praying for you, and that you'll be safe."

"We'll be praying for you, too, David," Mom said, holding my hand. Dad was strangely quiet, then he said, "You may never see us again, David." Though his words left me speechless, I thought, *No way, Dad! No way! God will protect you as He always has!* His next words seemed overly dramatic. "No matter what happens, David, I want you to follow Jesus."

"OK, dad," I said with the vast wisdom of my 18 years. "I'll be fine, and I'll be praying for you!" I disliked mushy farewells, and this was turning into one. I hugged them again. My eyes were dry, my heart unsuspecting, and time was a-wasting. I had urgent work to do on someone's. . .yard. With a wave, I turned, and stupidly, stupidly brimming with overconfidence, walked away, up the road, not even waiting for them to get in the car and drive away! Before I turned a corner, I looked back. They were standing together, wiping their eyes and watching me. I waved like I would see them at supper that night, then walked out of sight. It was the last time I would every see them, and I didn't even tell them how much I loved them… And now, now they were gone! As I wept, the Dean of Students, my pastor, and my favorite professor prayed for me, for my sister, for my three younger siblings who were safe at the mission school. "Lord," I thought as we prayed, "who's going to comfort them? Care for them, love them like Mom and Dad did?"

It was a long time before all of us would learn how brutally our parents died. The attack on Banmethuot began on January 31st at 1 a.m., when two Viet Cong soldiers knocked on missionary Carolyn Griswold's front door. She and her father lived next door to my parents, and when Carolyn opened the door to see who in the world would be knocking on her door in the middle of the night, she saw two Viet Cong soldiers. One of them told her to go upstairs to their bedrooms and wait. After they obeyed, he tossed a powerful bomb into the house and left. Seconds later the bomb exploded, and the house collapsed, seriously injuring Carolyn and pinning her under heavy debris and killing her father. The blast shattered the night, rudely awakening my parents, the Bible School Director Bob Ziemer and his wife Marie, and missionary nurses Ruth Wilting and Betty Olsen.

Over the next two days a fierce battle raged between the Vietnamese army base directly behind the mission compound, and the attacking Viet Cong. The U.S. army engaged Viet Cong forces in several other parts of the city. Though the Vietnamese army fired round after round of bullets and mortars at the Viet Cong holed up behind the mission houses, the fight was a stalemate. The remaining missionaries were trapped in their houses and could only pray and wait to be rescued.

As soon as there was enough daylight, my dad and Bob Ziemer began digging through the rubble of the Griswald's house to free Carolyn, who continued to cry out in pain. As they struggled to free her, bullets were flying in both directions around them. Eventually, the two men moved enough of the rubble to free Carolyn and move her to the nearby dispensary. Nurses Ruth Wilting and Betty Olsen —who had been present at the kidnapping of at the Leprosy Hospital six years earlier— took over Carolyn's care. Carolyn's father's body lay under a heavy beam the men couldn't move, and they had to leave his body in the rubble. For the next two days, the two nurses cared for Carolyn as well as they could, using the supplies from their dispensary to keep her alive and minimize her pain.

The battle for the city of Banmethuot raged for three days. Early on the second day, the trapped missionaries concluded that the Viet Cong would probably destroy the other three mission houses to improve their position. Though it was risky, dad and Bob Ziemer cleared out what had been a houses to serve as a bunker. As soon as it was ready, everyone but the two nurses and Carolyn, who was in the dispensary, abandoned the houses and sheltered in the bunker. Not long after and as they had predicted, the Viet Cong blew up the other three mission houses.

By the third day of fighting, the nurses reported that unless Carolyn received advanced medical care soon, she would soon die. Desperate to save her, Bob Ziemer and Betty Olsen decided to go with a white flag to the Viet Cong battlefront and appeal for permission to take Carolyn to the nearest hospital.

According to a witness who survived, when Betty Olsen and Bob appeared at the Viet Cong's front line with their white flag, the soldiers were initially surprised and didn't fire on them. An officer asked what they wanted, and as Bob was explaining, a soldier behind the officer shot Bob in the head and chest with a machine gun, killing him instantly. For some reason he spared Betty Olsen. Hearing the gunfire, nurse Ruth Wilting ran from the dispensary to the bunker. As she ran, a soldier fired on her with his machine gun, and she fell wounded into the bunker. Immediately after, the soldier who shot her ran to the bunker and tossed in a hand grenade. The explosion killed or severely wounded everyone in the bunker, including Ruth Wilting, a young tribal boy the missionaries were sheltering, and my mother and father. He then fired a row of bullets up my father's back as he tried to shelter my mother with his body. Bob Ziemer's wife Marie Ziemer was seriously injured by the grenade and deafened by the blast but somehow survived despite seventeen shrapnel wounds. When soldier who threw the grenade and fired on them saw she was alive, he ordered her out of the bunker. Somehow, she managed to crawl out. When the other Viet Cong soldiers saw how badly she was injured, they let her go. An hour later an American soldiers found her staggering down a nearby road and took her to a U.S. army hospital where she was hospitalized and survived. When the Viet Cong soldiers retreated, they took Betty Olsen prisoner, along with an American intelligence officer named Hank Blood. A month later she would die on the Ho Che Minh trail. He survived and at the end of the war was released from the "Hanoi Hilton" prison, along with 500 other American prisoners.

On the awful day that I learned of my parents' deaths, I did not know all these details. After I stopped weeping and calmed down, my pastor handed me an envelope and said, "David, our church bought you a train ticket to Nyack, New York, where your sister Judy is waiting for you to join her. Here's $20 so you can buy food on the way." In a fog of pain and bewilderment, I thanked my pastor and the men who had prayed for me, then walked alone to my dorm room.

I can't remember anything of that hundred-yard walk. When I got to my room I closed the door, got on my knees, and screamed at God, "Why? Why didn't you protect them? Where were you when they needed your help? You promise in the Bible to take care of those who love you!"

I had read Psalm 91 many times, and now the words in verses 3,4, and 5 seemed like lies, because the psalmist wrote, *"For He will rescue you from every trap and protect you from deadly disease. He will cover you with his feathers. He will shelter you with his wings. His faithful promises are your armor and protection."* Verse 7 even promises, *"Though a thousand fall at your side, though ten thousand are dying around you, these evils will not touch you!"* Now those promises sounded hollow, and God wasn't answering me.

In the silence of my room, I shouted at him, "How could you miraculously save my parents from death on previous occasions and abandon them now? What did they do to deserve this? And who's going to take the gospel to the B'nong people now?"

It was then that I heard God speak to me for the first time in my life. His words were so clear that to this day I can still hear them. He said,

"David, do you trust me?"

Through my tears I cried, "What does that have to do with anything? Of course I trust you! I've trusted you from the time I was six years old! What I need to know now is *why you didn't you protect them when they needed you most?*

After a long silence, God asked, "Do you trust me?"

Without even thinking, I shouted, "Of course I trust you! Haven't I dedicated myself to serve you as a missionary? Aren't I in school now for that? Just explain to me why you did this and what will happen now to my brothers and sisters!"

I was the oldest son. My sister Judy was one year older, but my brother Dale was 16, my younger sister Laurel was 11, and my youngest brother Tom was only eight. They had barely escaped the massacre because just three days before the attack they had taken a plane to Saigon and had continued on to the Mission school in Malaysia. Who would help them understand what happened now? Who would tell them why? I said to God, "I can't even talk to my younger brothers and sisters, let alone comfort them as an older brother!"

Then God asked me a third time, "David, do you trust Me?"

There followed a great struggle in my heart. On the one hand I loved God and wanted to please him and serve him. But on the other hand, I was heartbroken over the loss of the two most precious people in my life, and I couldn't conceive that any good could come out of their deaths. They were in their *early forties, in the prime of their lives and at the peak of their effectiveness as missionaries! They had learned French, Cambodian, Vietnamese, and were learning B'nong when they died.* Who was going to win the hearts of the B'nong people and bring them to faith in Jesus now? How did their deaths make any sense at all?

But even as I asked the questions and demanded God to answer me, I knew that demanding God to explain right then why He didn't protect them was not faith. It was the very antithesis of faith. Then God challenged me again. He said, "If it's really true that you trust me, then thank me!"

How do you thank God for taking away the people you love and rely on the most? I didn't know the answer, and I simply could not thank Him for taking them from me. But gently, tenderly, as I wept on my knees, God began reminding me of the great men and women of faith in the Bible, stories I had heard since I was a child. Stories about Abraham, Jacob, Joseph, Job, and David. They had trusted God through incredible suffering, and their suffering was far worse than mine. *Yet they trusted God without understanding why...*

There was one more thing I knew, and it troubled me deeply: If I didn't trust God, how could I serve him? I wanted to serve God more than anything else, and so as I wept, I finally said, "God, I can't feel thankful, I just feel pain. But because I want to serve you, I will say the words." I didn't know if God would accept that, but it was the best I could do. On my knees and heartbroken, I said to

God the hardest words I've ever spoken: *"Thank you for taking my mother and father."*

In that moment, God overwhelmed me with His love. I couldn't speak, only weep, but I felt His love so intensely that I knew that from that moment on, God would be both my father and mother and would never forsake me. When I finally got up off of my knees, I had a different heart.

Why do I write these difficult stories of long ago? In Psalm 71:16- 17, King David wrote, *"I will praise your mighty deeds, O Sovereign Lord. I will tell everyone that you alone are just. O God, you have taught me from my earliest childhood, and I constantly tell others about the wonderful things you do."*

I knew that's what God was asking me to do, and since then I have done my best to obey him.

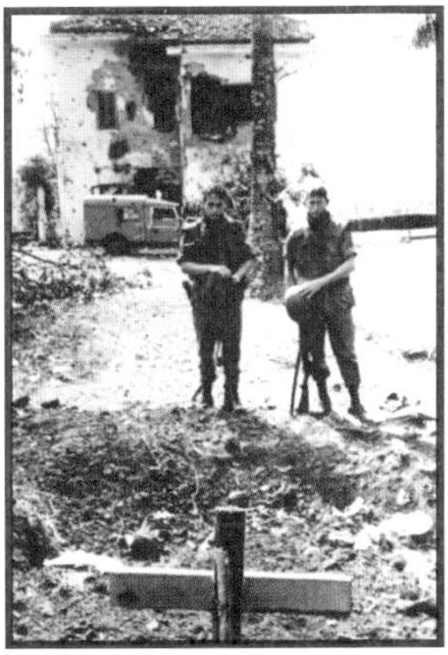

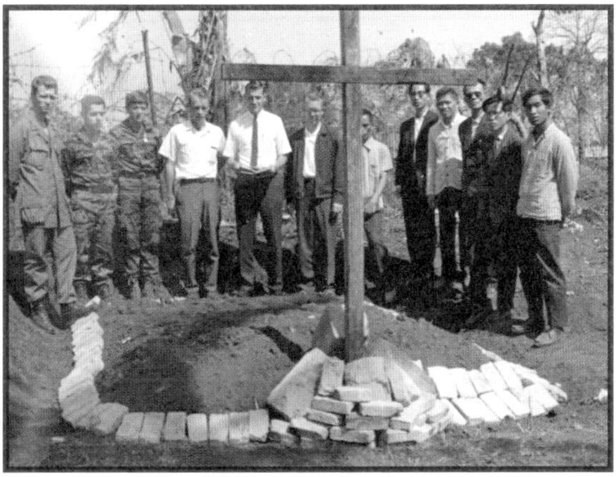

My mother and father and nurse Ruth Wilting were buried in the bunker where they fell. Missionary, Vietnamese, and Montagnard pastors officiated at the funeral.

In the years that followed my parents' deaths, God provided for all of my expenses at Geneva College, from complete strangers. This miracle of grace was a constant reminder of God's love for me. For my younger siblings, He provided a loving uncle and aunt— George and Harriett Irwin— who served as missionaries to Vietnam until 1975 when the war ended, and later to the Vietnamese diaspora in France. They loved us and cared for us as their own children.

At the end of my train ride to Nyack, New York, my sister Judy was waiting at the station. We fell into each other's arms and wept, still feeling broken and lost. But we also felt God's comfort and presence. After a week of mourning and learning to walk again by faith, I returned to Geneva College and my studies, and Judy returned to her classes at Nyack College.

In his recent memoir entitled, *On the Cruel Edges of the World,* retired missionary Reg Reimer wrote the following:

"Dick Philipps, Gene Evans, and I decided to fly immediately up to Banmethuot despite ongoing battles. I was 27 years old at the time. The large Banmethout mission station on the southern approach to the town consisted of four neighboring missionary houses, with a leprosy clinic and a large church off to one side. We were met *at the property by a a tribal pastor who had survived the attacks and a few other believers who helped us reconstruct the tragic events. I had never seen such abject discouragement as was etched on their faces. The missionary houses had been blown up by powerful satchel charges...The military had taken custody of the bodies of Leon Griswold and Bob Ziemer. Leon had been killed in the first house explosion. Bob had been greeted with bullets to the head and chest when he had emerged from a makeshift garbage-pit-bunker with a white cloth indicating surrender and a plea to negotiate. Immediately after, Viet Cong soldiers thew a hand grenade and sprayed rifle fire on the four missionaries who were in the bunker. Miraculously, Marie Ziemer survived. Hurriedly, US soldiers covered the bodies of the other three, Ed and Ruth Thompson and Ruth Wilting, with a shallow layer of dirt. It did not seem right to us that a garbage pit should be the burial place for our colleagues who had given their lives for the gospel... We carefully started digging. About a foot down we came to a plastic body bag. Removing debris around it, we saw that it was thrown over top of bodies. As we slowly pulled the bag to one side, it exposed the charred body of Ed Thompson, in a kneeling position with his arms wrapped around his wife Ruth below... Rifle fire had torn a row of bullet holes right down the middle of Ed's back. Alas, decomposition proved too advanced to allow us to disinter the bodies. We covered them with a mound of soil, tidied up the site, encircled it with bricks from the blown-up houses, and planted a wash line pole to serve as a cross. Then we surrounded the grave. Three*

missionaries, two Vietnamese pastors, some...tribal Christians, and a couple of American soldiers stumbled through the most moving committal service I have ever participated in," (pp.65-6).

Rediscovering Joy

After the death of my parents, life took on a new urgency. I decided to take courses in summer school so that I could finish my pre-med requirements and graduate with a Bachelor of Science degree in Chemistry in three years instead of four. It wasn't something God told me to do, and I didn't even ask Him, though I should have. Perhaps it was a way to deal with my loss and sorrow.

Once again, God provided for my needs through a combination of grants, scholarships, speaking honorariums, and the generous help of the Beaver Falls Alliance Church.

Nevertheless, the challenge of getting into medical school and finding a way to pay for my tuition seemed insurmountable. In response to my faith, God had provided for me during my college years, but my mother was no longer around to encourage me. Would God provide the hundreds of thousands of dollars I would need to stay out of massive debt while studying medicine? I filled out applications to six medical schools, all in Pennsylvania. The school I wanted to attend the most was the University of Pittsburgh School of Medicine, and it was considered one of the more difficult med schools to get into.

As I looked at the applications, I noticed they all had one question in common: "Why do you want to become a doctor?" They wanted an essay-type answer, preferably truthful. I was greatly perplexed by the question. It wasn't that I didn't know the answer— God had called me to be a doctor and a missionary to the poor, but if I wrote that as my reason, the professors might laugh and throw my application into the trash!

As I prayed about what to do, I remembered the story of Gideon and how he put out a fleece to confirm that he would really have God's blessing, and a plan formed in my mind. I would divide the six applications into two piles of three. On three applications I would write that I wanted to become a doctor because I loved the idea of caring for sick and poor people, while advancing medical knowledge in the developing world. On the other three applications, I would only write that I wanted to become a missionary doctor to serve among the poor people of the world and share with them the good news of Jesus. The question then became, in which pile would I put the application for the University of Pittsburgh?

After much soul-searching and prayer, I felt God wanted me to include the University of Pittsburgh in the pile where I would openly admit my goal to become a missionary doctor to the poor and share the gospel. Then I committed the matter to the Lord and mailed all six applications. Now all I had to do was wait for requests for interviews. In the weeks that followed, I heard nothing from the three schools in the "partial truth" pile, but two of the three schools that had received the whole truth about my call to medicine responded by asking for an interview.

One of the invitations was from Hahnemann University in Philadelphia. The professor who interviewed me was especially interested in my opinion about the Vietnam War but had no interest at all in hearing about my desire to become a missionary doctor!

My second invitation was from the University of Pittsburgh, which asked me to report to the Children's Hospital for an interview in two weeks with a Dr. W.B. Kiesewetter, the Chief of Pediatric Surgery.

On the appointed day, I drove my rusting VW bug into Pittsburgh from Beaver Falls, a 45-minute drive. As the hour for the appointment approached, a sense of panic gripped me. I countered it with prayer before leaving my car. I found Dr. Kiesewetter's office on the 11th floor of the hospital. When I opened the door and walked in, his secretary asked me to take a seat in her office. Ten minutes later her intercom buzzed, and she told me it was time to enter the professor's office. Dr. Kiesewetter was a trim, distinguished looking man with white hair and reading glasses perched precariously on his nose. As I entered, he looked up from reading my application, then stood and shook my hand. His smile was friendly but formal.

"I've been looking over your application, David, and I found it to be somewhat… uh… unique." I felt my stomach contract. "Tell me why you want to be a doctor, and why you think God has called you to be a missionary." I swallowed hard and told him about seeing a man die alongside the road in Cambodia when I was fourteen, and that I felt God had permitted me to see him to call me to be a missionary who could help people like him.

"How do you know it was God?" he asked.

"Well, He spoke to me in my heart," I explained. It sounded weak, but he nodded.

"Did you hear His voice?"

"Uh... no. He just spoke to me in my... uh...heart, and I knew that He wanted me to do... that:' It was March and the room was cool but sweat was already trickling down my ribs under my shirt. Dr. Kiesewetter nodded inscrutably and turned back to my application.

"If you become a doctor, then, you're going to preach to people?" I swallowed and said, "I want to share my faith in Jesus Christ with them if I can." I tried to stifle feelings of despair at the way the interview was going. Dr. Kiesewetter looked at me over the top of his glasses and asked, "What if they don't want to hear about Jesus?"

"Well, I would stop if they don't want to hear about...er... Jesus:'

"What do you believe about Jesus?" Dr. Kiesewetter asked, leaning back in his chair. "Do you think he was a good man who was misunderstood? That after he was crucified 2,000 years ago, He really came back to life?"

I swallowed and said, "I believe Jesus is the Son of God, that He came to earth to die for the sins of the world, including mine, and that after He died on the cross He rose from the dead." It came out in a rush, like I was reciting something I had memorized in Sunday school. Dr. Kiesewetter remained inscrutable and did not pursue it.

"I see that your parents are missionaries in Vietnam. Do you plan to join them?" He had stumbled onto the one subject I had hoped to avoid. I had no choice but to answer.

"Uh... my parents were missionaries in Vietnam, but they're not. anymore:' I explained weakly, hoping it would be enough. It wasn't.

"Where are they now?" I would have to tell him the truth... I took a deep breath I said, "They're in heaven. They were killed by Communist soldiers a year ago:'

Dr. Kiesewetter looked up sharply, then softened. 'Tm so sorry. Did it have something to do with the war?"

"Yes:' I said. "They were killed last year by North Vietnamese soldiers during the Tet Offensive:' My answer visibly surprised him.

"I'm very sorry, David. I guess I did read about that in the papers. Do you mind talking about it?"

"No, I don't mind," I said.

"How do you feel about their deaths?"

Hesitantly, reluctantly, and trying not to sound weird, I explained how since their deaths I had learned to trust God, and that I believed God had a purpose in their deaths that I would not understand on this side of heaven.

Dr. Kiesewetter asked many more questions about my family, how I was coping with my parents' deaths, and how their loss had affected my faith. Finally, he asked me if I believed the Bible and if so, why. His questions were not unfriendly, but they exposed me for what I was: a Christian who considered the Bible to be God's inerrant Word, and that God still uses it speak to those who read it. Never once did he indicate either disapproval or agreement.

By then the interview had lasted nearly 45 minutes, and all I wanted to do was escape! But then Dr. Kiesewetter removed his glasses and leaned back in his chair. A slight smile played at the comers of his mouth, and he looked at me directly.

"I haven't been entirely honest with you, David," he said. "I want you to know that I too, believe in the Bible." He chuckled at the look of surprise and relief on my face, then leaned forward and said, "Da- vid, I want to commend you for your courage today. I only wish that when I was in your position many years ago, I had had the courage to speak about my faith in Jesus Christ as openly as you have."

I didn't know what to say, so I just listened, gripping the arms of my chair.

"I want you in our medical school," he continued, "and I am prepared to do everything in my power to see that you are accepted."

In a daze I thanked him, shook his hand and stumbled back to my VW bug. How had it happened, I wondered, that out of the hundreds of doctors on the faculty of the University of Pittsburgh, a Christian doctor who loved God had been chosen to interview me?

Several years later, Dr. Kiesewetter told me that when the Dean of the medical school saw my application, he called him. The Dean knew that Dr. Kiesewetter was an outspoken Christian and was active in the Christian Medical Society.

"Bill," he said, "I have an application here for our medical school. This guy's so unusual I thought I'd better send him to you! You'll see when you get his application." That application was mine.

That year there were 2,200 applications for 100 positions in the first-year class at the University of Pittsburgh School of Medicine. Two weeks after my interview I received a formal notification that I had been accepted to the freshman class, starting the first week of September. It was a dream come true, but I still had no money!

About a week later, Dr. Kiesewetter called me on the telephone and invited me to come to his house the following Friday for dinner. After dinner we would go to a hockey game, and if we got back too late, I could spend the night with them. I immediately accepted and wrote down the directions to his home.

The Kiesewetter's house was in a lovely part of Pittsburgh, and when I arrived, I was amazed to see it was three stories high and beautifully preserved. After I rang the doorbell, Dr. Kiesewetter opened the door and welcomed me in. Never in my life had I walked on such plush carpets or seen such lovely furnishings. Dr. Kiesewetter introduced me to his wife, and I immediately sensed I had found a friend. Since dinner was ready, she led us directly to the dining room.

The sight of the formally set table triggered a wave of panic. Each place setting had two forks on the left, two knives on the right, several glasses and goblets, and two sets of plates! How would I know which utensil and plate to use, and for what? Sitting down, I barely averted dipping the end of my tie in a bowl of soup on my plate! After Dr. Kiesewetter thanked God for the food, Mrs. Kiesewetter asked if I would like white wine or red with my meal, and I felt my face turning pink. If I said yes, I would have to drink it. If I confessed that I didn't like alcohol, they might think I was a "holier-than-thou" guy. Mrs. Kiesewetter sensed my predicament and gently asked, "Are you accustomed to drinking wine with your meals? I know that not everyone is." I gratefully mumbled that I wasn't accustomed.

After thanking God for our dinner, Dr. Kiesewetter selected a spoon for his soup, giving me a clue about which spoon to use first. The dinner went smoothly, and I began to enjoy myself. After dinner we headed downtown to watch the Pittsburgh Penguins play another team. I had never seen ice hockey, and the Kiesewetter's had season tickets for seats in the second row, on center ice. I couldn't believe how violently the players turned and spun and crashed into each other on ice skates, all at incredible speeds! The game was fast and violent, and the skill of the players was amazing. Dr. Kiesewetter kindly explained the rules as the game progressed.

Afterwards we returned to the Kiesewetter's home for ice cream. Dr. Kiesewetter turned to me and said, "David, the reason I asked you to come this evening was so Mrs. Kiesewetter could meet you." He paused and looked at his wife as if to confirm something. "Now that she's had a chance to meet you, we would like to invite you to come live with us while you're attending medical school."

All the air went out of my lungs, and for a moment I thought I'd misunderstood him! Live with them? In that house? But as I played his words back in my mind, I realized that he was serious. These people hardly knew me, yet they were offering to let me live in their palatial home during my four years of medical school! For a moment I couldn't think of anything to say. "I think that would be wonderful," I finally blurted, fighting back tears. "I'm so surprised I don't know what to say!"

"Of course, we would want you to eat your meals with us when we're home," Mrs. Kiesewetter explained with a smile, "and we would expect you to help in the yard and around the house." I nodded my complete agreement.

"Having you stay in our house will help us, too," Dr. Kiesewetter added, as if I needed convincing. "We're often away on trips, and this way the house won't be empty." I assured them I would be happy to take care of the yard work and anything else they might want me to do.

And so, in the space of a few hours, the problem of my need for food and lodging while I was in medical school was settled. As I headed my VW bug back to Beaver Falls, I sang praises to God at the top of my lungs!

A few days later and after I returned to earth, I began wondering how I was going to purchase textbooks and pay the tens of thousands of dollars I would need for my tuition. Once again, I prayed and asked God to provide. Two weeks after our memorable evening together, Dr. Kiesewetter phoned me. He knew of a group in Philadelphia called the Pennsylvania Medical Missionary Society. This organization provided grants to medical students who were planning to become missionaries. If the student served overseas for at least 10 years, the grant became a gift. Dr. Kiesewetter explained that he had called their president and asked her to send me an application. He added that the organization would probably pay for my tuition only, but suggested that when I filled out the application, I include the cost of books too. Dr. Kiesewetter then mailed my application to the organization with a strong letter of recommendation.

One month later I received a response, and as I read it d my hands began to tremble: the Pennsylvania Medical Missionary Society had agreed to pay for my tuition and my books, and *for all four years*!

There remained in my life only one troubling uncertainty. During my years at Geneva College, I had started looking for a partner in life. I was certain that I would find her during college, since bachelorhood didn't appeal to me. Finding the right girl, however, turned out to be more of a challenge than I had imagined. To begin with, I was still trying to figure out the American system of courtship. The social structure at the mission school was designed to discourage teenagers who lived together from sunup to sundown from getting into really serious romances.

During my senior year of high school in America, I had dated several girls in our church youth group, but my efforts clumsy and painful! After several evenings of strained conversation and awkward blunders, the young ladies didn't encourage me to try again, probably concluding that I was nice but strange!

In college, however, the business of courtship was a serious matter. My mother had warned me to be very careful and had strongly counseled me to ask the Lord to help me find the right girl. I dated only Christian girls and was confident that I would recognize the right one when I saw her. Several times I got into relationships that seemed at first promising, bud didn't last. When a girl I was interested in found out I was planning to become a doctor, the friendship warmed up— until she learned I was planning to be a missionary doctor. The one exception was a beautiful young woman who after dating me long enough to hear my story and hear about God's call on my life, fell in love with me. But when it became apparent that God had not called her to become a career missionary, I had to decide. She was of the opinion that my call to a lifetime of missionary service would be enough for both of us, and that if our relationship progressed God could work it out. The last thing I wanted to do was hurt her, but when I told her as gently as I could that our love for each other would not be enough, she wept bitterly. Missionary life would require many sacrifices, most of which she couldn't understand. I was careful not to do that again.

What made that time of my life a lonely time was that after my parents' deaths in 1968, my sister and I were the only members of our family who lived in America. Our wonderful aunt and uncle who had adopted us, remained in Vietnam until seven years later. After our parents' deaths in 1968, my sister Judy and I appealed to our mission to help us finance our travel to Vietnam so we could and spend the Summer with our aunt and uncle and our younger siblings. Our mission regretfully declined, stating that they had instead established a fund for our younger siblings to attend college.

Seven years later after Vietnam fell, our aunt and uncle moved to France with our younger siblings to minister to the thousands of Vietnamese refugees who fled to France. Soon after, my sister Judy married a man from upstate New York.

Sixteen years after our parents were martyred, the five of us children came together for the first time, at our brother Dale's wedding. As we talked and tried to catch up on each other's lives, Dale, Laurel, and Tom asked why Judy and I didn't come to Vietnam to comfort them the Summer after our parents were killed? Why did we just forget about them and go on with our lives? When the dust settled and the truth came out, we wept together and hugged for a long, long time. To this day, we remain close and get together often.

In 2002, the five of us made serious plans to visit our parents' grave. But when we applied for visas, the government of Vietnam refused and asked *what crime our parents committed that resulted in their deaths!!* It was shocking evidence that it was too soon to attempt a return visit.

During my third year of pre-med, I finally began to consider a life of celibacy. Previously the idea had seemed ridiculous, but as I focused all my efforts on qualifying for medical school, I wondered if it was God's plan for me. In my heart I hoped I would someday find the girl o8f6 my dreams and that she would want to spend her life serving as a missionary with me, in some desperate part of the world. But nothing I had tried had worked. Thoroughly discouraged, I decided to leave the matter in God's hands.

By this time, I was attending summer school so I could finish the last requirements for a Bachelor of Science degree in chemistry. I had already been accepted to the University of Pittsburgh School of Medicine for the fall of 1969, but it was conditional on earning my degree. My younger brother Dale had just graduated from the mission school in Malaysia and was returning to the States, so I drove to New York to meet him and my older sister, Judy. From her I learned that one of our former classmates at the mission school was getting married in a few weeks and had invited all of her former classmates to a party, including us!

As far as parties go, it was pretty tame, other than the fact that everyone sat around talking at once. After loading up my plate with cookies, ice cream, and grabbing a soft drink, I sat on the floor between my younger brother and older sister. Minutes later I noticed a very attractive brunette sitting across the room. I thought, "This is supposed to be a Dalat School reunion, but I don't recognize her at all!" I leaned over to my sister and whispered, "Who is the girl sitting over there?" She started laughing and finally told me it was Becki Mitchell! At first, I laughed out loud, because she looked nothing like the Becki Mitchell I remembered.

A few minutes later she noticed me staring at her, so I took that as my cue, got up, and sat next to her. To my surprise, she really was Becki Mitchell, was friendly, and impossibly beautiful! As we talked, I realized that despite all our years together at the mission school, I hardly knew her. Now she had charm, intelligence, and was, well… intoxicating! Forgotten were the days when she outran, outjumped, and outclimbed me. To my surprise, she told me that she was studying to be a missionary nurse!

When it was time to say goodbye and go home that night, I complained to my sister, "It just doesn't seem fair! The most interesting girl I've met in years is studying in a nursing school in Tacoma, Washington, while I'm starting medical school in Pittsburgh!" There was clearly no future in that! But as I drove back to Pittsburgh with my younger brother, I couldn't stop thinking about her. During the next week as read my Bible and prayed, I asked God to show me what I should do. By the end of the week, I had a clear answer from God: PURSUE HER!!!!

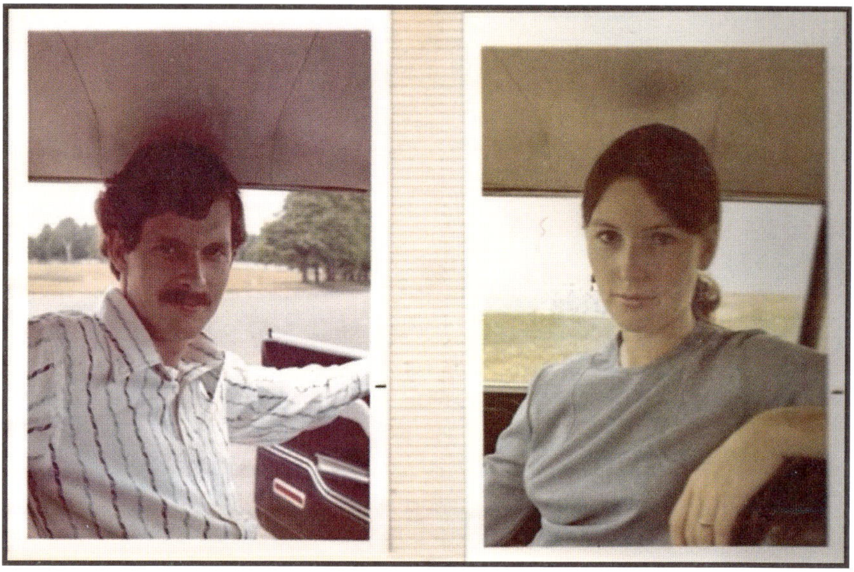

Becki and me, after our first fight together.

The following weekend I decided that my brother Dale and I really needed to visit our sister Judy again in Nyack. I was taking several night school courses that didn't end until 6 p.m. on Friday, so as soon as I got out, we climbed into my VW bug and drove until after mid-night. At 9 a.m., I dialed Becki's number and asked if she would go out with me for dinner that evening. Thinking I was still in western Pennsylvania, she was puzzled, until I told her I had driven half the night to be with her!

That was the beginning of a special friendship that quickly grew into romance. Both of us had lost missionary parents and understood the suffering and challenges to faith that came with that. Both of us had struggled to understand God's purposes and had chosen to trust Him. Finally, both of us had chosen to hold tightly to the admonition of Proverbs 3:5-6, *"Trust in the Lord with all your heart, and do not depend on your own understanding."* Finally, both of us had parents had disappeared from our lives. The only difference was that I knew my parents were with the Lord and were buried in Banmethuot, Vietnam, while Becki didn't know if her father was dead or alive. Our shared suffering only drew us closer. Although the eight-hour drive in my VW bug was long, it was pure joy for me to drive to Nyack and back another five times that Summer!

Within two weeks of our first meeting, I knew God had brought us together. I didn't know if she felt the same way, and it seemed a bit rash to ask for her hand in marriage so soon, especially since she had two more years of school before she would earn her B.S. in Nursing. I still had four years of medical school looming ahead.

In early September we kissed and said goodbye, this time with many tears. Becki drove her aging Ford Fairlane by herself from Nyack,

N.Y. to Tacoma, Washington, and I got ready to start medical school. Every week we wrote letters and called each other. Medical school made my undergrad studies seem like a picnic. During my first year I spent so many hours sitting at my desk that I developed pressure sores on my butt and had to sit on a pillow! When I did well on my mid-term exams, the pain was well worth it!

Soon after, I learned that during our Christmas break we would have ten days off from med school. A friend of mine wanted to go to California for Christmas, so the two of us decided to take his car and share the driving and costs. The evening my last class ended, my friend and I left Pittsburgh, swapping places at the wheel every two hours. The 30 bologna sandwiches I had prepared for our trip were tasty at first, but by the second day we couldn't stand them!

Fifty or so hours after we left Pittsburgh, we pulled up to the main bus station in Sacramento, California, where Becki and I had agreed to meet. As I walked into the bus station and scanned the room, my heart was racing. At first, I didn't see her sitting with her back to the door I had entered, and my heart sank. Then I saw her. She was wearing a long, black raincoat and boots, and was looking down, as though praying. Afraid it wasn't her; I shuffled to where I could glance at her surreptitiously. When our eyes met, that beautiful woman jumped up, threw her arms around my neck, and kissed me so enthusiastically that a few of the people in the waiting room whistled and clapped!

Becki had borrowed her uncle's fancy car so she could meet in Sacramento, so over the next 3 hours while I slept in the back seat, she drove us north to her uncle and aunt's home near Redding, California. That night I slept like a log, and the next morning after a breakfast of delicious pancakes that her aunt prepared, we drove north to Klamath Falls, Oregon where more of her aunts and uncles welcomed us. Becki's uncle was a hard-working logger, and he eyed my soft hands with a snort of disdain! Eventually he decided to overlook my deficits, and we enjoyed a wonderful Christmas together.

On our last evening together, Becki and I drove to the top of a hill overlooking Klamath Falls. A light snow and moderate fog gave the city lights below us a magical glow. One of us was enjoying the moment; the other was terrified! I was at a crossroads in my life, and this beautiful girl had the power to crush me like a bug or make me forever happy! The only sound on that silent night was our breathing. Then I held my breath and asked Becki to marry me.

I had expected her to hesitate or shake her head, either in shock or astonishment. Surely, she would want to think about it for a while before answering! She might even want to pray about it for a week or suggest we decide about marriage *after* I graduated from med school in three and a half years. When in the next breath she answered "yes!" I nearly fainted!

"Are you sure?" I asked. She was laughing at me. "Of course, I'm sure, you idiot! I've been sure of it since the night we met at the party in Nyack, when you didn't recognize me! After I got home that night, I wrote my mother that I had met the man I was going to marry! Since then, I've been waiting for you to wake up and propose to me!"

Before we said goodbye and I headed back to med school in Pittsburgh, we agreed to wait to marry until Becki graduated from nursing school. Those would be two and a half of the longest years of my life!

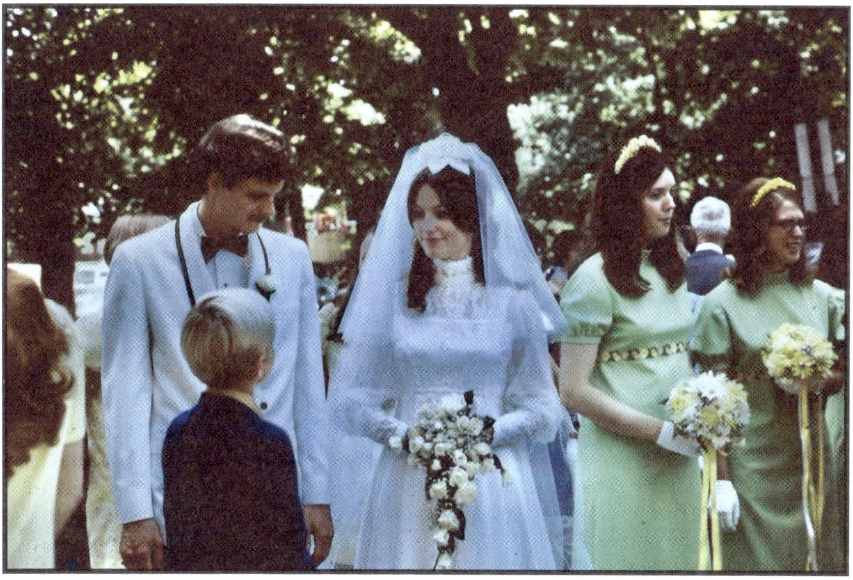

Married at last!

After I got back to Pittsburgh and resumed my medical studies, the months seemed to drag on at a snail's pace. Our weekly letters and phone calls confirmed our love for each other but also helped us focus on finishing our schooling well. Becki graduated from nursing school in early June 1972. On June 26, 1972, we finally got married in Nyack, New York! Dr. and Mrs. Kiesewetter gave us a wonderful wedding present by paying the airfares for Becki's mother and her youngest sister Geraldine so they could fly from the mission school in Malaysia and attend our wedding in Nyack. God's blessings to us as a couple were just beginning.

After Becki's father was kidnapped in 1962, her mother Betty waited in Vietnam, ever hoping and praying that he would be found or that someone would turn up who knew what happened to him and the other two missionaries. During those years, Betty served among the Montagnards in Banmethuot, and Becki and her three younger siblings grew up, graduated from the mission school, and returned to the U.S.

Betty had long been fluent in Vietnamese, but during her years in Banmethuot while she waited for her husband Archie to be found, she learned the language of the Raday tribe and began visiting their villages, befriending them, and sharing the gospel with them. One day a lady from one of the villages she visited said to her, "Do you know why I started listening to you?" Surprised, Betty said, "No!"

"Well," the Raday woman said, "I often watched you when you drove from Banmethuot to our village to talk to us about Jesus. One day when it was raining hard your car even slid into the ditch! I was so impressed that you would come alone, even when the road was slippery with mud! I thought, 'There must be something very important this lady has to say to us.' So, I came to hear, and I saw God's love in you. Jesus lives in me too now!" Betty never stopped befriending people, no matter who they were, and while she waited and prayed for her husband to be found and returned, she led many Montagnards to faith in Jesus.

Becki's Mom is Imprisoned in Hanoi In March of 1975, and while Betty and other missionaries were still ministering to the Montagnard tribes, the North Vietnamese army launched a second surprise attack against south Vietnam. Weakened and disheartened by America's withdrawal and internal corruption, South Vietnam's army collapsed in disarray and panic. The South's major cities were quickly overwhelmed, including Banmethuot.

When the city fell, Betty and other Western missionaries were captured and forcibly marched north on the Ho Chi Minh Trail, along with thousands of Vietnamese prisoners. After a week of walking from dawn to dusk and sleeping at night on the ground, Betty came down with malaria and collapsed. There were no medicines for her and prisoners who were too sick to walk were left on the trail to die. That would have been Betty's fate, but Vietnamese prisoners who knew her took turns carrying her in a sheet, until military trucks showed up and carried the prisoners the rest of the way to Hanoi.

Betty and six or seven other missionaries were imprisoned in the notorious "Hanoi Hilton." After treatment antimalarial medications, she slowly recovered. The communists were convinced that the missionaries were spies and agents of the U.S. government, and with almost daily interrogations they did their best to prove it. Betty, however, was so gentle with her replies and so determined to share the gospel with her captors, that her main interrogator gradually started to ask her questions about Jesus!

Betty's greatest disappointment was that her interrogators steadfastly insisted that they had no record of Archie's capture or whereabouts. Neither did they know what happened to Dr. Ardell Vietti and Dan Gerber, the other two missionaries who were kidnapped with her husband.

After seven months of imprisonment, God answered our prayers and the prayers of Christians around the world, and the North Vietnamese released Betty and her missionary colleagues and flew them to Bangkok. The day Betty arrived in Bangkok, she collapsed from cerebral malaria and was rushed to a hospital where she nearly died. She was so malnourished that she looked like a survivor from Dachau. After a week of aggressive treatment for malaria and malnutrition, she recovered enough to be released from the hospital. Rather than fly directly back to her home in Oregon, Betty and her 17-year-old daughter Geraldine flew to Albertville, France to spend a week with Becki and me, where we were studying French. Our reunion was overwhelmingly joyful, but also tearful, as Betty explained that she had heard nothing more about her husband Archie's disappearance or whereabouts.

When months later someone asked if she was happy to be free, she replied, *"Free yes, but there is a purpose for everything that comes into our lives. The Lord takes us through testing and trials and comforts us so that we can comfort and reach out to others with the comfort He comforted us with."* It was an answer we would always remember.

After just six months in the U.S. with her children and extended family, Betty accepted a position to serve as the head dietician at the Dalat School for missionary children in Tanah Rata, Malaysia. She served at the mission school in that capacity for nine years, then moved to Greensboro, North Carolina, where thousands of Raday Montagnards had settled after fleeing Vietnam after the war. Betty never stopped sharing the love of Jesus and the gospel message with her beloved people, and died on June 28, 2017, at the age of 96, surrounded by her children and confident that she would at last be reunited with her beloved Archie.

William Taylor, Antonia van der Meer, and Reg Reimer write, *"The cross directs our gaze from contemplating our own anguish and suffering to the suffering and transforming God who shares in our suffering. When we look at the cross, we realize at once that God suffered in a way that none of us has or will ever suffer. On the cross, Jesus gave us His all and His utmost so that we may live. By so doing, He incredibly demonstrated His overwhelming love for us. Thus, the death of Jesus Christ on the cross brings us face to face with the wonder of God's sacrificial love so much that we are strengthened to deal with our suffering with courage and determination,"* (p.127).[3]

Betty Mitchell suffered greatly during her lifetime, but instead of weakening her faith, suffering only strengthened her faith in Jesus. How could this happen? God said to His people in Isaiah 48:10, *"I have refined you, but not as silver is refined. Rather I have refined you in the furnace of suffering."* Those who knew and loved Betty, including all four of her and Archie's children, were awed and profoundly influenced by her life of suffering and faith.

In the years that followed my admission to the University of Pittsburgh School of Medicine, God provided so wonderfully that by June,1972 when I graduated and received my MD diploma, I had no school debts. As I walked up the steps and received my MD diploma, I wished my parents could have been there to celebrate with me. But I was not alone. I was blessed and grateful that Becki was there, applauding with tears in her eyes, along with retired missionary Gene Evans and his daughter Jodi. Gene Evans was special to our family, both because he and his wife served at Dalat School while we attended, and because he was one of three missionaries who stood with Montagnards and Vietnamese pastors at the bunker-grave where our parents fell.

---

3 Quote from *Sorrow and Blood: Christian Mission in Context of Suffering, Persecution, and Martyrdom,* by William Taylor, Antonia van der Meer and Reg Reimer, 2012.

Serve *Where*?!?

Growing up in Southeast Asia seemed to Becki and me the perfect preparation for serving the Lord as missionaries. Between the two of us, we had lived in the cities of Dalat, Banmethuot, Bangkok, Kratie, Phnom Penh, Tanah Rata, and Penang. We were familiar with Asian food, Asian cultures, Asian history, Asian's predominant religions, and Asia's geography. We even had a head start on learning some of Asia's languages! Naturally, we assumed that God's plan for us would be to return to serve Him as a doctor and nurse in Asia!

In addition to my conviction that we would best serve God in Asia I was also in a hurry, driven by a secret fear that Jesus might return to earth with His angels and take all of us to heaven before I had a chance to do anything important for God! Apart from that secret fear, I also wanted to be serving God wherever in He put me and in every stage of my life. Becki and I became active in our local church in Pittsburgh in establishing a ministry to young couples. We also helped reawaken the Christian Medical Society at the medical school where I was studying.

By my third year in medical school, I knew what specialty I was drawn to the most: it was general surgery and would require five years of arduous residency training. I considered applying for a position at the University of Pittsburgh, but by the spring of my third year I had developed such virulent hay fever that Becki and I decided to head west, closer to where her family lived and well out of the pollen zones. The summer before my fourth year of med school, we drove to the west coast so I could interview at surgical residency programs in California and Oregon. After numerous interviews, the program that interested me the most was at Mercy Hospital, in San Diego. As my second choice for the match I listed a Seventh Day Adventist hospital in Los Angeles called "White Memorial." In March of that year, I matched with my first choice: Mercy Hospital in San Diego. At the time, it was the largest and busiest hospital in the city. After graduating from medical school, Becki and I rented a U-Haul trailer and headed for San Diego. Once settled, Becki got a job as a nurse in a NICU at San Diego's Children's Hospital, and in early July of 1973, I started my surgical residency.

It was a great and challenging year, but as I prepared for my second year or training, a vague feeling of dissatisfaction began to grow in my heart. At first, I couldn't put my finger on where it came from. Our marriage was happy, I loved being a dad, I was appreciated by my superiors and colleagues at work, and I was active in our local Alliance church. In every respect, I seemed the model of Christian faithfulness. But I did not feel spiritually ready for what lay ahead.

Those who knew of my parents' deaths in Vietnam at times treated me as though I had been martyred! When my mother-in-law, Betty Mitchell, spent a year in San Diego during her furlough, I realized that she knew and loved God in a way that I did not. There was a power in her life that I lacked. It was a holy power that put others first—a power to love unlovable people, a power to be meek and at the same time courageous. Her example served to heighten my dissatisfaction.

My hunger to experience God more intimately grew so intense that one Sunday evening I wept over my spiritual coldness. I knew what I wanted, but how could I become more intimately acquainted with the God I loved and wanted to serve? I didn't even know what to ask Him. One night I heard God speaking to me in my spirit, asking me to give Him control not only over my daily life, but also over our future. Could He take my life and do with it as He wished? Could He ask me to do anything, anytime, anywhere? Would I serve Him joyfully in conditions that He would choose, and endure hardship? Would I serve him in obscurity? In poverty? In sickness? Would I accept humiliation and serve Him without holding back?

That evening at the altar at the front of our small Alliance church, I got on my knees and gave my whole life and future to Jesus, adding this one condition: "Take my life and make it yours. Take all of me, only fill this void in me with more of You! Please let me have more of your Holy Spirit." I sensed then that God had heard me, and that a spiritual transaction had taken place.

As that week unfolded, I felt a rekindling of the grace God gave me the day I mourned the death of my parents and God overwhelmed me with His love. It was as though spring had returned to my soul! I felt free to talk to my fellow interns and even my patients about Jesus.

In that first week I had led several patients to faith in Jesus. The dissatisfaction I had felt was replaced by a feel of expectation and intimacy with God that I had not experienced before. God was doing something exciting in me! Several of my Christian friends my pastor identified it as "a fresh filling of the Holy Spirit."

During the latter part of our first year, Becki and I bought a small house in a burgeoning suburb of northern San Diego on 1/8 of an acre. The development was called Mira Mesa, and it was one of 500 new homes. At the time, rental costs were so high that buying a house and making the payments cost less than renting! Friends of ours bought a home in the same development, and as we spent time together, we realized that there were no churches within ten miles. We shared a common burden to establish a church in our community. Our pastor in downtown San Diego encouraged us to go ahead, even though we were laymen and didn't yet have a pastor to lead us. We first met in homes, then in a school, praying and asking the Lord to help us. Within two years, our church grew from four to 40 souls, many of them new believers. After two years, God provided a pastor to lead us. Our involvement in planting the church was a great stimulus to our spiritual growth, our knowledge of God's Word, and our experience in leading people to faith in Jesus.

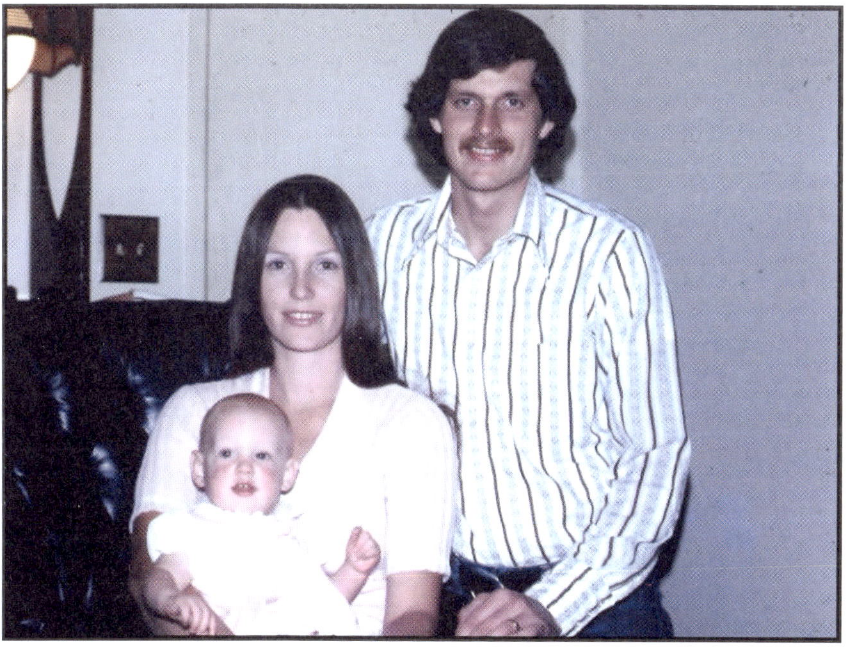

In 1974, God blessed us with our first child—a beautiful little girl we named Rachael Joy. From the beginning, she lived up to her name! Soon after her birth, the American Board of Surgery came to review surgical residency programs in San Diego. There were only two in the city, one at the University of California in San Diego in a modest county hospital, and our program at Mercy Hospital, the largest hospital in town. To our shock and surprise, at the end of its review the American Board of Surgery withdrew its accreditation! That meant that all six of the surgery residents in our program would have to find positions elsewhere. Our program director assured us he would help us and was confident that if I applied for a third-year position at one of the other general surgery programs in California, I would be able to continue. To insure that would happen, Becki and I got on our knees and asked God for a miracle. But as I called training programs in California and around the country, I couldn't find any openings— unless I was willing to start over as a first or second-year resident! By the time the academic year ended, my surgical career was over.

I was crushed, and I couldn't understand what God was doing and why He was turning my dream to serve him as a surgeon into a nightmare! Added to our bewilderment was the concern that if we stayed in the U.S. too long, the attractions and obligations of living in a materialistic culture would grow on us until we were too entangled to escape. We had encountered other Christian physicians and nurses who confessed that at one time in their lives they had planned on becoming missionaries. But because of financial, professional or marital concerns or concerns about raising their children overseas, they eventually decided to stay home. We were determined not to join their ranks, but God wasn't making it easy! It was one thing to trust in the Lord as he opened doors, but why would God slam a door in my face when I was earnestly seeking to obey Him? I would not find that out until many years later.

After several months of praying and seeking God's will, Becki and I contacted the Christian & Missionary Alliance, the mission both of our parents had served with. I explained to the mission that my training program in general surgery had closed after two years, and that the doors to continue seemed closed. Did the Alliance have medical work overseas that could use a less than half-trained surgeon and a fully trained nurse? When they answered "yes" and that they had an opportunity in Cambodia, our hopes soared! The Alliance asked us to fly to New York for a pre-appointment interview, which we did. At the end of our interview, the mission leaders explained that World Vision was building a pediatric hospital in Phnom Penh, Cambodia, and they were looking for missionary doctors and nurses who would be willing to learn Cambodian and serve long term. Would we be willing to serve with World Vision in Cambodia? It sounded too good to be true, and after praying about it we accepted the invitation. World Vision explained we would need to arrive in Phnom Penh in July of 1975 so we could attend the opening of the hospital.

We immediately began preparations to move halfway around the world. Then in August, Cambodia was in the clutches of an extreme Marxist Communist named Pol Pot. He called his movement "Khmer Rouge," which is French for "Red Cambodians." Aided by Communist North Vietnam's army that swept to victory in South Vietnam that same year, Pol Pot surrounded Cambodia's capital city. Under near-impossible conditions, World Vision completed the construction of the Children's Hospital, but in April the Khmer Rouge overran the weak Cambodian army, took over Phnom Penh, and ordered all foreigners—including World Vision— out of the country. Once again, Becki and I had nowhere to go. Several weeks later, the Alliance offered us three different ministry opportunities. The first was to work at a leprosy clinic in Thailand that was on the verge of closing. The second was to work at a hospital in Irian Jaya that was run by another mission organization; the final one was to serve at one of two possible places in Africa. In our minds, Africa was simply out of the question, but the opportunity in Irian Jaya, formerly known as "New Guinea," sounded exciting. With our mission's encouragement, we set about filling out the application forms for the mission hospital in Iran Jaya. The Alliance was already supporting other missionaries in Irian, and they were willing to support us financially and loan us to the other mission. However, as we worked our way through the application process, our responses to some of the other mission's questions revealed that we had significant doctrinal differences. In the end, the hospital in New Guinea informed us they would not need our help! Once again, we were stunned and bewildered. God seemed to be bouncing us around like ping pong balls! The rejection closed the third door to, leaving us with our mission's only remaining offer: Africa!

God had worked financial and spiritual miracles to prepare us for missionary service, but the collapse of my surgical residency and a succession of closed doors left us emotionally drained. Our mission was offering us an opportunity to serve in Africa, but it was the one continent we could not see ourselves serving in!

About this time Scott Wesley Brown's song, "Please Don't Send Me to Africa" became quite popular in Christian circles. The lyrics, which were a musical prayer to God by a fearful Christian, were uncomfortably amusing. To a degree, they expressed some of our reservations about serving in Africa!

"Please don't send me to Africa, I don't think I've got what it takes! I'm just a man, I'm not a Tarzan, I don't like lions, gorillas or snakes! I'll serve you here in suburbia, in my comfortable middle-class life, but please don't send me out into the bush, where the natives are rest- less at night!"

Of course, the lyrics of the song were mocking the week-kneed faith of many American Christians, but our laughter was hollow. It was at that uncomfortable moment that we were given two choices: we could serve at a 40-year-old mission hospital in former Belgian Congo, assisting two other missionary doctors, or we could establish a medical clinic at a place in Gabon—a country we had never heard of. The place in Gabon was called "Bongolo." Both options sounded dubius, but because God sometimes calls His servants to go to dubius places, we realized we needed to do some basic research about Gabon and then hear or see a sign from God that the bewildering dance was over.

Our first search was for Gabon, which we found below Africa's "armpit" just south of Cameroun and opposite Kenya, on Africa's east coast on a map of the world. Bongolo wasn't there, but the town of Lebamba was there in fine print. Once again, we got on our knees and asked God for faith, forgiveness and fortitude, and clear direction to both of us as to where God wanted to send us. A week later as I was finishing out my last few days of residency at Mercy Hospital, I decided to eat my lunch on the roof of the hospital. As I was munching my sandwich the Lord said to me just as clearly as if someone had spoken to me out loud, "I want you to go to Gabon!"

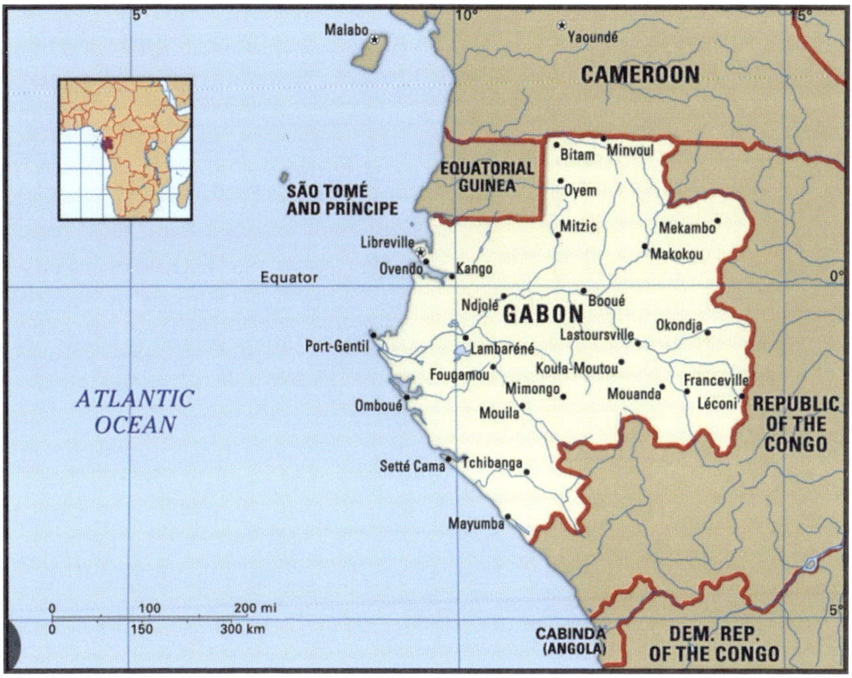

Later that day when I arrived home, Becki opened the front door with Rachael in her arms and before I could say a word said, "Guess what? I know where God wants us to go! It's Gabon!" Step by step, with patience and foreknowledge, God was leading us away from Cambodia, away from Asia, and to the continent, the country, and the location he had prepared us for: Bongolo, Gabon.

At the time we said *'yes:* we knew nothing about God's work in Gabon, except that it was an equatorial country in West Africa where Alliance missionaries had been serving for a long time. We had never heard of Don and Dorothy Fairley or any of the other missionaries who had begun the work in the 1930's and had served there until they retired. And we most certainly had never heard of Bongolo Falls and its horrible curse!

In September of 1975, Becki, Rachael and I said tearful goodbyes to our friends in San Diego and flew to Paris, France. The next day, we boarded a train and traveled to the town of Albertville in the French Alps where there was a French language school for missionaries headed to French-speaking countries. The Alliance had reserved an apartment for us, and the school had a lovely cafeteria that served

French food every evening. We were only on our own for morning and noon meals. The evening meals were simple and quite French. The first time the kitchen had served us each an entire fish, complete with staring eyeballs, fins, and scales, we grimaced but followed the example of our enthusiastic French hosts! Our view from the school included snow-covered mountains all year around, and we quickly fell in love with Albertville's abundant fresh vegetables, crisp French bread, and delectable pastries. Our teachers spoke little English and were Christians who routinely drank wine in moderation, though that was not an option for us! To our initial surprise, they used real wine for communion on Sundays, which upset some of our sterner colleagues from other mission organizations so much they decided to hold their own services! During the year we studied French with wonderful Christian instructors who helped and encouraged us with grace and humility. By the end of the year, Becki and I were conversing comfortably with French people, though at times they would suddenly cover their mouths and giggle!

Our next challenge was applying for a five-month course in Tropical Medicine at a famous institute in Antwerp, Belgium, and finding an apartment. I drove up from France and paid in advance for a small apartment near the Institute. Then I wired the address to our mission and asked them to send our next support check to our new address in advance. The day before the check was supposed to arrive, missionary friends of ours ran out of money and needed gas money to get back to Brussels, where they lived. The next day we arrived in Antwerp, and our mailbox was empty. We were penniless, Rachael was crying with hunger, and we didn't know a soul in the city! All we could do was pray, so we got on our knees and asked God to help us. After we finished praying, I opened my empty wallet and went through it one more time. Suddenly, I discovered a tiny pocket that I had never seen before. As I opened it, there was a crisp, new, $5 bill! It was a Sunday, and all the grocery stores were closed except a tiny stand in the nearby train station. We had just enough money to buy a can of oatmeal, a can of powdered milk, and a bag of sugar. Becki made oatmeal, added the milk and sugar, and Rachael ate it happily. There was enough for Becki and me that night, and the next day we ate oatmeal for breakfast and lunch and supper before we ran out of everything. The next morning when we checked our mailbox, our check had arrived!

A few days later we found a nursery for preschoolers run by Catholic nuns. Rachael loved the school and the nuns, but two weeks later developed a serious limp. When we asked her if it hurt, she shook her head. It took X-rays and a week of prayer before we discovered that her favorite teacher at the nursery was a young nun who limped! Once we explained to Rachael that she didn't have to limp to be her friend she was cured! What a relief!

Two weeks later we started our studies in Tropical Medicine. We both took the same courses, but to my chagrin, Becki outscored me at exam time! In April of 1977 and during the Easter break, we traveled to England and purchased a new Land Rover for $15,000, thanks to the gift of an elderly saint back in America who knew our parents and was prayerfully following our progress. In March, we signed up to travel to Gabon on a freighter that offered a deal we couldn't resist, which was to sail to Gabon with our Land Rover for half the cost of flying!

The Alliance gave us a green light to buy our tickets, so in early April we drove to Marseille, France, boarded the ship, and watched as a crane swung our truck up onto the rear deck of the ship. Carolyn Thorson, a nurse who was also assigned to our future team in Bongolo signed up for a similar deal with a Toyota Landcruiser she had purchased in Europe. As our ship pulled away from Marseille, France, we were so excited that we waved goodbye to the dock workers!

But our euphoria soon tanked when over the next two weeks our ship sailed to three different ports in the Mediterranean and loaded freight for Africa. The last stop was Valencia, Spain, where dock workers pumped thousands of gallons of Spanish wine into vats in the ships hold. Our voyage to Gabon was only supposed to take three weeks, but after two weeks we were still in the Mediterranean! A week later we finally sailed past the Rock of Gibraltar and into the Atlantic Ocean. The weather was spectacular, and every day we watched porpoises frolic alongside the ship for miles at a time. In the evenings, brilliant sunsets faded into velvety, star-lit skies.

Two days later we docked in the port of Dakar, Senega, and set foot on the continent of Africa. After two more days we were on our way again, only to drop anchor off the coast of Sierra Leone for two days to pick up additional crew members.

By this time, we were beginning to tire of our cramped quarters. There were only two single beds in our cabin, and a long narrow sofa. Since we didn't want Rachael to fall out of bed at night, I slept on the sofa. To keep our sanity, in the evenings we helped Carolyn make Scrabble and Clue games out of cardboard that we played until they fell apart!

Two days later our ship anchored a half mile off the coast of Togo. When we asked the captain why our ship wasn't docking, he sighed and explained that Nigeria's sudden wealth from newly discovered oil wells had caused a huge back-up of ships waiting to unload orders of building supplies, generators, computers, vehicles—the list was too long to even explain. As a result, both Nigeria's only major port and Togo's port were so backed up that 50 ships were always anchored offshore both ports, waiting to unload orders from all over the world. Our ship would unload Nigerian orders at Togo's port so they could be trucked across the border into Nigeria. Several days later the ship's air-conditioning failed, and the temperature in the cabins climbed to 100 degrees Fahrenheit.

Two miserable weeks later it was *finally* our ship's turn to dock in Togo's port and unload its cargoes for Nigeria. After that our ship headed south, and four days later we arrived at the port of Dakar, Cameroun. With hours of docking our ship began pumping the thousands of gallons of wine it had taken on in Valencia into tanker trucks on the dock. It was somewhat entertaining to watch as the crew filled the tanker trucks to overflowing that pulled up to the dock. As wine overflowed down the sides of the tankers, the dock workers and drivers rushed madly to the undersides to drink the wine spilling off dusty fenders and running boards! To the captain and crew's great amusement half of the dock workers were soon too drunk to stand. Some of the drivers barely managed to drive away without running into each other or the nearby warehouses!

After two days of pumping wine, our ship continued south to our next destination, Libreville! We were already a month behind schedule. The next morning as Becki, Rachael, Carolyn and I enjoyed our last breakfast onboard, the captain entered with the shocking news that our ship would have to wait three weeks to get a berth in Gabon's small harbor! Aghast at the thought of another three weeks on the freighter, we begged the captain to let us get off with our suitcases.

We were anchored less than a half mile from the coast and could even see cars driving on Libreville's roads! The captain understood and promised to radio the customs police and ask them to come out in their launch to stamp our passports. Our waiting finally over, we happily packed our bags.

Around 1 p.m., a customs launch motored out to our ship and pulled alongside. Several uniformed policemen climbed aboard and went to the captain's cabin. Soon we heard angry shouting, doors slamming, and feet pounding down the ship's metal stairs. As we rushed to the railing to see what was happening, the policemen climbed back into their launch and sped back to the port! When we asked the captain what happened he glumly explained that the police could not let us get off the ship because it was a national holiday of some kind and their boss had taken the rest of the day off! Incredulous, I asked the captain, "How can a country's customs department simply take the afternoon off? Will they come back tomorrow?"

The captain shrugged and said, "This is Africa, not Europe, and it's the way things work here! Our ship is on the waiting list for the few docks they have, and because there are many ships ahead of us, we can't afford to sit here and wait for them to let you off! We'll travel a day south to Pointe Noire in the Republic of Congo where we can load hardwood logs into our hold. After that we'll come back to Libreville." It was shocking news and a hard lesson. Worse yet, we had no telephone number for the mission that would enable us to call and explain what was happening. As we glumly watched the coast of Gabon disappear, we wondered why the Lord would delay us for yet another two weeks.

A day and a half later we reached Pointe Noire, a port city on the coast of the Gabon's southern neighbor, the Republic of Congo. In Don Fairley and Harold Pierson's day, the Republic of Congo was called "French Congo." In 1977, the Republic of Congo had become a communist state, and because Americans were not welcome, we were not allowed to leave the ship.

As our ship unloaded containers onto the dock, two Swiss passengers got on board for the ship's eventual return to Europe. That evening as we ate in the officer's cafeteria, they told us a chilling story. They had had a business in Pointe Noire and had lived in the country for twenty years. Six months previously their twenty-year-old daughter flew from Switzerland to visit them. One evening, she and her French boyfriend went for a walk in the park next to the ocean. An unidentified man suddenly ran up behind them in the dark and struck her on the head with a machete. She fell to the ground, bleeding and unconscious. Her boyfriend rushed her to the best hospital in the town, where she regained consciousness. A French doctor examined her, pronounced her wound superficial, sutured her scalp wound, and sent her home.

The following week she began complaining of headaches and developed an unexplained fever. Then she began having seizures. A day later, one side of her body became paralyzed. Her parents evacuated her by plane to Switzerland, where she was diagnosed with a brain abscess. The machete had not just cut her scalp but had penetrated into her brain, bringing contamination and resulting in an intracranial abscess. Had the doctor in Pointe Noire examined her wound more carefully and taken an x-ray, he might have discovered that the machete blow had penetrated her skull. As a result of his sloppy medical care, the injured woman had developed a brain abscess that left her partially paralyzed. Her doctors didn't know yet if she would recover completely or would be left with permanent disabilities. Her parents sold their business and were now leaving Pointe Noire. After listening to their story, we wondered what disasters might in store for us! It was a serious reminder to stay close to Jesus.

On May 15, 1977, fifty-two days after boarding our ship, we finally docked at the port of Libreville! Our field chairman, Melvin Carter, came aboard and welcomed us with questions: *"Where were you all this time? Why didn't you tell us you were delayed? We've been tearing our hair out worrying about you!"* Nobody from the mission had heard from us for two months, and our leaders back in the U.S. were wondering if we had been taken hostage by bandits, fallen off our ship and drowned, or had gone AWOL! We sheepishly apologized for failing to keep our leaders better informed! It had never occurred to us that the people who were responsible for us might be worried when they didn't hear from us and we didn't show up for nearly two months! The Lord had many more lessons to teach us, but thankfully, none would require us to twiddle our thumbs on a freighter for fifty-two days!

Chapter Three:

THE ADVENTURE BEGINS

God's Yoke

Once we were on land, Melvin Carter began the process of helping us register our Land Rover, apply for drivers' licenses, and purchase food supplies for living down-country. The road from Libreville to Bongolo is 540 kilometers (336 miles) long. Until 2010, the first 74 miles of the trip were paved, and the rest was laterite. Back then Land Rovers didn't have air conditioners, and we had to drive with our windows open to keep cool. That worked well in the rainy season, but in the Dry Season if we were following another car by even 400 yards, we would eat red dust! More than once, we arrived at our destination with ghastly, red-toothed smiles! The alternatives were to reduce your speed or pass the car ahead at wild speeds through choking clouds of red dust! During the rainy season the dust was replaced with an abundance of red, slippery mud. This led to many memorable experiences— but I'm getting ahead of our story.

During our first trip down country, Melvin Carter led the way in his Toyota, and we followed three hundred yards behind. Some of the bridges on the last part of the trip were so broken that we had to pray for courage to follow him!

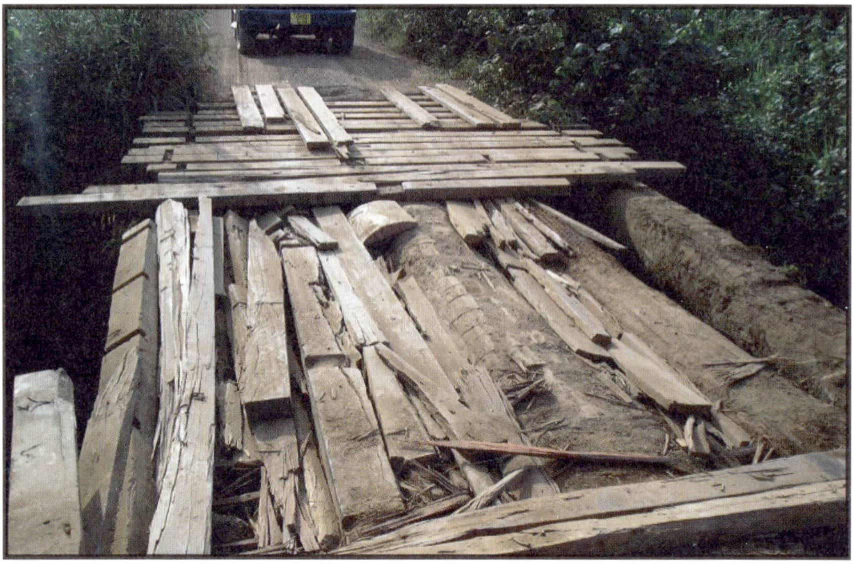

A bridge on the road to Bongolo

On the first day we drove two thirds of the way and stopped for the night at the mission station in Mouila where Melvin and his family lived. The next morning, we continued our trip and three hours later arrived in the small town of Lebamba. The population of the town back then, was less than 2,000 souls, and that included Bongolo and the village called Dakar. Bongolo was three miles west of Lebamba on a rarely graded dirt road. The last hurdle was the Louetsi River, which in the rainy season could swell to 100 feet across.

When for the first time we pulled up to the river, we discovered a hand-pulled ferry that previous missionaries had welded together. It had a clever pully system that enabled the ferry to slide across the river with the help of the current. How could it be, I wondered, that after forty-three years of continuous occupancy, nobody had thought to build a bridge? In retrospect, I blush at my naiveté. At least I had the sense not to voice my thoughts!

After we drove onto the ferry, the hired boatman pulled us across. We watched in amazement as the boatman turned the ferry slightly, enabling the current to push the ferry across to the other side with little effort on his part. A mind cleverer than mine had designed it. When we reached the middle of the river, the soft rumbling sound of a waterfall drew our gaze upriver, where for the first time we saw Bongolo Falls. It was indeed "modest." Perched on the lower left side was a small, square orange brick hut that we subsequently learned housed Bongolo's 30-year-old hydroelectric plant, completed in 1945 by Don Fairley and Furman Lentz. More than three decades later the plant's water-powered generator was still bringing light and 5,000 wats of steady electricity to Bongolo's five mission houses, the Bongolo Dispensary, and the Bongolo Church, 24 hours a day.

The other river-crossing service was a 30-foot dugout canoe that a hired man crossed regularly with pedestrians. During times that the ferry sprung a leak and had to be pulled out of the water for repairs, the only way to cross the river was in the 30-foot dugout canoe.

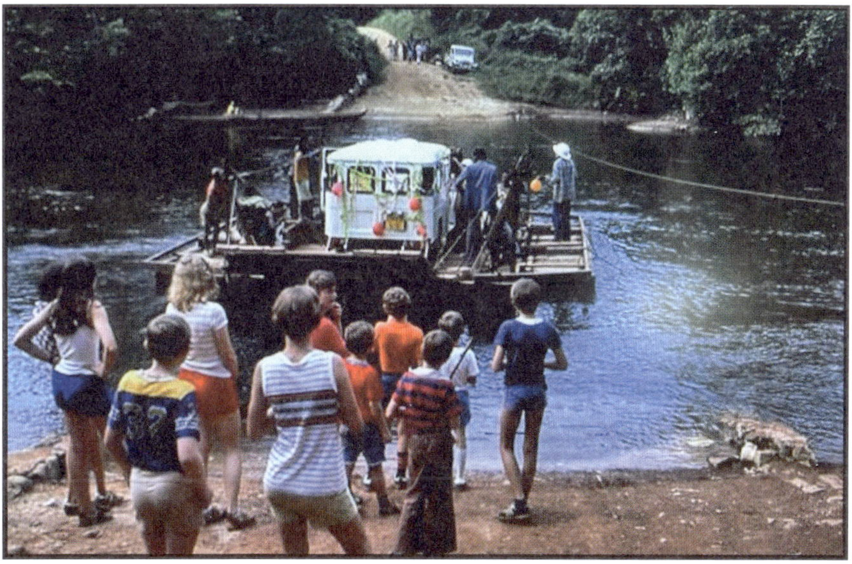

The "De Lux" Ferry still in use in 1977. In this photo kids from the mission school

After crossing on the ferry, we drove up a dirt road that paralleled the river for half a kilometer before passing a large white church on our right. The rough dirt road continued up a hill and past a large brick house 50 feet up a hill on the left. We later we learned that Don Fairley built the house in 1938, and that it was only forty feet from the fearsome cliff of death.

The road continued up the hill and finally leveled out in front of a large, whitewashed brick building that we later learned was called

"The Foyer." It, too, was built by Don Fairley, and was serving as the dormitory for the missionary kids who attended the elementary school on the station. Melvin stopped at the Foyer, and as we stepped out of our cars we were quickly surrounded by an excited and welcoming crowd of missionary kids, dorm parents, schoolteachers, and nurses. Minutes later several excited African yard workers showed up and pumped our hands enthusiastically! Everyone wanted to see Bongolo's first doctor and nurse couple and join in welcoming us!

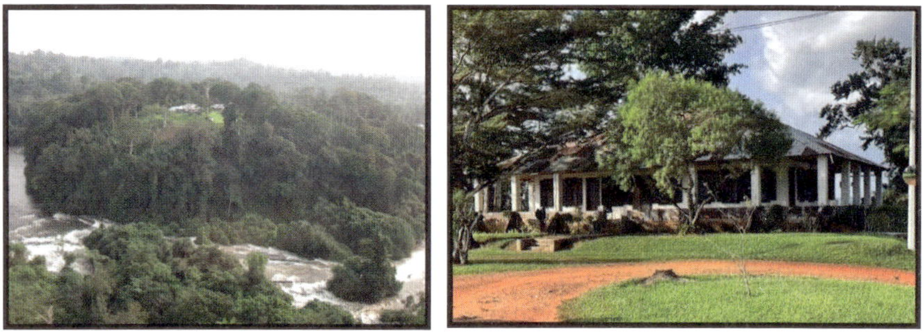

Two views of House 5, which Harold Pierson completed in 1939, after four years. The Thompsons lived in it from 1977 to 2013. The caves the Thompson boys later discovered where the leopards may have lived in were located near the top of the vine-covered limestone cliffs behind the Thompson's house.

Half an hour later our Field Director had us follow him up the hill to the house we would live in, called "House 5." It was surrounded on three sides by jungle. As we began unpacking our bags we heard the constant sound of rushing water from the whitewater rapids below. House 5 was the only house made entirely of hardwood boards and was completed in 1934. The Pierson family lived in the house for just one year before moving 150 miles to the west to bring the gospel to the Bapounou people. Over the decades that followed, at least four other missionary families lived in House 5 before we came.

All of the mission houses were surrounded by beautifully landscaped lawns, flowering trees and shrubs, and a variety of fruit trees. Because of Bongolo's tropical climate, the grass had to be mowed every ten days to keep it from taking over and hiding snakes.

The next day Melvin and the missionary nurses who arrived before us took us down the hill to a football field size plateau next to the Bongolo Church, a lovely structure that could seat a thousand people! On the other end of the plateau were two small buildings that served as the Bongolo Dispensary. In between the dispensary and the church was Bongolo's Elementary School for the Christians in Dakar. Once we learned the tribal language, Bongolo became our second home and workplace.

The next day we visited the Bongolo Dispensary. Twenty years before our arrival, missionaries had built the main building out of burnt bricks. Later, the Bongolo church added a 20 x 40-foot patient ward using mud bricks. As we entered the dispensary, a small crowd of patients in the waiting area jumped up and began cheering! Men, women, and children crowded around us, excitedly shaking our hands, laughing with joy, and asking us questions we couldn't understand! A small, young white woman who turned out to be the head nurse for the dispensary eventually appeared from inside and greeted us. She and her husband were missionaries from Holland. Her name was Sarah Luteijn, and she had been running the dispensary for several years while training two African nurses' aides. It was a joyous welcome, and our field director used the moment to introduce us to the crowd as "Docteur et Madame Thompson."

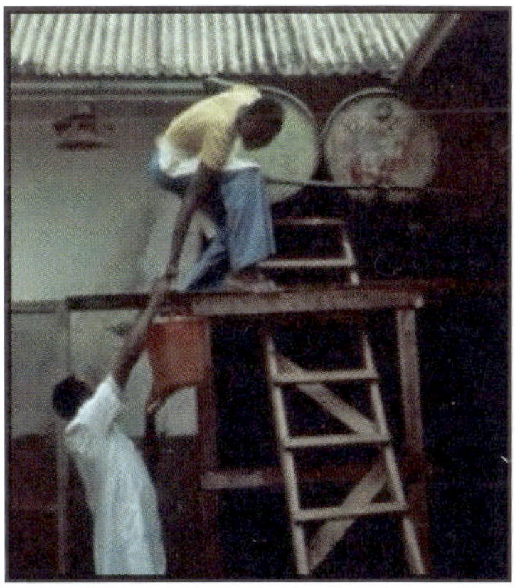

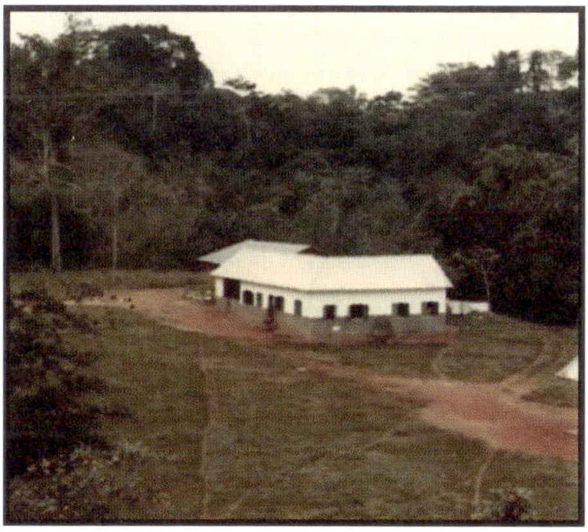

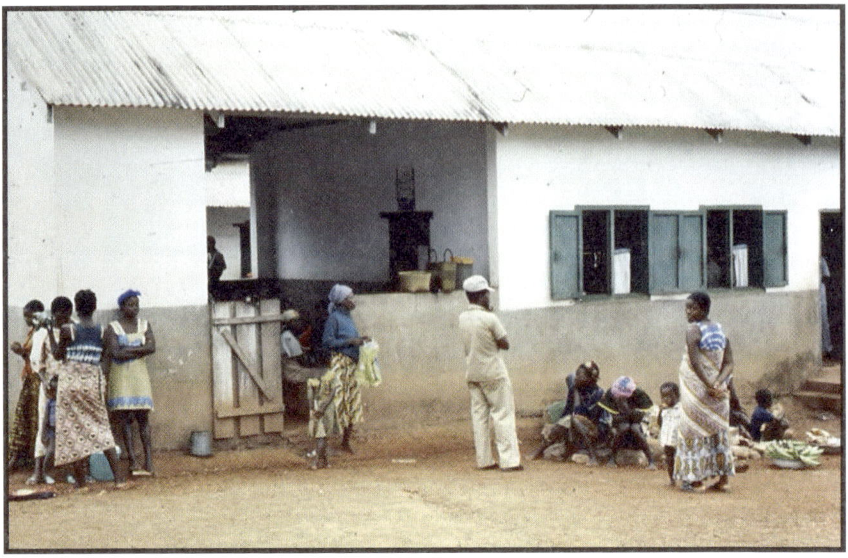

The Bongolo Dispensary in 1977 when we first arrived.

One day the dispensary would serve as the first phase of Bongolo Hospital, but the crude medical facility we saw that day was less than wonderful. Its walls were faded and smudged. It was furnished with a few wooden tables and cupboards made of locally cut boards and shipping crates. The pharmacy shelves had only a few bottles of medicine.

Other surprises were a waiting room littered with goat droppings and cement floor, stained brownish red by the dirt and mud patients brought in each day on their feet. We also wondered why the outside walls of the building were only painted white from the bottom of the windows to the roof and were marked with a curious, horizontal brown streak that encircled the building. The brown streak turned out to be the work of 50 or more goats that slept under the eaves every night and rubbed their itchy butts on the walls!

The water system that made handwashing possible in the dispensary's two sinks consisted of two 55-gallon drums on a small platform under the eaves. When it rained, which was often, rainwater from the roof filled the barrels. During the three-month dry season, patient's family members had to carry water from the river in buckets and fill the drums so we could wash our hands. The only signs of advanced technology were 40-watt light bulbs hanging from the ceilings. The dispensary also had an ancient wind-up telephone that was connected by a single strand to the missionary nurses' house, and to our house.

Pastor Ndongo Philippe was the pastor of the 700-member Bongolo church. Several days after we arrived, he came to visit us. Speaking French, he expressed thankfulness to God that we had finally arrived and apologized that there were so few people from the church to welcome us. "After all," he said wiping his eyes, "we have been asking God to send us a doctor for twenty years!" His comment left me sobered and mindful of the confusing path God had led us on. In the months and years that followed, Pastor Philippe would become one of our most trusted and faithful counselors.

During our first week in Bongolo, we concentrated on settling in and getting used to our new surroundings. Bongolo station did not have enough houses for our growing medical team, that eventually included six single nurses. Our house had four bedrooms, so we were asked to share two of our bedrooms with two of our missionary nurses until other lodgings could be built.

The official language of the people in Gabon was French, and though most of the time we would use French in our medical work, the majority of the people at the time spoke only Yinzebi. Becki and I wanted to begin working in the dispensary immediately, but the Mission had arranged for a veteran missionary who was translating the New Testament into Yinzebi to begin teaching us the Yinzebi language, at least the greetings and tribal customs. We were grateful for her orientation and were soon greeting the people in their own language. About that same time our field director, Melvin Carter, came to see how we were doing.

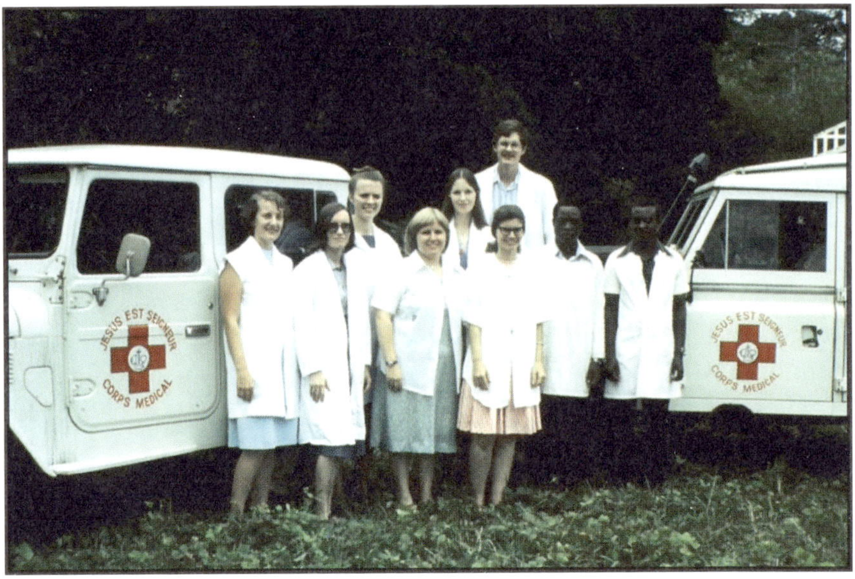

We called ourselves "The Jesus Is Lord medical team!"
Norbert was on the far right, and Marcel was in front of me.

Thinking that after our six-week orientation course was completed, we shared with Melvin our plans to begin providing medical care to the population. He listened patiently, but when we were done said, "I think you're going to have to put your plans on hold:'

"Why?" I asked.

"You must first learn the Yinzebi language," he said. "That means spending six hours a day until you pass your exams. For most people, that takes 18 months to two years:' Melvin's words hit us like a bomb!

"Why?" I said, "That's going to take another 18 months, and we've already spent a year learning French and another seven months studying Tropical Medicine! Many of the people here speak French!"

Our director sighed. "We're not asking you to do anything that we don't require of all of our new missionaries. If you want to have an effective ministry, you must learn the 'language of the heart, which here in Bongolo is Yinzebi.

The discussion that followed was tense and unhappy. Our Field Director ended by saying that for the next 12 to 18 months, those of us who were new to Gabon would be spending six hours a day and six days a week studying Yinzebi!

The problem was that I was already being called down to the dispensary for emergency cases several times a day and night. The people had heard there was a doctor in Bongolo, and even though we didn't have a hospital, if they or their children were seriously ill

or injured it was far better to show up at our dispensary than rely on the Ngangas, risk treatment at the small Lébamba hospital, or travel 250 miles north to Schweitzer Hospital. Each time the nurses sent word that an urgent case and come, I simply couldn't sit in my house and study Yinzebi! Added to our frustration was the lack of equipment, the lack of a laboratory and an X-rays unit, and only a few medicines. At the very least we had to stock our pharmacy with a basic medicines and supplies!

A few weeks later, a veteran missionary named Julie Fehr invited Becki and I to visit her. She lived among the Mitsogo people thirty kilometers northeast of us in a village called Guevede. As we sat in her simple kitchen poured out our complaints about the unfairness of our situation, she listened quietly.

When we finished griping, she sat quietly for a moment, then said, "David and Becki, I'm sure you're having a tough time, but I wonder if you really understand your position as new servants in the Kingdom. You're here to learn, and this is the best opportunity you will ever have to get close to the Banzebi people. After all, you're not just here to take care of their sicknesses and injuries, but to lead them to faith in Jesus so one day they can live forever! Maybe you should accept the requirement that you learn the culture and the language of the people you came to be serve as a gift from the Lord!"

We both sensed that God was speaking to us through Julie, so we sat quietly as she continued. "Let me share something from Proverbs that has been of great help to me. *Proverbs 13:14 says, 'The instruction of the wise is like a life-giving fountain; those who accept it avoid the snares of death.'* Here's one more word I think applies to you," she added, "and it's a quote I've found very helpful. 'In the way of acceptance lies peace.'" Her words settled into our troubled hearts like rain on parched ground.

At the end of our visit, we thanked Julie for her hospitality and wise counsel and headed back to Bongolo. A week later the Lord spoke to me from Proverbs 13:10: *"Where there is strife, there is pride, but wisdom is found in those who take advice."* I was the one causing strife, and it certainly wasn't because I was humble!

But the challenges didn't stop. In fact, they were endless, and the road to obedience took many unexpected turns. Six months into our language studies we began seeing an increasing number of children under five dying from measles, pertussis (otherwise known as whooping cough), polio, dysentery, and malnutrition! The anguish of the mothers was unbearable, and the numbers were increasing so sharply that our team decided to make an emergency order of vaccines from Europe for measles, pertussis, and polio, as well as some of the newer medications to treat malaria. While we waited, we continued our Yinzebi studies and did everything we could to save the children who came with diseases we could treat. But many we couldn't help, and those children died.

As soon as our vaccines and medicines arrived by air from Europe, I dropped everything and drove to Libreville and purchased basic medicines and coolers. Then I filled them with ice and drove back to Bongolo. A day or two later, we divided our team up and began vaccinating children at our dispensary and in every village in the province we could reach by car.

Becki and I had brought a small camping tent, so we used it as our "portable clinic" in the villages where we vaccinated. As soon as we would arrive in a village and pitch our tent, mothers would show up with their children. When we announced that we were vaccinating children under age 10 for just 25 cents a child, the crowds doubled! We didn't vaccinate for free, because we had learned that the people thought that free medicines were worthless! Over the next two months, our teams vaccinated thousands of children and stopped the epidemics in their tracks. We later learned that more than 500 children under the age of five died that year in our district, most of them before we began vaccinating. Without our vaccination campaign, the number of deaths would have doubled.

Six months later our team carried out a survey of 100 houses in our area and learned that over the previous five years, four out of every five children under five had died. Equally shocking was that one out of every 50 maternal deliveries in the rural villages ended in the death of the mother. In 2023, the number of maternal deaths in the U.S. was 18.6 per 100,000 live births. The maternal deaths of the women in our survey were more than 100 times more frequent than in the United States!

Though Becki and I were gradually able to work out a schedule that allowed us to study the language three days a week, there were still days when I simply could not stay at home. Trying to help critically ill or injured patients without even a simple laboratory, X-rays, and an inadequate supply of medicines was frustrating, time-consuming, and too often impossible. By responding to emergencies, we could at least try to help. Perhaps a third of the time my efforts made a difference.

The situation came to a head one day when our field director came to Bongolo and complained sharply that Becki and I were not even close to studying Yinzebi 30 hours a week as we had promised. I was going several times a week to the nearby village to converse and write down new words, but Becki had a 3-year-old and our newborn son to take care of and could only study at home.

After sitting us down our director said, "David, if you and Becki don't start spending six hours a day learning the local language, the Mission is prepared to send you home." I sighed and said, "We are doing our best to learn this language, but I cannot refuse to help a dying man, woman, or child if my presence can make a difference. What would you do?"

That night, Becki and I talked far into the night. As we talked, the Lord reminded us of His instruction in Hebrews 13:17: *"Obey your leaders and submit to their authority. They keep watch over you as men who must give an account. Obey them so that their work will be a joy, not a burden, for that would be of no advantage to you."* God's Spirit reminded me of the covenant I had made with Him at the altar years before in San Diego—the promise to go *wherever* and do *whatever* He told me to do. That night we asked the Lord to forgive us for complaining about our leaders and our language requirements and purposed in our hearts to renew our efforts to learn the Yinzebi language.

Eighteen months later, God enabled us to pass our Yinzebi exams. We will always be grateful to Melvin Carter, Julie Fehr, and our mission executive committee for insisting that we take the time to learn the Yinzebi language and culture, while at the same time giving us the leeway to treat the sick and dying children that desperate mothers brought to us nearly every day. The ability to speak and understand the people in their own language helped us immeasurably, gave us important insights into their cultural and economic challenges, and made it easier us to serve and understand the Yinzebi people with love.

Lamentations 27:27-29 says, "*It is good for a man to bear the yoke while he is young. Let him sit alone in silence, for the Lord has laid it on him. Let him bury his face in the dust—there may yet be hope!*" In Daniel 12:10 God said to Daniel about future sufferings, "*Many will be purified, cleansed, and refined by these trials!*"

Divine Treasure!

We had been in Gabon only about three months when Melvin asked me to take a week off from language study and help transport in our new Land Rover several veteran missionaries returning from furlough in the U.S. who needed to travel back to their assigned posts in eastern Gabon where their cars were in storage. The distance from Bongolo to eastern Gabon was considerably shorter than the northern route. Ray and Maurine Holcomb were returning from Canada with their three boys. Veteran missionary Ron Israel, who was with his wife Joan and was in charge of the dormitory for the missionary kids attending the school in Bongolo, volunteered to drive the mission's 10-year-old, five-ton Dodge truck to Moanda with the Holcomb's crates and packed barrels. In our new Land Rover, I would transport some of the Holcombs and Enid Miller, a single Bible translator.

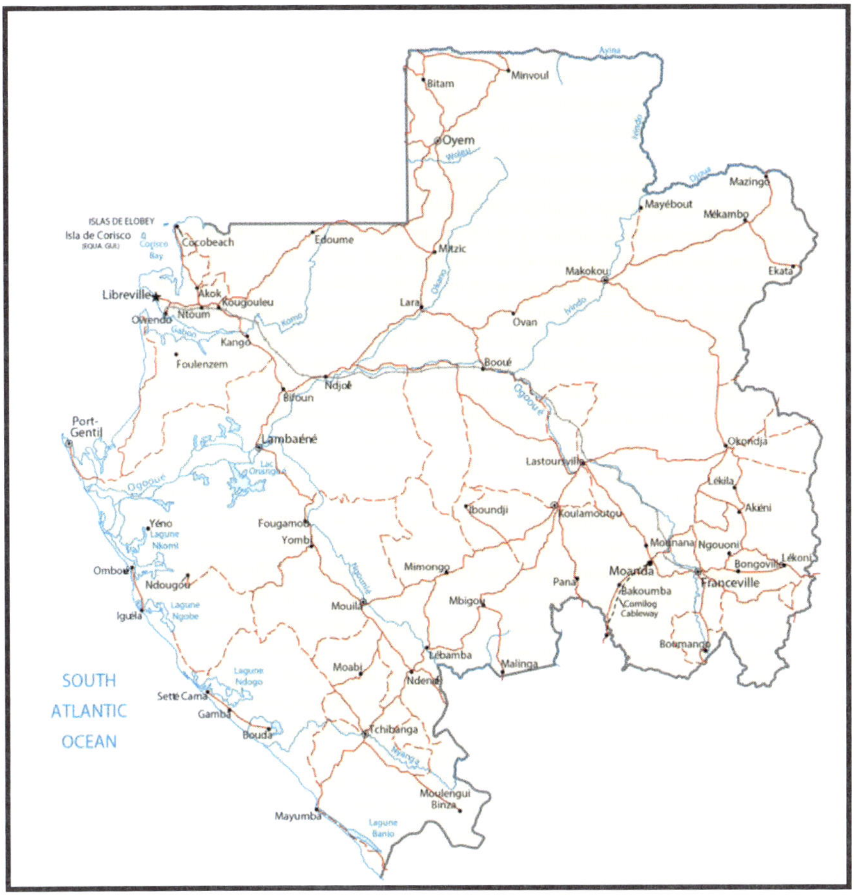

Road and river map of Gabon (roads are drawn in red and rivers in blue).

Our three vehicles left Lébamba at 7:00 am and snaked slowly north- east through Gabon's rain forest on a rough laterite road towards Mimongo. From Mimongo we continued on to the town of Koula Moutou (see map). The road was dusty, and the log bridges were poorly maintained and sometimes treacherous. Some of them had logs that had rotted and fallen through, leaving dangerous gaps. In the rainy season, the trip would have been impossible, but since it was the dry season, the road was dusty but only occasionally difficult.

After nine hours, all three vehicles made it safely to Koula Moutou, where Wayne and Donna Webb would live and minister for the next four years. The m ission house h a d been closed for a year, so everything in the house was covered with dust. We were too tired

to care, and after a meal prepared from cans shook out our bedding and slept! The next morning the rest of the convoy continued on to the city of Moanda, arriving around 2 p.m.

Moanda is Gabon's manganese mining center and one of Gabon's five largest cities. We all pitched in to unload the Holcomb's crates and 55-gallon drums from the Dodge truck. Afterwards, Ron and Wayne headed back to Koula Moutou in the Dodge, where Ron would wait for me to join him the next morning. That afternoon many of Moanda's Christians came by to welcome the Holcombs back. Around 4 p.m. we were visiting with some of them when Wayne opened the front door and walked in! His sudden appearance startled us, since he and Ron had left for Koula Moutou in the Dodge hours earlier.

Wayne quickly explained that fifteen miles outside of Moanda a front wheel bearing on the truck had burned out, rendering it undriveable. The Mission h ad purchased the seven-year-old truck from the Peace Corps five years earlier, with no spare parts. Ron had stayed with the truck to protect it from thieves. The question on all of our minds was where in the middle of Africa were we going to find a front wheel bearing for a seven-year-old American truck? To our knowledge and true to missionary tradition, it was the only remaining 5-ton Dodge truck in the entire country that was still running! After we ran out of ideas, we bowed our heads and asked God to help us find a solution to our dilemma.

We had no sooner finished praying when Ray Holcomb said, "Wait a minute, wait a minute! The Peace Corps used to have a base near here, and they had those same 5-Ton Dodge trucks!" He explained that years earlier the Peace Corps had established a large base just outside of Moanda as part of a project to build schools

in the surrounding villages. At its height, the Peace Corps base had ten volunteers and at least four 5-ton Dodge trucks. In 1971, there was a rift in relations between the U.S. and Gabon's government, and Gabon's president had abruptly ordered the Peace Corps to leave Gabon. Their departure was bitter, and the American volunteers were ordered to pour sand in the engines, rendering the trucks useless.

After a few years, ten-foot-high grass and vines covered the camp. As was customary in rural villages, every Dry Season the villagers set fire to the tall grass beyond their gardens to reduce the hordes of mosquitos, insects, rats and small animals that made their homes in the tall grass near the village. The rusting Peace Corps trucks were eventually reduced to blackened hulks and were completely hidden by the tall grass.

The village was only a few miles outside Moanda, and Ray thought it might be possible to locate the old Peace Corps camp. If we could find one of the trucks and recover a front-wheel bearing, we could take it to Ron in the morning and fix the truck! It seemed far-fetched, but I was not in a position to offer advice.

Ray rummaged through his stuff and found a good flashlight, a Coleman lantern, and his toolbox, so we loaded them into the back of his Land Rover. I volunteered to join him, suspecting that it might be a fun. It turned out to be one of the wildest adventures I would ever experience!

Ray drove his truck straight to the village on the outskirts of Moanda and stopped close to where an old man was sitting next to a fire in front of his house. The old man watched us suspiciously as we approached. Ray tried to explain our mission, but the old man smoked his pipe and said nothing. Switching from French to the local tribal language, Ray greeted the man again. This time he looked up and gruffly asked what we wanted. Ray quickly explained that we needed help to find the old trucks the Peace Corps had left in the brush behind the village.

After another puff on his pipe the old man said, "Tomorrow!" When Ray explained it was urgent, the old man said roughly, "Not tonight!" There was no point in arguing, but Ray wasn't ready to give up. By then, all of the other houses in the village had closed their doors for the night.

After a moment of reflection Ray said, "We'll have to find it ourselves. I'm sure I can find the old trucks, but we'll need the lantern."

We walked back to his truck and lit the lantern. The old man watched as we walked past him and through the village but stayed in his chair smoking his pipe.

I was prepared to work all night helping Ray take apart whatever pile of junk we found, but as he followed a path into thick, tall brush and grass I began to doubt the wisdom of continuing. Wasn't this country famous for its venomous snakes? I had seen a Gabon viper in the San Diego Zoo years before, and even behind two panes of glass it was fearsome. Now I was crashing around in snake heaven in the dark! And what about cobras? They loved this kind of brush! But Ray didn't seem bothered. I meekly followed him around in the fading light. Thirty feet behind the village we found ourselves walking through vegetable gardens, over crude stick fences, and along barely visible paths that Ray could somehow see in the light of the lantern.

When he thought we were close to the old Peace Corps camp, Ray abandoned the path altogether and headed directly into the ten-foot-high grass! In the stillness of the night, we sounded like elephants crashing around. In my mind, I could already see my epitaph: "David Thompson: 1948-1977. Trampled by enraged buffalos— after being bitten by poisonous snakes!"

Ten heart-pounding minutes later we bumped into a high-tension line pylon. To be on a life-threatening safari in the African brush and run into an electric pylon was culture shock to the extreme. What was a pylon doing out here? But at least it represented safety from snakes! Ray suggested that we *climb up* the pylon to see if we could see something from higher up! I was only too happy to get out of the tall grass and out of the reach of vipers, but now we were climbing towards high tension power lines! By this time, the sun had gone down and everything outside the range of our lantern was inky black.

When we had climbed twenty feet up and were trying to see what was below, the lantern's light blinded us. Ray finally took it from me, held it over our heads, and peered into the brush below. Unfortunately, all we could see was very tall grass. Discouraged, we climbed back down and contemplated our next move. Ray thought we should strike out in another direction, but before we could take another step, we heard a new and truly ominous sound: the voices of angry men shouting!

At first the men's voices were distant, but within seconds we realized they were rapidly coming toward us from several directions at once and were very angry! I did not need to understand their language to realize that we were in serious trouble. Seconds later ten men burst through the tall grass and surrounded us! As Ray and I stood frozen, the men shouted and slashed furiously at the brush with their machetes! Their chests were heaving and sweat poured off their faces! The two crazy white strangers who had been sneaking nefariously in their backyards were now at their mercy! It had to have been the one of the most bizarre and incomprehensible experiences of their lives! I know it was for me!

As the junior missionary, I thought it best to let Ray to explain what we were doing. The Lord must have given him courage, because while my mouth was frozen open, he began speaking to the men in their tribal language. This both surprised and calmed them. Ray quickly explained that we were looking for what remained of the old Peace Corps trucks so we could fix our old Peace Corps truck that had broken down. As he talked, the men gradually lowered their machetes and listened. When he promised to pay them something if they helped us find one, their hostility evaporated, and they quickly fanned out to look for burned Dodge truck carcasses.

Within minutes, they found one and called us over. While I stayed with the men, Ray ran back to his Land Rover to get his tools. The men cleared away some of the underbrush around the blackened truck, using their machetes. The tires had long since burned away, leaving only the rims. A few minutes later Ray got back with his tools and a jack. We used a jack to raise up one end of the front axle out of the dirt. The bolts on tire rim had rusted solid, but by using a steel chisel Ray was able to loosen them and pull the wheel rim off the axle. Then, under the light of our lantern, he reverently lifted out an almost-perfect front wheel bearing, still slippery with grease! It was too much to believe! We had found the right part, and it still had grease on it!

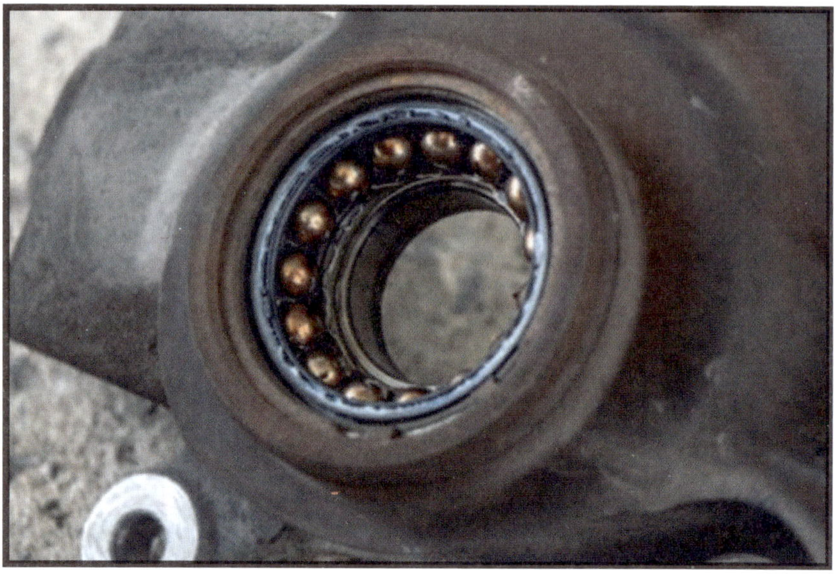

A wheel bearing

Ray thanked the men and paid each of them the equivalent of $5. Though we couldn't be certain until the next day if the bearing was the right part, the circumstances around finding it were so remarkable that we returned to Moanda, singing God's praises loudly and off-key!

In foreknowledge, our Heavenly Father hid and perfectly preserved an American-made front wheel bearing in the heart of Africa for our nearly extinct truck. Not only that, but he protected it through multiple fires. When Ray Holcomb and I came looking for it in the dark and stirred up a hornet's nest of angry of villagers, our Father protected us and put it in the villagers' hearts to help us— two white strangers—to find God's hidden treasure. Truly, there is no God like Jehovah!

Early the next morning, Ray and I headed down the road towards Koula Moutou with the wheel bearing in hand. Fifteen miles later, we found Ron Israel sleeping in the Dodge. When we told him how we had found the replacement wheel bearing he was incredulous, then shouted his thanks to the Lord! He had already removed the broken bearing, so all he had to do was see if the new one fit. As we held our breath, he slipped the bearing over the end of the axle and dropped it into place. It fit perfectly!

The next day we began our trip back to Bongolo. Ron drove the Dodge, and I followed far enough back to avoid choking in his dust. It was extremely hot, and neither of the vehicles had air conditioning. By nightfall we had guzzled all of our drinking water. We stopped for the night in a small village where there were Christians. They greeted us warmly, but when they realized that we were planning to sleep in our vehicles, they made a great fuss and insisted we stay in their home! They didn't have filtered or boiled water, but they did feed us a delicious meal of sweet potatoes, manioc, and chicken. Unfortunately, we were so thirsty we could hardly taste the food, and neither of us had the courage to ask them to boil water for us over an open fire for twenty minutes until it was safe to drink! Rather than risk dysentery, we went to bed with dry throats.

In the morning, our hosts boiled water for instant Nescafe coffee and seemed surprised that we drank so many cups of coffee! We thanked them sincerely and tried to leave some money to pay for their hospitality, but they would have none of it and after a prayer of blessing, sent us on our way.

Back on the dusty road and motivated by thirst, we drove without stopping to and pulled into Bongolo around 5 p.m. Cold water never tasted so good! By the grace of God we didn't develop kidney stones, at least on that trip!

I've often marveled at the way God provides and overcomes the attacks of Satan. To this day I'm still amazed that in the middle of the African rain forest, God perfectly preserved for seven years the exact wheel bearing we would need to repair our aging truck. He then led Ray Holcomb and me to the right village, and when we couldn't find the burned trucks, sent angry villagers to help us locate it! Anyone who thinks that was mere coincidence has their head in the sand.

It was for these kinds of experiences that the Apostle Paul wrote, *"And my God will meet all your needs, according to His glorious riches in Christ Jesus"* (Philippians 4:19). How often we forget that there are no coincidences in God's world, and that there is nothing, absolutely nothing, that He doesn't know and can't do for his children!

The Suffering South

In 1913, Dr. Albert Schweitzer started building a hospital in a small logging town called Lambaréné. The town was on a large island in the middle of the massive Ogoué River, Gabon's largest. Over decades, Schweitzer staffed his hospital with European doctors and nurses, many of whom were devout Christians. Schweitzer himself was a humanitarian and rejected both the divinity of Christ and the truthfulness of the Bible. Nevertheless, until his death in 1965, his hospital provided the only Western medical care in the interior of Gabon and saved the lives of thousands of people, both African and foreign, including many missionaries and their children.

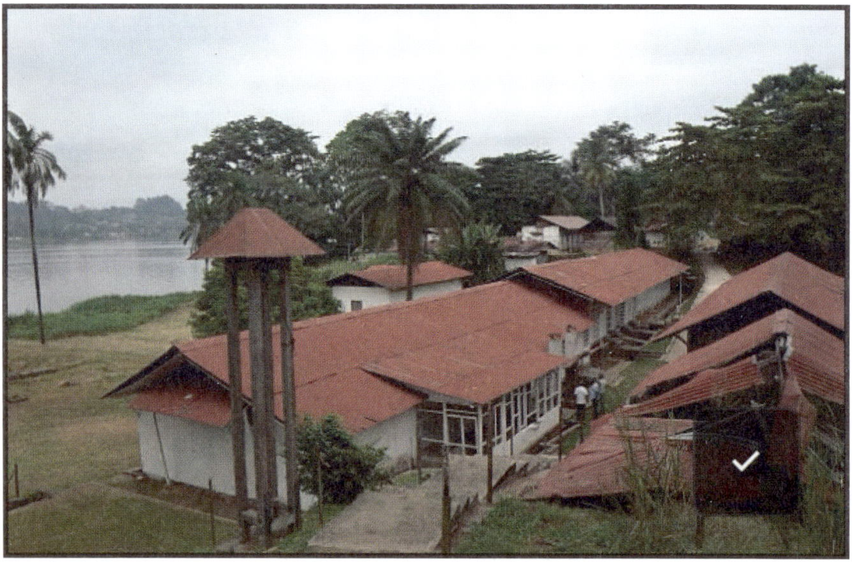

Schweitzer Hospital, 1940's

In the early years and before roads were built, the missionaries serving in Bongolo could only travel to Schweitzer Hospital on the rivers. They made the exhausting trip either to give birth to their babies or treat their more serious illnesses and injuries. During the 9-month rainy season the trip by boat was harrowing, took two to three days, and required them to hire a team of villagers to carry their heavy launch around treacherous falls and rapids.

The majority of Gabon's southern population lived hundreds of away from Schweitzer Hospital. Villagers who fell critically ill or were seriously injured were doomed to permanent disabilities or a slow, painful death. It was not until the 1950's that Gabon's French colonial masters bulldozed roads into the interior and established ferry crossings on the major rivers. Even then, two-thirds of Gabonese children were still dying of malaria, malnutrition, whooping cough, dysentery, and polio. Gabonese women in the south died horribly from obstructed labor, sleeping sickness, tuberculosis, and animal attacks. Many developed inguinal and abdominal hernias from carrying 50 to 75-pound loads of the food they grew in their jungle gardens on their backs. The women were also prey to animal attacks from leopards, wild buffaloes, and elephants that at times stripped their forest gardens bare. Men mostly died from lethal animal attacks, strangulated hernias, and logging accidents.

The Ngangas took advantage of these realities by insisting there were *no* natural deaths. They talked with the spirits the people worshipping, and the spirits told them that every death was caused by the sorcery of a secret enemy. By consulting the "good spirits" Bwiti and Mwiri, the Ngangas claimed inside knowledge about who was responsible for each and every death. The Ngangas boasted they could answer *why* people and their children experienced accidents, illnesses, or death, giving them a stranglehold on truth. Even Jesus didn't provide these kinds of answers, and at times new Christians were enticed to go to them for answers.

For a fee, the Ngangas also offered "protection" in the form of sacred objects, called "fetishes." Clients were instructed to tie them around their necks or bury them under their beds to protect them from evil spirits. But the fetishes did not protect them from being falsely accused of sorcery by the all-knowing Ngangas. This gave the Ngangas limitless opportunities to draw power from the people, enrich themselves, and learn of their clients' deepest secrets.

During the first year that the Fairleys and Piersons lived in Bongolo, Chief Boudiongo became a Christian and burned his fetishes, though as was often the case, he had to do it more than once before his confidence and faith in Jesus grew strong enough. To his credit, he was the first Banzebi to publicly declare his faith in Jesus and was eventually baptized.

Ten years later, Boudiongo suddenly developed a strangulated hernia that resulted in a bowel obstruction. Simple hernias can usually be reduced by firmly pushing on the skin over them until it slips back into the abdominal cavity. But when that doesn't work, the trapped intestines swell and become "strangulated," resulting in intestinal blockage, vomiting, and within hours or days, death.

When Boudiongo fell ill the Christian community immediately began fasting and praying for his healing, but a day later he was worse. Knowing well what the eventual outcome would be if he didn't have an operation, six strong rowers in his village made him as comfortable as possible in a dugout canoe and headed for Schweitzer Hospital. They set off at a tremendous pace and rowed all night long without stopping. In 36 hours, they travelled 350 miles and portaged around two waterfalls. But by the time they reached Schweitzer Hospital, Boudiongo was comatose. Dr. Schweitzer and his team immediately started IV's and took him to the operating room, but he was too far gone. He died on the table and was buried the next day in Lambaréné.

Chief Boudiongo's death was a great loss to the young Bongolo church and sent shockwaves through the Christian community, which by then had grown to more than 500. His death made it abundantly clear to Africans and missionaries alike that Schweitzer's hospital in Lambarene could not meet the needs of critically ill or seriously injured people who lived in the south.

Boudiongo's death was only one of many during the Bongolo church's early decades. On many occasions God responded to the Christians' prayers with relief and healing. But as was the case for Chief Boudiongo, not everyone was healed, and the Christians were a tiny fraction of the people living in the south. The rest of the population could only rely on the sorcery of the Ngangas, and when they failed— which was most the time—someone else would have to die! The suffering of the people in the south became so great that by 1950, the Christians were begging their missionary friends to build them a hospital like Schweitzer Hospital and staff it with not just nurses, but doctors. Unfortunately, in the 50's and 60's very few doctors were applying to the Alliance to serve as missionaries, and the few who did were sent to older mission fields and to countries with greater populations.

By 1945, the Bongolo Church had outgrown the temporary buildings the early pioneers had constructed out of local materials. Don and Dorothy Fairley translated the New Testament into the Yinzebi language, taught many of Bongolo's children to read, and discipled many. Their disciples then took the gospels to more than twenty surrounding villages. Two of their disciples were Boudiongo's sons who in time served as pastors in the Bongolo church.

In the early 50's, the Fairleys and other missionaries who joined them established a Bible school on the campus and began training pastors. Around the same time, Fairley designed and built a magnificent church building that could seat 1,000 people. Don supported the tall, steeped roof with soaring hardwood rafters that seemed impossibly slight and roofed the building with aluminum roofing tins shipped from the U.S. The design of the building allowed cool breezes to flow from both sides through multiple arched windows. With funding from their supporters in the U.S., Don and Harold Pierson's team of carpenters and masons finished the building in under a year.

Today the original Bongolo church building is more than

70 years old. Despite the pummeling of hundreds of violent rainstorms every year, the building has remained strong and beautiful, a silent testimony of the strength of Christ's church. Since it was finished in the 1950's, four generations of African Christians have grown up in it. Best of all, God's word is still preached.

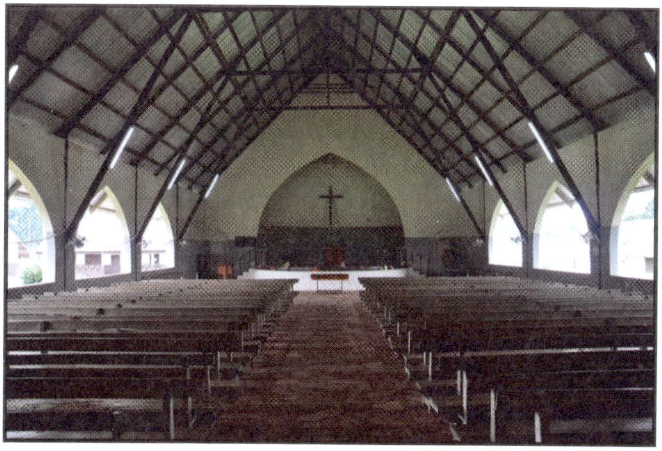

Bongolo Church, built by Don Fairley with manpower only, in 1954. The photo was taken in 2023.

Two of Chief Boudiongo's sons served as the church's first pastors. Boudiongo's oldest son served only briefly, but his youngest son, Sylvain Kivy, pastored the church for two decades before moving to Gabon's capital to establish the first of many Alliance churches in the city that followed. But I am getting ahead of my story!

In the mid 50's and in response to the cries of the Christians for medical care, the Alliance appointed missionary nurses to serve the tribes in south Gabon. These courageous and mostly single women included, Mary Lou Stuckey and Irene Piper, who served the Banzebis and Bavoumbou tribes near Bongolo; Anita Reader, who served the Mitsogo and Massango people east of Bongolo; and Betty Keifer, who ministered to numerous Bapounou villages to the west of Bongolo.

Another nurse who was serving at the Bongolo dispensary when we arrived was Sarah Luteijn, from Holland.

All of these courageous women raised funds from their supporters to build small clinic buildings, purchase medicines and medical supplies, and basic medical equipment. In addition to treating the sick they proclaimed the gospel and made disciples, trained assistants, for decades provided the only healthcare for thousands of villagers and fiercely opposed the Ngangas. Without the possibility of C- sections, access to X-rays, laboratory tests, or access to doctors for medical advice, these courageous women set simple fractures, treated leprosy and tuberculosis, drained abscesses, delivered babies, sewed up lacerations, treated malaria, and saved the lives of countless children. Their prayers for the sick, their medical skills, and their compassion brought uncounted blessings to those living near them. But for the majority of sick men, women and children living in south Gabon, there were only the Ngangas.

Final Plans

As newly arrived missionaries, our introduction to the Bongolo dispensary in early June of 1977 took place the day after we arrived. Up until then, missionary nurses had been doing what they could for the sick and injured for twenty years. While we were still studying French and Tropical Medicine in Europe, our Mission informed the Gabonese Church leaders that they had finally found a doctor for

Bongolo! They added that if the Bongolo Church wanted a hospital for him to serve in they would have to provide significant resources for construction. To show their commitment, the people in the Bongalo church donated money and volunteer labor and built a forty-foot by twenty-five-foot mudbrick building next to the dispensary to serve as a small, two-room, ward. On the day we arrived, the dispensary was treating thirty outpatients a day and twelve straw-covered cots in the ward were being used for people who were either too sick to come every day for treatment or lived far away and had no other place to stay.

The nurses consulted with patients four at a time, and of course, nothing was confidential! After a nurse took a brief history, examined the patient, and wrote in the patient's a brief prescription, all four patients moved to an adjacent bench to be served their medicines. Each room in the dispensary had a 40-watt light bulb hanging from the ceiling, and two of the three rooms in the mud-brick ward had lights. The small room used as a nursing station and procedure room, did not merit a light bulb.

The mud-brick hospital ward was furnished with twenty low, wooden beds and stained, straw-filled canvas mattresses. Every patient's medical record was written in a 25-page school notebook that cost 25 cents. After a consultation, a nurse would write in the notebook the date, tentative diagnosis, treatment orders, and any nursing notes. Patients had to purchase their own notebooks and could take them with them home after they were discharged.

There was one outhouse for everyone and a separate, mud-brick communal kitchen that was about eight by ten feet, with 4-foot walls and a two-foot gap at the top to allow smoke from the open fires to filter out the open windows. Each patient's helper cooked meals over small fire on the dirt floor of the kitchen, and each patient had to have a family member to look after them, cook their meals, and wash their laundry. Since the helper usually slept in the same bed as the patient and since sometimes the whole family came along, family members sometimes slept under the bed (if there was room), or on the floor. The crowding required quite an adjustment on our part! During our first year there were nights when 40 people slept in the small ward!

Later that week, I learned from our field director that our Mission Headquarters in the U.S. had agreed on a plan for the new medical work. As was often the case, the Gabonese Church leaders had a plan too that was quite different from the Mission's plan, but since the Mission was providing the doctor, the nurses, money to build, and housing for us, everyone understood that the Mission's plan would prevail. Our Field Director called our team together and explained that our mission leaders had decided that since there was already a hospital just four miles away in the town of Lébamba that had 24 beds, it made no sense for the mission and the church to build a hospital in Bongolo. Their plan was to have us work in Lébamba's government hospital, once an agreement with the government could be signed. We were stunned and bewildered, and Melvin answered our complaint that it was not the plan we had agreed to by apologetically shrugging and turning his palms up!

Soon after, Melvin drove with me to Libreville to visit the Minister of Health and ask his permission for our team to work in Lébamba's government hospital. The Minister received us courteously and listened as Melvin explained that our mission had sent an American doctor and five missionary nurses to Bongolo. Would it be possible for our medical team to work in the Lébamba hospital alongside the government's health employees? The minister was astonished by Melvin's question, and almost speechless. After asking why we might want to do that and hearing Melvin's explanation, he shook his head and stated that the population of Bongolo and Lébamba would be better served if the Mission established its own hospital! Our field director explained that the mission wasn't willing to establish its own hospital. When Melvin tried to argue, the Minister of Health said flatly, "Your doctor and nurses may NOT work in the Lébamba Hospital! Build your own!" And that was the end of our discussion! The next day Melvin sent a report to the Alliance with the news that the Minister of Health had refused to let our team work in the Lébamba Hospital.

Even before traveling to Libreville with Melvin for the meeting, I had visited the Lébamba hospital to meet the hospital director. He was a Gabonese nurse practitioner who had been in charge of the hospital for four years. He introduced himself as "Dr. Bayonne," which surprised me considerably. No one had informed us there was a *doctor* in Lébamba! Later I would learn that he was a nurse practitioner, not an M.D., but I didn't know that during my first visit to the hospital.

Dr. Bayonne, as he called himself, took me on a tour of his twenty-four-bed facility. As we walked between the run-down buildings and stepped around trash and animal dung, I could hardly restrain myself from commenting. There were plastic bags everywhere, no trash cans were visible, there was one, small outhouse for 24 patients plus the staff, and there were no showers or sinks with running water for hand washing. Similar to Bongolo's dispensary, patients had to carry water in buckets, but instead of the relatively clean water of the Louetsi River, their source was a muddy stream fifty yards awa1y3. 4The wards smelled of urine and unwashed bodies, and the walls were spotted and smeared with dried blood. There were no mattresses on any of the beds, and the patients' "sheets" were pieces of cardboard or straw. I saw no charts or medical records of any kind, and the few nurses we saw were not in uniform and had learned on the job. The final straw was when "Dr. Bayonne" stopped by the bed of a severely burned patient who was lying on blood-stained pieces of cardboard and without any bandages over his burns. The man sat miserably on his bed, waving flies away with a piece of bloodied cardboard. Cleaning the patient rooms and finding cardboard to lie on was left up to the patients and their families. By the end of the tour, I was so angry I was shaking.

Mr. Bayonne then showed me his operating room, which I was grateful to see, was the cleanest room in the hospital. He explained that he was averaging twenty C-sections a month under spinal anesthesia, a truly astonishing number for a 24-bed hospital! I would later learn that he performed an average of 10 C-sections a month and based his decision to operate on the word of the hospital's two informally trained midwives.

When I asked Mr. Bayonne how he sterilized his instruments he showed me a gas oven and opened the oven door. Inside was a stainless-steel tray with perhaps ten stainless steel instruments on it. Between cases a nurse would wash his instruments (with soap, I hoped) and then put them in the oven for 30 minutes. I was tempted to point out that dry heat required 1-2 hours and 180 centigrade (356 degrees Fahrenheit) to sterilize clean instruments, but he didn't seem interested in anything I had to say, so I said nothing.

At the end of the tour, I told Dr. Bayonne that our mission had recommended that I work at his hospital, along with our five American nurses. He was quite surprised at the suggestion, then said, "If that happens, I will be the Medical Director and will have to approve all of your medical decisions to make certain they are correct." I didn't trust myself to even answer.

Back in Bongolo I asked to meet with the Church leaders and discuss with them the Mission's plan. I had some ideas about the best way forward, but I wanted to hear from them. When I told them about my tour of the Lébamba Hospital and what Mr. Bayonne had said to me, they roared with laughter! Then they asked, "If you and our missionary nurses work at the Lébamba Hospital, how could you take care of the patients like they do at Schweitzer Hospital? How would you even win one person to believe in Jesus?" They had known all along that Mr. Bayonne wouldn't agree to any arrangement that would diminish his prestige. What the church leaders proposed was that we place the entire medical team in Bongolo, enlarge and improve the dispensary, and work towards building a small, Christian hospital. I couldn't have agreed with them more.

Shortly after our that meeting, we asked the church leaders if they thought it would be OK for our medical team to do a survey of 100 homes in Bongolo and Lébamba to find out what the most important medical needs were. They agreed to it, so a few weeks later we split up into several teams and visited 100 homes in our area. The results were deeply troubling, and we shared them with the church leaders and with Melvin.

- Nearly in everyone in every household had intestinal worms and scabies!
- One out of every 40 women who delivered in their homes died in childbirth.
- Four out of five children under the age of five were dying from measles, malaria, whooping cough (Pertussis), polio, and dysentery.
- The major cause of death in men were strangulated hernias and trauma.

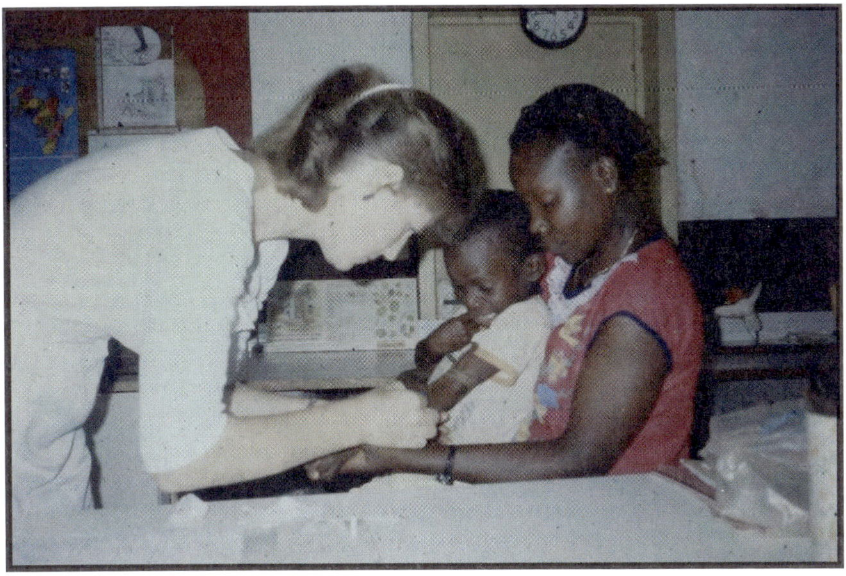

Becki starts an IV for a sick child

After weeks of conversations with our mission leaders, the church leaders, and the mission, we agreed to the following plan:

1. We would build our own hospital in Bongolo, as God provided.
2. We would begin a vaccination program in all of the surrounding villages in our province to control ongoing epidemics of measles, polio and whooping cough.
3. We would open a nursing school to train and disciple Gabonese nurses for our own hospital.
4. We would open and operate three satellite dispensaries in impoverished outlying villages that someone on our team (preferably me) would visit every two weeks.
5. We would build a surgical and maternity building with an operating room and a delivery room, with separate wards for maternity and surgical patients.

In an amazing campaign, women's groups in Alliance churches across America raised $50,000 so we could start.

On November 22, 1977, just six months after our arrival, Becki went into labor with our second child. Months earlier we had decided to trust God for her delivery. God had already provided a missionary midwife—Joyce Strouth—to be a member of our medical team, and she expertly performed Becki's prenatal visits. We didn't have an operating room yet, should Becki need a C-section, but because the delivery of our daughter in 1973 had lasted only two hours, after praying we decided to birth our child in our bedroom, with me assisting our midwife.

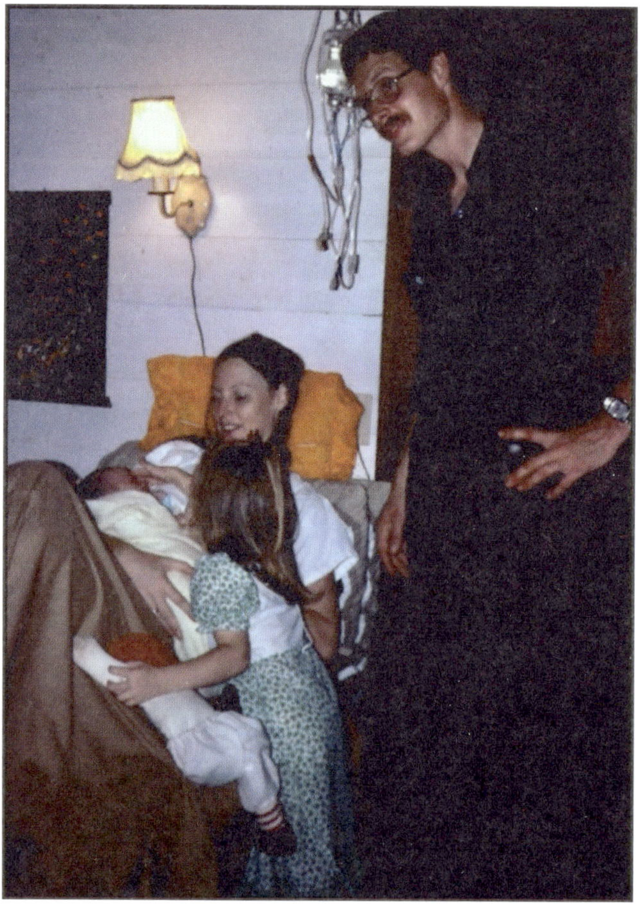

On November 23, 1977, Becki gave birth to our son Joshua in our bedroom

Becki's labor started in the early afternoon of November 23 was over by 6 pm. Our second child was a healthy baby boy that we named Joshua David Thompson! By then his big sister Rachael was three years old. We were deeply thankful to the Lord that Becki's labor and delivery went forward smoothly and without any complications.

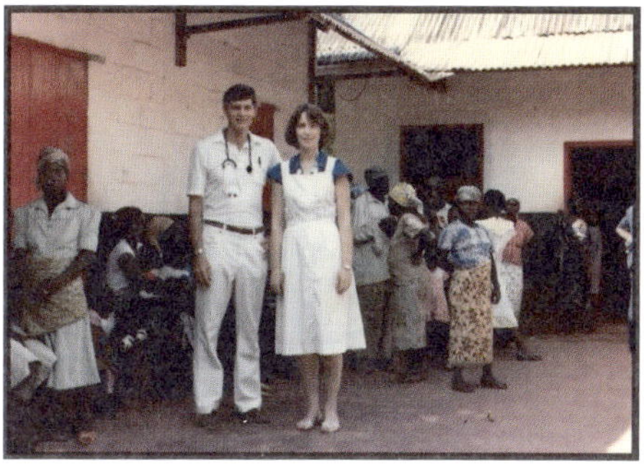

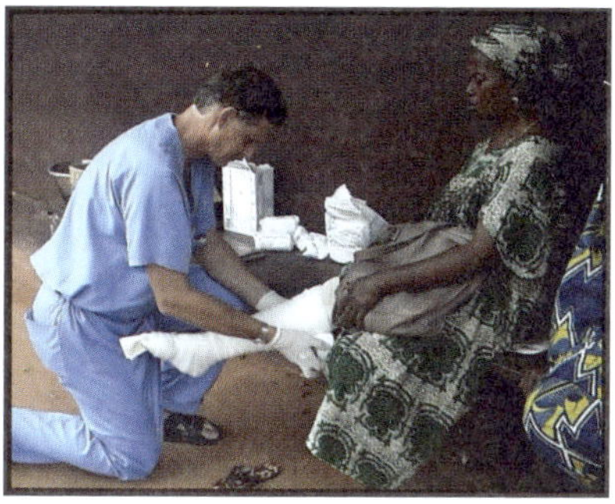

Becki and me caring for patients in the dispensary

Ambulance Duty

We had been serving in Bongolo for about a year when a man with a bowel obstruction came from a village seven kilometers away. His abdomen was quite distended, and he staggered slightly as he got out of the pick-up truck that brought him. The nurses gave him a bed and called me.

When I arrived, a fourth-year American medical student named Sam Zylstra was already examining the man's bloated abdomen. Sam and his wife were old friends, and the couple was spending what would turn out to be an adventurous month with us in Bongolo. The man had been vomiting for the past 24 hours and had not had a bowel movement or passed gas for the previous six hours. The most common cause of bowel obstructions in Gabon was strangulated hernias, but our patient didn't have a hernia. We started an IV to rehydrate him and began discussing what we should do next. The normal treatment would have been to pass a nasogastric tube down into his stomach and hook it up to suction, but our tiny hospital didn't have either a nasogastric tube or a suction machine!

An unresolved bowel obstruction is a serious condition, and if untreated can lead to death within one or two days. It can have many different causes. An X-ray of our patient's abdomen would have been helpful, but we didn't have an X-ray unit yet. Our only option was to evacuate him to the nearest hospital that had a qualified surgeon.

That would usually be Schweitzer Hospital, but when I proposed taking him there, the patient refused. Instead, he wanted us to take him to the provincial hospital in Tchibanga, 100 miles to the west (see map). That was considerably closer than Schweitzer Hospital, and there was supposed to be a surgeon there.

Tchibanga is in the tribal area of the Bapounou people, and our patient was from the Banzebi tribe. But before he would go anywhere, he wanted to discuss the matter with his extended family back in his village. By this time, it was getting dark, and we still had to cross the river on the hand-pulled ferry. The trip to the patient's village would take another thirty minutes of driving in the wrong direction. If we refused his request and he didn't go to either hospital, he could die. Sam and I reluctantly agreed to drive our patient and his wife back to their village.

We laid our patient on a mattress in the back of my Land Rover, crossed the river in the dark on the ferry, and drove to the patient's village. Within minutes of pulling up to his house a crowd of family and friends surrounded us. Cars rarely ventured into the village at night, and when the news got around that one of their neighbors was on a mattress in the back of a vehicle and might need surgery, some of the women thought we had brought him home to die and started wailing!

The village chief calmed everyone down and called us all into the meeting house. I explained why we had brought the man back to his village instead of keeping him at the hospital and that he needed to go to a hospital that had a surgeon. By then, the family had laid our patient on a mat in the middle of the floor. About fifty people crowded into the meeting house with us. The chief asked me in French to explain what was happening, and because I wasn't fluent enough in Yinzebi, a young man translated for them as I explained why we needed to take their friend to Tchibanga for an operation. A great hubbub ensued as various family members voiced their objections. Some were afraid he might die on the way, while others complained the trip would cost too much. When I explained I would not be charging for the trip, a murmur of approval spread across the room. Some seemed to think the Nganga should be asked to get involved, but since his treatment had already failed, the suggestion was greeted with silence.

It had been a long day for us, and we had hoped to be on our way after a fifteen-minute delay in the village. We still had another four hours of night driving on an unfamiliar road. As the villagers continued talking, we stepped outside for a breath of fresh air. The night sky was like black velvet, studded with millions of diamonds. Under normal circumstances it would have been breathtaking, but right then I was tired and frustrated by the delay.

Half an hour later, the meeting finally broke up and several of the relatives helped the sick man back onto the mattress in the back of the Rover. The village had decided who would advance the money to the family and who would accompany him. It seemed that at last, we might get on our way, but once again, I was wrong! The patient's relatives came running with baskets of pots and pans, food, bedding and clothing. Last of all, one of the patient's wives got in. As I pre- pared to close the back door, an argument suddenly erupted! Two women were arguing with the patient's brothers, and soon everyone was talking at once, and the conversation was too rapid for me to understand. The wife who had already climbed into the car now climbed out. I moved away from the door and asked a young man who spoke French what was happening.

"Well," he said with a smile, "they're arguing over which of the two wives should go with you. The one who stays home will have to do all the work at the house and feed the children, and the oldest wife is insisting that she should be the one to go!"

Before I was able to say or do something I would regret, the older wife climbed triumphantly into the car. We were finally ready to roll! It took us half-an hour to get back to the main road.

Around 1 a.m., Sam and I found ourselves on a new section of road that had been recently graded. What a relief to drive 50 kilometers an hour on smoothly graded dirt! But an hour later the road abruptly changed, and we found ourselves bouncing over enormous ruts and driving around 10-inch boulders. Then suddenly, the road ended in a tangle of brush! Either the city of Tchibanga had been swallowed by the jungle, or we had missed a turn! With a sigh, we turned around.

A half hour later we found the turnoff we had missed and got back onto the main road. At 2 a.m. we saw a hunter walking along the road and asked directions. He confirmed we were on the right road. An hour later we crested a hill and saw the lights of Tchibanga below.

Once in town we drove around for twenty minutes before locating the hospital. There were only two nurses on duty for the entire, 60-bed hospital, and the one we found first was half drunk. Thankfully, he managed to give our patient a bed and called the doctor. We could hear the doctor complaining about being awakened at such an early hour, but I eventually overheard him tell the nurse to pass a nasogastric tube down to our patient's stomach and connect it to suction. After he hung up, the nurse explained what the doctor had ordered and that he would see us in the morning. Sam and I would have preferred to see the doctor right then, but there was nothing more to do but find a place to sleep. The nurse suggested that we try the local Alliance church, which was not far away.

It was 3:30 a.m. when we drove up to the darkened church and parked. The only light was a nearby streetlight, and even the dogs were sleeping. As we were quietly arranging our sleeping bags in the back of the Land Rover, the pastor of the church suddenly appeared and asked who we were. After I explained to him that we were doctors and had brought a patient from Bongolo, he introduced himself as Pastor Joel and insisted that we sleep in his guest room! We tried to talk him out of it, but he wouldn't hear of us sleeping in the Rover. He awakened his entire family, including all six of his children, and had them clear out a nearby shed and bring a double bed frame from somewhere! Clouds of dust billowed out the door and windows as the children hastily swept the room! Two of the older children appeared from nowhere with a double mattress, sheets, and a mosquito net. After everything was in place, the pastor brought us a kerosine lantern. Then we all went to bed. Sam and I were asleep in minutes!

We slept until 8:00 a.m. when bright sunlight streamed through the shed's only window. Pastor Joel had one of his kids bring us a bucket of warm water so we could wash up. Then he invited us to breakfast. Ten minutes later when we entered the small parsonage at the back of the church, the family had set their small table with their best dishes and a tablecloth. We were eight people knee-to-knee around the small table, and two of the children had to share a chair. As we bowed to give thanks, I noticed something out of the corner of my eye. The door to a bedroom on my right was partly open. There was no bed or mattress in the room that I could see, only a blanket on the floor. Suddenly I understood. At 3 :30 in the morning, the pastor and his wife had given us their own bed, bedsheets, pillows, and mosquito net, and had spent the rest of the night on the floor with nothing but a blanket! I couldn't believe it, and I blinked tears from my eyes quickly so nobody would notice.

Breakfast consisted of French bread dipped in hot "coffee." The pastor apologized that they were out of instant Nescafé coffee but offered instead hot water mixed with sweetened condensed milk. Everything tasted delicious! Pastor Joel's family gave new meaning to the writer of Hebrews who wrote in 13:2, *"Don't forget to show hospitality to strangers, for some who have done this have entertained angels without realizing it!"* We certainly weren't angels, but we were treated as though we were.

After breakfast we thanked Joel and his wife and tried unsuccessfully to give them a gift for their trouble. Sam and I then drove to the hospital and checked on our patient. The doctor had not yet seen him, but the nasogastric tube had drained about a quart of fluid and our patient already looked better. We later learned that he didn't require surgery and recovered from what was probably a large tangle of intestinal worms.

As Sam and I drove home, we marveled at God's ways. The kindness we had shown to the sick man had been returned to us by a wonderfully generous pastor and his family. We should have been tired, but our hearts were too full of joy to notice!

Saving Norbert's Marriage

I met Norbert the day after we arrived in Bongolo. He represented the second generation of Christians in south Gabon. His parents were among the first generation of Christians and were discipled by the early missionaries and their helpers from Ngoma. Norbert's parents sent him to get an education in Bongolo's elementary school, which for years was the only one within 100 miles. The school was taught in the Yinzebi language rather than in French, but when the government opened schools in nearby Lébamba and throughout Gabon, students were taught in French. In 1948 Norbert graduated from sixth grade and could read the New Testament in Yinzebi, but not French.

This made it impossible for him to transfer to the government high school and continue his education.

Nevertheless, he was bright and a hard worker, and he soon got a job in Lébamba as a storekeeper. In the evenings he studied French with some of his friends, as well as simple math. He worked in the store for eight years, learning to speak, read and write French on his own.

When he was twenty, he married a young woman from his home village of Idembe, just 10 kilometers from Lébamba. He gave a large dowry to his wife's family, but in the Banzebi tribe dowries are for the life of the parents, so he continued saving a good part of his earnings and giving it to his in-laws.

During the eight years Norbert worked for the storekeeper, his employer never missed a franc. This was unheard of, but though the storekeeper valued Norbert for his honesty, he didn't take him with him when he moved to a bigger town. Hearing there were high-paying job opportunities in logging north of the Ogoué River, Norbert left Bongolo and moved his family to the town of Ekouk.

Cutting trees in the African rain forest was dangerous work. The Green Mamba lives in trees and is one of the deadliest snakes in the world. Since birds are its primary food source, the snake's venom must kill its prey in seconds. It's also deadly on the ground, where it can outrun a grown man! Black mambas live on the ground and are just as fast. A bite from either snake is fatal, and victims stop breathing in minutes.

Gabon Vipers are deadly too, but they live in dense underbrush. If disturbed, they strike people in their ankles or legs. Without antivenom, after a Gabon Viper bites a victim's foot or leg, the victim's leg swells massively, causing shock and slow death several days later.

During his years working as a logger at Ekouk, Norbert had many close calls with poisonous snakes but was never bitten because the Lord protected him. His hard work and reliability caught the attention of the French foreman, and he was eventually promoted as an assistant foreman. But Norbert and his family were the only Christians in the camp, and there was no church in the town of Ekouk. Every Sunday Norbert held an informal church service in his home, but though he read the Bible, taught his children, and taught them to pray, he and his wife were unable to keep their children from taking on some of the customs of the pagans around them. That included their fear of sorcery and an even greater fear of Bwiti and Mwiri. Determined to save his children, Norbert and his wife moved back to Bongolo.

Soon after his return Norbert visited Irene Piper Shank, the missionary nurse in charge of the Bongolo Dispensary. She had started training one or two nurses a year, but when Norbert asked if he could be one of her students, she accepted with the understanding that when he finished, she would not be obliged to hire him. Two years later Norbert graduated, and Irene didn't have the money to pay him. After praying for guidance, Norbert offered to work in the dispensary without pay.

To feed their family, Norbert and his children cleared a large garden in the forest a mile from Bongolo. In the dispensary, Norbert's nursing skills, faithfulness, and gentleness brought in more patients, and Irene was eventually able to pay him.

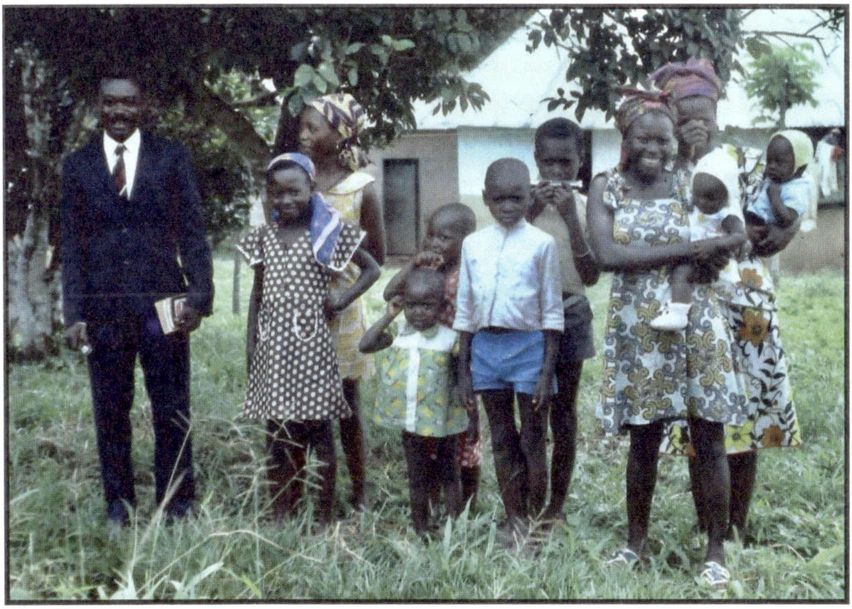

Norbert and his family. His wife and oldest daughter are holding their two grandchildren.

A week after Becki and I arrived, Irene and her husband left Bongolo and moved to the Democratic of Congo to teach at a Bible school. That left Norbert and a Dutch missionary nurse named Sarah Luteijn to run the dispensary. We soon got to know Sarah, Norbert and another male nurse that Sarah was training named Marcel.

One day four months later, Norbert came to work with a long face. Since he was usually cheerful, I asked him what was bothering him. The story he told me was so strange that I found it hard to believe

Surprised I asked, "What's happening with your wife?" Norbert had seven children, was a good father, and had always been faithful to his wife. Norbert sighed and said, "My wife's uncle has decided to break up our marriage and force her to return to her parents with all of the children." He was nearly in tears. Obviously, this turn of events was a strong possibility! Shocked, I asked, "Why would your wife's uncle want to break up your marriage?"

"Revenge," he replied.

"Against you?"

"No, against my uncle who lives in the same village." Since he didn't seem to mind my prying, I persisted.

"Why does your wife's uncle want revenge against your uncle?"

Norbert explained that before moving to Ekouk to work in the lumber industry, he and his wife had cleared roughly two acres of land for a garden near their uncle's village. Among other things they had planted several palm trees. The trees grew quickly during the years they were in Ekouk, and the palm nuts the trees produced fell to the ground and produced more trees. When Norbert and his wife moved back to Bongolo so he could train as a nurse, both his uncle and his wife's uncle claimed the plantation as theirs and began tapping the trees for palm wine. Tapping palm trees was risky work for older men past their prime because it required them to climb to the top of the trees, force a thin and sharpened bamboo tube into the heart of the trunk, and collect sap into a gourd over several days. After several days the tree tapper would return, collect his sap-filled gourd, and spit into it so the sap would ferment. After a few days the sap would turn into wine.

One day Norbert's uncle climbed a tree that his wife's uncle had previously tapped. Just then his wife's uncle arrived, and when he saw that his rival was stealing his palm wine, he climbed the tree too. The two men started fighting, and Norbert's uncle knocked his rival out of the tree! When his rival hit the ground, he broke his leg! Both men were lucky to be alive, but though there were plenty of palm trees to go around, a war between the two families ensued!

Norbert was the only wage-earner in both families, and his meager income at the dispensary supported his wife, his eight children, and his wife's uncle. In Banzebi culture when a man marries, he agrees to pay his in-laws a dowry until the in-laws are completely satisfied or die. By this time, Norbert and his wife had been married for more than ten years, and every month Norbert was paying dowry money to his wife's family. But there was more. According to local custom, Norbert's wife's family had the power to break up the marriage at any time and for any reason! Without consulting their daughter, Norbert's wife's family decided to get their revenge by breaking up their daughter's marriage and taking custody of the children!

By the time Norbert explained all this I was depressed too! I said to him, "Why doesn't your wife refuse? Doesn't she love you?" Norbert pondered the question, then said, "I think so, but it's not our custom for a man to tell his wife that he loves her, or for a wife to tell her husband she loves him." I was flabbergasted!

Finally, I said, "If you don't mind telling me, Norbert, what problems are you and your wife having in your marriage?"

Surprised by my question Norbert said, "We're not having any problems, except between our uncles!"

By now my biblical worldview was making it difficult to comprehend such a marriage. Then Norbert explained, "Gabonese husbands and wives rarely if ever express love for one another, but that doesn't mean they're not devoted to each other. We have to balance our loyalties between our families and our marriage partners."

It was clear that Norbert didn't want his wife to leave, but neither did he want her to be a pariah in her own family. I could see the dilemma he was facing, but I was disturbed that as second-generation Christians Norbert and his wife were even *considering* agreeing to this evil plan!

Norbert asked if he could have the next day off from work so he could talk with his in-laws, and I gave him permission, promising that our entire missionary staff would be praying for him and his wife. The next day as Becki and I stayed home to study Yinzebi, I remembered my promise and prayed for Norbert and his wife. But by late afternoon, he had not returned from his uncle's village.

The next morning after I made rounds on our inpatients and I saw a few outpatients, Norbert was smiling.

"What happened?" I asked.

"Well," he said, "when I got to the village neither family was expecting me. I asked both families to meet in the presence of the village chiefs to settle the problem. At first, they refused, but the Lord was with me, and they finally agreed." As Norbert talked, several of our missionary nurses joined us to listen.

"We met in the meeting house in the center of the village. One family sat on one side, and the other family sat on the other side. The village elders sat at the end of the room to hear the matter. I spoke first, explaining again what had happened when the two uncles fought and how my wife's uncle broke his leg when he fell from the tree. Then I told them that my wife and I had had nothing to do with the fight. I said, 'We didn't even know that our two uncles were fighting over our palm trees, so we don't understand why we and our children should be punished for what happened! Besides, we don't want to break up our marriage!' The Lord helped me to present my case."

As we listened breathlessly, he continued. "The two sides argued back and forth for hours. Finally, the elders made their decision. I will have to pay my wife's uncle a month's salary. My side of the family didn't want me to pay anything, but because the Lord was with me, the village elders made them agree. Isn't this a wonderful answer to prayer?"

I failed to see how losing a month's salary was wonderful, but God had certainly intervened to save Norbert's marriage, and we rejoiced with him and his wife!

What the episode revealed to me was that three decades after the gospel came to Bongolo and brought Christ's kingdom to the Banzebi tribe, the marriages of the Christians were still being controlled by a culture that prevented spouses from loving each other more than they loved their blood relatives! The fact that even Christian parents would agree to give up their children according to pagan dictates was appalling! The curse of Bongolo Falls was by now a forgotten legend in the Christian community, but the pagan world view that put loyalty to blood relatives above loyalty to one's spouse and children was still dragging demonic curses into Christian marriages!

Of course, the lifting of the curse had brought great changes. After the birth of a child, Christians no longer handed their newborns to a Nganga to hold up to the sky as an offering to the demon gods, as was the custom before the gospel came. But they were still bowing to the pagan tradition of granting their unbelieving relatives the power to break up their families!

It would take another decade before the biblical teaching of pastors and missionaries on the topic of Christian marriage would significantly challenge these practices. God's truth and Holy Spirit had to first change the hearts of Christian men to obey God's word and *"love your wives, just as Christ loved the church and gave himself up for her."* Until men who had been baptized and took communion announced to their extended families that they were followers of Jesus and loved their wives more than they loved their blood relatives, *their families would remain prisoners of the curse.*

Until Christian wives chose to obey the command *"Wives, submit yourselves to your own husbands as you do to the Lord* and obey God's Word, they would be at the mercy of their pagan relatives.

Only God can transform an evil culture and make it conform to His Word. When we first began giving transfusions to save the lives of women who bled massively after delivering a baby, the culture of the curse said a married man couldn't donate his blood to save her life! Neither could a wife give her blood to the save the life of her husband who was bleeding out from an injury! Marriage under the curse was a financial contract that took power and love from husbands, wives, and their children, and gave it to pagan relatives. That a man and a woman could become "one flesh" was anathema to pagans. It was time for ancient pagan teachings about marriage, love and child-rearing to die and be buried forever, and for Christian love to be born in transformed hearts!

From that day forward, my hope for Norbert's family and for the families of all of our nurses was that their children would grow into adulthood and faith as wards of their parents, and that all of

Bongolo's Christian husbands and wives would learn what it meant to openly love each other!

The Perfect Outhouse

A great deal of work had to be done to turn the Bongolo Dispensary into a hospital. Though we had committed to study the Yinzebi language until we learned it, I was convinced that some hygienic improvements simply couldn't wait. One problem that couldn't wait another year for a solution was the hospital's inadequate sanitary facilities. Our one and only latrine was a mess, with huge, blue-green flies careening around in dizzying circles whenever someone entered.

It also gave off an appalling stench! The Africans preferred to use the fresh-smelling forest, but because people drank water from the river and heavy rains washed everything into the river that didn't have roots, something had to change!

When I explained to our patients that they were spreading diseases and parasites by not using the hospital's outhouse, they asked me if I myself had ever used it. Since I had not, the discussion came to an awkward end. One Gabonese characterized the problem with typical African candor, saying, "When you squat down, hundreds of those big flies suddenly fly out of the hole, making a loud, buzzing noise as they bump into you." Just thinking about it was enough to make me queasy!

Besides the revolting flies, a close inspection of our latrine revealed an alarming weakness in the central floorboard that had a hole in the center for the passage of… well, whatever! If that weakened board ever broke while someone was standing or squatting on it, the result would be terrible!

I thought about the problem for days. The floorboard with the hole in it would have to be replaced, and while I was replacing it, why not make it into a three-hole, sit-down outhouse? The idea of a multiple sit-down outhouse appealed to my Western sense of propriety and efficiency!

My plan was to build the frame for an eight-foot-long box that was open at the bottom. It would be fifteen inches high, enclosed on the front and back, and its top would have three large holes, spaced a foot apart. The result was pure genius: a bench toilet with three openings in the top, each with a hinged lid!

Between language lessons, I set to work with enthusiasm, using our own toilet seat as a model to trace holes on the top of the bench. I filed and sanded the edges of the holes until they were smooth and comfortable to sit on. Next, I cut a lid for each hole and attached it at the back with a hinge. This would keep the holes closed when not in use and limit the smell and flies. When the three-hole bench was completed, I brought it down to the hospital on the roof of my truck.

Norbert helped me unload the thing, though he was obviously surprised by the design. He didn't say much as we carried it down the path. It was a struggle to pull the weakened one-hole-board out of the floor, and of course the flies went crazy! When we placed the three-hole bench over the opening, the result was a masterpiece of innovative carpentry. I threw several cups of DDT powder into all three holes to discourage the flies, then showed Norbert how the lids over the three holes opened and closed. Finally, I demonstrated how patients could sit comfortably when they did their business, like one would on a porcelain toilet. Norbert didn't say much but seemed to understand. I took one last glance at my handiwork before heading back to my language lessons.

About a week later, I decided to inspect the outhouse with Norbert. For some reason he was reluctant to come, and I soon understood why. When I opened the door, I could not believe what I saw! The place was a disaster! Not only were there more blue bottle flies than I had ever seen in my life, but there were excrement and pee all over the top of the bench, even on the lids and between the three holes and I had made!

"Norbert," I asked, "how is it possible for the patients to make such a mess?" Obviously embarrassed, Norbert explained that the patients were not used to sitting down when they pooped.

"But how can they make a mess around the holes when they're sitting down on them?" I persisted.

"Well, doctor," he explained hesitantly, "they're not used to sitting down to poop, and they think it's unnatural."

"Unnatural?" I almost shouted, "I've done it all my life, as do most of the people in the world! How could it be unnatural?"

"Well, doctor," he continued, looking down at his sandals, "it's not that the people don't appreciate what you've done. It's just that the holes are too wide for the people when they squat." Squat?! People were SQUATTING over my finely crafted toilet holes!? Then Norbert put the final nail in the coffin. "And the children almost fall in," he said, his tone apologetic. "Also, when people climb up on top of the bench, some who are taller have hit their heads on nails in the roof," he added.

Nails in the roof? I looked up. Sure enough, some of the roofing nails protruded through the thin wooden rafters. If I were to stand on the bench my head would probably hit a nail! I winced. People were climbing up on *top* of my bench and squatting, and when they stood up to leave, the taller ones were getting poked in the head by rusty nails…

By this time, I realized that my idea to teach Gabonese patients to relieve themselves in a whole new way was an absurd failure. The next day I grimly removed the 3-holed bench—this time with the help of a hired worker— and nailed a new, sturdier board with a single hole back in the middle of the floor, the way our African patients preferred. I would eventually win by introducing porcelain toilets, but it would take decades of humble and gentle persuasion!

The Goat War

Soon after my experience with the outhouse, I took on the goats. The goats were one of the first things we noticed when we arrived in Bongolo. They were everywhere—running freely over the Mission property, pooping on our porches, on the floors and benches in the waiting areas, even standing defiantly in the open church windows at times! About 100 goats considered the dispensary to be their home, and everywhere they went they left their greenish brown droppings. Their droppings were especially dense on the steps in front of every doorway and on the paths from those doors, making it inevitably that goat poop would be tracked into every room of the dispensary and the ward. By the end of each day, the goat droppings would dry and be swept out of the dispensary in clouds. Eventually goat dust settled and coated everything! A better scenario for introducing tetanus into open wounds could not have been devised! I took it as my solemn duty and obligation to rid the dispensary of this plague!

During our first few weeks, I observed the goats carefully. Although they were surrounded by acres and acres of fresh grass and succulent vegetation, they continually wandered through the dispensary courtyard, rubbing their butts on the outside walls. Every building in Bongolo had a brownish, four- inch-wide line running around its base, thanks to the goats! In open surrender, the dispensary committee had ceased to paint the lower four feet of the outside walls of the building. It was clear that something had to be done.

I started by asking my staff to throw stones at the goats whenever they saw them around the buildings. They were less than enthusiastic, and by the end of the first week, I was the only one carrying on the fight. For months, whenever a goat came within range, I interrupted whatever I was doing to stone it. The goats soon learned to scatter when I appeared to be looking for a stone. In order to inflict pain, I had to be more subtle. Whenever I saw a goat, I would casually glance around until I spotted a stone. Feigning complete indifference to the goat, I would saunter over to the stone, then in a blur of motion, I would pick up the stone, pivot and hurl. This technique reduced my accuracy to almost zero. Not appreciating the seriousness of the problem, the Gabonese—and even my staff— thought the routine was quite comical.

After six months of battle, the goat deposits remained as abundant as ever. The goats were simply staying out of range when I was there and returning with a vengeance at night. Unwilling to accept defeat, I resorted to modern technology: I bought an air-powered pellet rifle. Conditioning was the key to the problem, I decided. I had to somehow condition the goats so that they would associate the hospital grounds with stinging pain. In order to succeed, I reasoned, I would have to consistently apply the conditioning.

It occurred to me that an occasional goat might die, but by this time, nothing would have cheered me more than the sight of goat carcass- es all over the hospital lawns. That would, of course, create major palavers! The goats represented wealth, and every goat belonged to someone. How the Gabonese kept them straight I'll never know, but they knew which goat belonged to whom. Before escalating to the air gun, therefore, I consulted our local pastor.

Pastor Philippe advised patience, but I suspected that he was thinking more about saving his goats than helping me with the problem. However, when he realized that I was serious, he agreed to announce in church the following Sunday that if people did not remove their goats from the hospital plateau within one week, the doctor would begin shooting them! The next Sunday morning he made the announcement. After a moment of shocked silence, a murmur of disapproval filled the air. Every eye turned to see my stern face. When the pastor rang his little brass hand bell for order, the service resumed.

The goat-owners had one week to corral their animals. A few of the more sincere ones actually came and caught some of their goats. This required two highly athletic individuals and several lengths of expensive rope. The rope only temporarily slowed the goats slightly, however, since they could chew through them in less than thirty minutes. As soon as they escaped, they returned to the hospital. The net effect being zero, I waited with growing relish for the week of grace to end.

Monday morning dawned bright and clear, a perfect day for hunting goats! I made my rounds at the hospital and consulted patients all morning. In the afternoon, I returned to the hospital with my air rifle and a pocket full of pellets. The ensuing hunt was emotionally cathartic. In the glory of seeing bawling goats run into each other as they tried to get away, my months of frustration were forgotten! I hadn't realized how stupid they could be! It took each goat four to five hits before it associated the pain with the pale man standing nearby in white holding an odd-looking stick! After another two or three hits, they realized they could escape the pain if they left the area at high speed. Within twenty minutes, there wasn't a goat in sight, except for three carcasses lying on the ground. Unfortunately, all three dead goats belonged to Pastor Philippe…

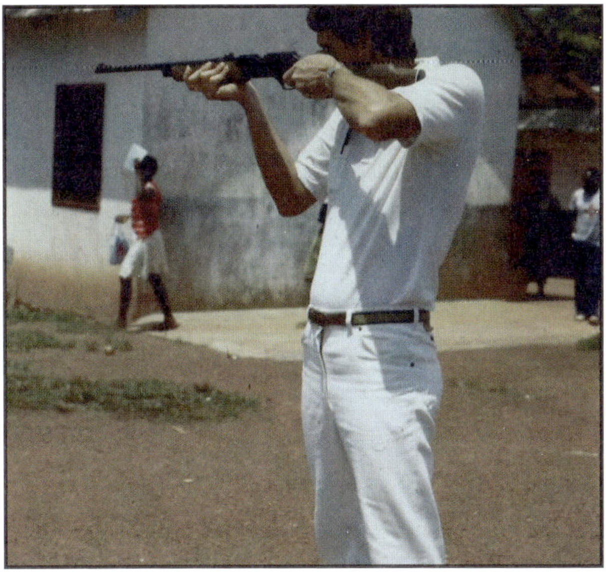

A solution (a pellet gun)!

Much to his credit and to my relief, Pastor Philippe accepted his loss as the price for having a doctor and a hospital. But though the battle was won, the war was not. The goats returned the next day and had to be reconditioned. By the end of two weeks, only a few of the more stubborn ones remained around the hospital. They had somehow figured out the range of my weapon, and as soon as they heard me pumping the gun they would scurry out of range.

The goat war considerably disrupted my hospital routine. I took to carrying my gun on rounds, already pumped up. If I saw a goat in range, I stopped whatever I was doing to get it in my sights, sometimes even shooting out of the windows of the wards! The children at the hospital joined in the game, running up breathlessly to tell me that a goat was hiding on the other side of the building or behind a bush! When I flushed it out and zapped it, they celebrated with laughter and joy! By the end of a year of battling them (yes, that's right—a year), I began to smell victory. There remained, however, a few clever goats that refused to concede. They would stay away during the day but return at night when they knew I was not around. In the morning when I came down to work, the sight of their droppings all on the benches in the waiting area yard still made my blood boil.

By this time, I knew what the offending goats looked like, and one late afternoon I decided to go after them. I found them browsing in the forest on the other side of the church. They heard me coming and scuttled into the thick underbrush. I was wearing my hospital whites but decided to go in after them anyway. Carefully working my way through the brush, I circled around behind them, hoping to flush them into the open where I could get a clear shot. They wisely chose to stay hidden.

I moved closer, stepping up onto a fallen tree. Just twenty feet away I saw an inviting, furred rump. I brought the gun to my shoulder, sighted down the barrel and began to squeeze the trigger. Suddenly my legs were on fire! In my excitement to shoot the goats, I had stepped onto a column of army ants! Army ants have a wonderful ability to incite frantic and bizarre motions in large animals and humans. At that moment, the only thing in the world that mattered was to get my pants off and pull the ants off that were burying their jaws into my flesh! Thrashing and leaping about in the underbrush, I finally managed to do just that. It took about two minutes to tear the big ants off and another five to find all the little ones. Fortunately, no humans had witnessed my antics.

After I got my pants back on, I stepped out of the forest with both my dignity and resolve back in place. As I came around the corner of the church building, I saw the receding rump of a white goat. I threw the gun to my shoulder and fired. To my surprise, the goat dropped in its tracks. I walked up to it just in time to see it take its last breath. With amazing accuracy, the pellet had entered the goat's skull from behind in an unprotected spot.

Two days later, Pastor Philippe dropped by our house for a visit. We exchanged news and chatted for a few minutes before he fell silent, began to rub his hands and clear his throat. Obviously, there was something he wanted to say.

"Do you remember the goat you killed the other day, doctor?" he asked finally. I told him that I remembered. He cleared his throat again.

"It was Lebongo Antoine's animal." I didn't know Lebongo Antoine very well, except that he was a head schoolteacher in the local elementary school. He was known for his heavy drinking and his bad temper. Whenever he came to the hospital, he was rude, unless he received preferential treatment. He had always been respectful to me, however. The pastor continued.

"Lebongo was very angry that you killed his animal. Last night he drank too much and told his drinking buddies that he is going to get revenge." I was not afraid of Lebongo Antoine. What could he do to me?

"He told them he was going to do something to your children." A chill crept into my heart. Our daughter Rachael was five and Joshua was two.

"How serious is he?" I finally asked.

"We don't know," the pastor answered, "but the whole village knows about his threat, and everyone is angry with him. He won't do anything openly, but he's a difficult man and at the very least he will put a curse on your children." Assuming that as a Christian I was automatically protected from evil spirits and understanding very little about spiritual warfare, I was not too concerned.

"What do you suggest I do?" I asked. "Should I go and apologize?" The pastor didn't think I should apologize. After all, hadn't I shot everybody's goats? Hadn't I warned everyone first?

"Perhaps," he suggested, "you could just frighten away the goats for a week or so until things quiet down. In the meantime, you will have to trust God for the safety of your children."

We prayed together and the pastor left. After he had gone, Becki and I got on our knees and recommitted ourselves and our children to God, placing us all under His protection. I did not see Lebongo Antoine again before returning to the United States later that year, because shortly after that incident, the church leaders used their influence to send him to a church school in another town eighty kilometers away. It was not, however, the last I would see of him.

And what about the goats? They are still a problem. Every goat born in Bongolo seems to have to learn the hard way that to linger at the hospital is to sometimes experience inexplicable discomfort. The goats have not wearied of reproducing, but I have wearied of the battle. Perhaps the time has come for newer technology. A laser goat vaporizer would suit me just fine!

Saving Veronica

Several months later I was awakened by someone pounding on our front door. We had no telephones or CB radios at the time, so when there were emergencies during the night the nurses had to walk a quarter mile up the hill with a kerosine lantern and pound on our front door until I answered. When I opened the door, I saw a middle-aged man wearing a battered felt hat and holding a kerosene lantern. The flickering light cast deep shadows across his anguished face. In broken French he explained that his daughter was dying.

As we drove down the hill to the hospital, the father explained his daughter's symptoms. It sounded to me like a severe case of malaria. When we pulled up in front of our small mudbrick ward, the windows were tightly shuttered to keep out the mosquitoes and bats, making the air inside hot and heavy.

Veronica lay on a brightly colored cloth her mother had spread on the bare boards of the bed. In my zeal for cleanliness, I had thrown away the blood-stained straw-filled mattresses we found when we arrived in Bongolo, but new foam mattresses had not yet arrived from the capital city. Veronica was about nine years old, but she was so thin I at first thought she was five or six. I surmised that she had been ill for a long time. As I asked her parents questions about the history of her illness, she looked at me solemnly and with a mixture of trust and fear. We had no separate examining room in the small ward, so virtually everyone in the children's ward watched my every move. When I listened to her heart and lungs, everything sounded normal, except that the right side of her chest was noticeably quieter than the other. The six-bed ward had one 40-watt bulb hanging from the rafters, but in the dim light I could see nothing to pin a diagnosis on, other than her fever of 104 degrees and a slightly enlarged liver. I had already learned that many African children had enlarged livers from chronic malaria, so I was not too concerned. I decided to treat her for malaria and instructed Norbert to give her aspirin to control the fever. As I drove the quarter mile to our house, I wondered why Veronica's father had seemed so concerned. After all, malarial fevers were common in Gabon. As I climbed between the clean sheets, the cool night air flowed through the screened window, but it took me a long time to stop trying to solve Veronica's problem and fall sleep.

In the morning when I came around to see the hospitalized patients in our tiny ward, Veronica was no better. For the next three to four days her fever spiked to 104 degrees Fahrenheit every afternoon. Thinking she might have typhoid fever, I started her on an antibiotic, but 48 hours later she was worse. Her struggle to live hovered over us like a black cloud. It was clear that unless we found the cause of her fever soon, she would die. I didn't share that thought with her father, but even he could see my utter frustration. Our excuse for a hospital was so pathetic that we couldn't even take a simple x-ray! All we could do was pray, and before I went home, I laid hands on her and prayed that God would heal her.

The week before Christmas our family was trying to prepare for our first Christmas in Africa. Veronica's mysterious fever made it hard for me to focus on decorations and presents for the kids, though we had un-boxed our scrawny, three-foot artificial tree we had brought with us from Europe, along with a single string of lights. Our daughter Rachael was thrilled, but little Veronica was slowly dying, and my heart was too heavy to celebrate.

During our Wednesday night prayer meeting, our missionary team prayed that God would hear our prayers for Veronica and heal her. We also prayed that her entire family would come to know Jesus. I pleaded with God each morning, asking him to show me what I was missing.

At 2:00 a.m. I was awakened again by shouting and pounding on our front door. Once more, Veronica's father stood outside, accompanied by one of our African nurses. Tears were streaming down his face, and once again, he pleaded with me to come to the hospital and save his daughter. The nurse confirmed that the situation was indeed grave, so I threw on my clothes and drove us all down to the hospital. As I entered the mudbrick ward, the other patients and their families were awake and watching Veronica as she gasped for air, holding the right side of her chest. As one nurse held a lantern so I could see better, I listened to her lungs with my stethoscope. This time I found something new: she had no breath sounds at all over the entire right side of her chest! When I tapped that side with my finger, it wasn't resonant like the left side. Obviously, she had fluid in the space around her collapsing right lung. I mentally kicked myself for not having thought of it before!

To confirm my diagnosis and prepare Veronica's parents for what would come next, I took a syringe and needle and gently inserted the needle into the right side of Veronica's chest, between her ribs. When I pulled on the plunger, the syringe filled with thick, light brown fluid. To fully drain the liquid around her lung I would need a chest tube the size of my little finger. Unfortunately, our order for chest tubes and other critical supplies was still months away. After a frantic search, one of our nurses found a yellowed nasogastric tube in a box full of medical junk, and a surgical clamp. There was no way to know what the tube had been used for in the distant past, but I thought it might work to drain the fluid from Veronica's chest.

After washing the tube with soap and water I let it boil for 20 minutes in water over a kerosine burner. With every minute, Veronica's breathing was becoming more difficult. When the tube and instruments were ready, I t1o6o0k Veronica into the small nursing station and quietly explained to Veronica's mother and father what I had to do next to save their daughter. The result was pandemonium! Up to this point, Veronica's mother had remained calm and had encouraged her daughter to be brave, but now she was wailing and throwing herself on the floor in the traditional manner of mourning the death of a loved one! Her husband dragged her out of the nurse's station, and the other patients in the ward were tried to calm her down.

Realizing that the little girl's life hung in the balance, I asked Veronica's father to stand in the doorway and keep his wife out, and laid Veronica on the table. I quickly injected a local anesthetic into a space between two of her ribs and with a scalpel blade, swiftly made a quarter-inch incision. Then I pushed the tip of a curved Kelly clamp forcefully into the space until it popped into her chest. Veronica screamed in pain, then stopped when she saw thick brown fluid oozing out around the clamp. I pulled the clamp out, quickly grasped the end of the tube with the clamp, and jammed the end of the tube through the hole in her chest. Veronica screamed again, then coughed violently, forcing the pus in her chest to pour through the tube into a basin.

As soon as her mother saw what was happening, she stopped trying to get past her husband and stared in amazement. The heads of half of the people in the ward suddenly appeared around the curtain, and despite a most unpleasant smell, appreciative murmurs filled the air. No physician ever had a more encouraging audience than I did that night, especially as Veronica's breathing gradually eased. I taped a compress around the tube draining her chest, making it air-tight and letting it drain into a bucket. Then we put her in her bed. Norbert wasn't working that night, but because his house was near the dispensary I asked him to check on her during the night and went home. Norbert later reported that Veronica slept the rest of the night.

The tube in Veronica's chest drained brown pus for two days be- fore I took it out. My guess was that her illness started with amoebic dysentery that spread to her liver and created an abscess. When the abscess in her liver ruptured through her diaphragm (a common complication) the infection spread into her chest.

Amoebic dysentery is common in rural Gabon in areas where people prefer to relieve themselves in the rain-washed forest behind their houses, instead of in smelly outhouses. When the rains come everything infectious ends up in the streams and rivers. We treated Veronica with the appropriate antibiotic for amoebic infections, and ten days later she went home, already gaining weight and smiling.

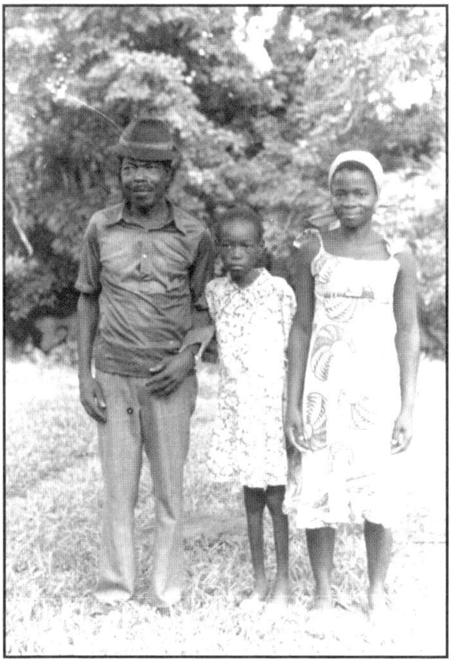

Veronica a month later, with her mother and father.

Veronica a month later, with her mother and father.Another reason that Veronica was smiling when she left was because she gave her heart to Jesus, and so did her mother. Her father never did, but whenever he saw me in town, he would remove his battered hat and proclaim to everyone within earshot that I was the doctor God sent to save his daughter from certain death! With each telling, the story got better, but since he gave God the glory, I didn't object. As Veronica's story was told and retold, our fame began to spread. Eventually we were inundated with more surgical cases than I was equipped to treat or had beds for. Most came believing that if I set my mind to it, I could cure anything. At times when I expressed surprise at people's faith in my abilities, they would respond, "Oh, your God will show you what to do. We've heard the stories!" In the face of such faith, what else could we do but smile and carry on? After all, they were right!

Veronica's recovery lifted the cloud of gloom from our Christmas celebrations and gave me a deeper understanding of the joy that Christ's coming brings to our lives. With only a few presents, we experienced the first of many warm and wonderful Christmases in Africa. Our joy did not come from gifts or partying, nor from the few traditional trappings we managed to bring. It came instead from the joy that comes from helping desperate and impoverished people regain their health, find the Savior of the world, and discover that God truly loves them. And with every healing associated with the name of Jesus, the curse of Bongolo Falls grew weaker.

The Extra Mile

During our first four years in Bongolo, a couple named Ron and Joan Israel served as dorm parents for eight to ten missionary children who attended Bongolo's elementary school for missionary children. The teachers lived on campus too, which was a huge blessing to us once our children were old enough to start school. We were also blessed to have short term and long-term missionaries serving with us who had a wide range of mechanical, electrical, maintenance, and building skills. One of them was a single Dutch single missionary named Daan, who eventually married one of the teachers.

One day I returned early from the Independence Day celebration in Lébamba. When I stopped at the hospital to see if the two or three nurses on duty were doing OK, they told me that a woman in labor was in trouble and was lying on a path "not far" from the hospital. The woman's mother had brought them the news that her daughter had collapsed on the way and was requesting someone to go and get her with a car.

Realizing that I would need help to carry the woman and that almost all of the hospital and missionary staff except Daan were in Lebamba, I drove up the hill and asked Daan if he would drive his pickup out the back road where a woman in labor had collapsed. The back road had started out as a logging road that snaked through the forest for fifteen miles before it joined a main road. It was poorly maintained and had at least five log bridges that periodically collapsed and had to be rebuilt.

Daan immediately agreed to help, so we put a canvas stretcher in the back of his pickup and headed down the road. After five minutes of driving, we came to a collapsed log bridge, so we left the pickup and continued on foot with the canvas stretcher. Thirty minutes later we found the woman lying on the path and moaning and in labor. She was dehydrated and in the early stages of a complication called, "eclampsia" and that if not treated can be deadly to both the mother and the baby. We helped her onto the stretcher and started off, with Daan taking the lead. The temperature was in the 90's, with Gabon's usual 99% humidity! Though much of the trail was shaded, sweat was soon pouring off us. The woman must have weighed close to 200 pounds, and as I struggled to keep up with Daan and hold up my end of the stretcher, I couldn't keep sweat from dripping onto the woman's face! The smart thing would have been to switch ends so I would be dripping on her feet, not her face! Fortunately, the Lord helped me keep up with Daan and eventually the woman's mother covered her daughter's face with a towel.

A more serious problem was that every ten minutes I had to stop and catch my breath. Since most mornings at 6 a.m. I ran a mile, I thought I was in pretty good shape. That turned out to be very different from carrying a heavy woman on a stretcher during the hottest part of the day! To Daan's great amusement, my suggestions for rest breaks gradually increased to every five minutes. Fortunately, we arrived at to the log bridge soon after, but carrying the woman down into the stream, across it, and up the steep bank on the other side nearly finished me off! Ten minutes after the stretcher and her mother were in the back of the truck we were at the hospital, and the midwives took over. Later that day they helped her deliver a healthy baby.

On another day when Daan was away in Libreville a problem arose that forced me again to man up! I was finishing up a hernia operation when a heavy rainstorm rolled in with thunder and lightning. A bolt of lightning struck somewhere up on the hill above the hospital where the mission houses were located, and our electricity went out. With Daan away, it was up to me and the station yard workers to find the problem. First, however, I had to finish the operation. We kept flashlights in the operating room for such events, so as one of the nurses held a flashlight from the head of the operating table I finished the operation with my nurse assistant. As we closed the skin, our midwife opened the OR door and said, "Doctor, there's another woman in labor, and her baby is in trouble! She needs a C- section right away!"

I didn't want to attempt a C-section with a flashlight, no monitors, and no suction, so I told the surgery team to clean up the OR and get it ready for another case while I figured out the electrical problem. I stripped off my operating gown and gloves and hopped on my trusty motorbike. It was still raining lightly, but I was able to check the power lines running down to the hospital and up onto the mission station and look for downed or tangled power lines. A few minutes later the yardmen and I found where a broken branch had fallen on two power lines and caused a short. With help from our yardmen, we removed the fallen branch and untangled the power lines.

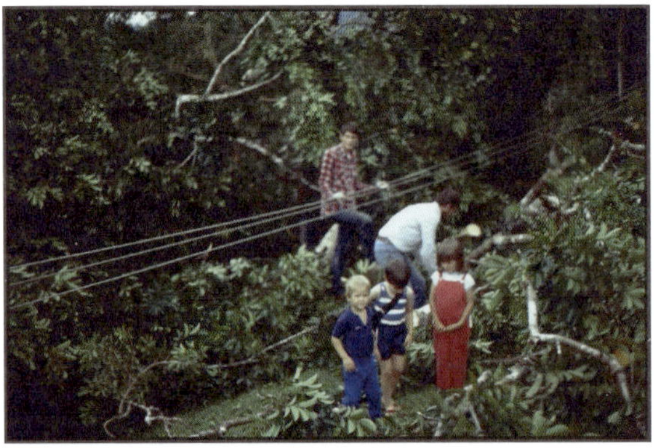

The author dealing with a similar episode of downed power lines.

In the event of a major short circuit, our hydroelectric plant across the river was designed to shut itself off and couldn't be turned back on without going across the river and manually resetting the main circuit breaker. The oar to our dugout canoe was kept in the station's maintenance shed, so after grabbing it, I balanced it on the handlebars of my motorbike and rode down to the river's edge. The canoe had two inches of rain in it from the storm, but I didn't have time to bail it out, so I paddled across the river with water sloshing over my shoes.

The river below Bongolo falls is seventy-five feet wide during the rainy season and has a swift current, so it took ten minutes to row across and run 30 yards up a path to the hydroelectric hut. Everything related to the turbine and generator seemed fine, but the main circuit breaker was off, so I flipped back on and breathed a prayer of thanks when the lights came back on. I ran back down the path to the canoe and rowed to the other side, thinking to myself that in my wildest dreams I had never thought I would be paddling a dugout canoe across an African river so I could do an emergency C-section! Once the canoe was chained up, I jumped on my motorbike and raced up the hill to the hospital. Untangling the power lines and getting the power back on had taken thirty-five minutes, and by now I was worried for the mother and baby.

Once I got to the hospital, I kicked off my muddy sandals, put on clean OR slippers, scrubbed my hands and arms, and pulled on sterile gloves. With the help of the surgical nurses, I administered a spinal anesthetic, and within minutes the young woman felt nothing from her toes to her diaphragm. After pulling on a sterile gown and gloves, I sliced opened the woman's abdomen and uterus and pulled out a healthy, squalling, baby boy! We all cheered and thanked the Lord! By the time I had sutured the mother's uterus, abdomen, and skin back together, the midwife confirmed the baby was healthy and doing well.

Several years later, it was time for Daan and his wife to return to Holland for a year and reconnect with their supporting churches. By then the missionary school had closed, and Ron and Joan Israel were serving in Libreville. So that year I was left in charge of the hydroelectric plant, the pumps at the river that filled our water tower, the station workers who mowed the lawns and cleared trees that fell down, the maintenance of the lawn mowers when one of them broke down, and making sure we always had gasoline and diesel fuel for the lawn mowers and the back-up generator! I was also supervising the remodeling of our medicine ward! The list of my duties seemed endless!

Two weeks after Daan and his wife left for Holland, the bottom of the mission's dugout canoe rotted out. Daan had put together what I called a "Micky-Mouse canoe" to use while we waited for a local canoe maker to finish making a new canoe out of a tree. Daan had made an interim canoe using a 10-foot by 8-foot tarpaulin, a piece of plywood, two innertubes, and a rope! First, he laid the tarpaulin flat, then placed a rectangular piece of plywood just long enough for two inflated innertubes to rest on next to each other. Next, he punched holes along the edges of the tarp and reinforced them with aluminum grommets. Finally, he threaded a rope around the edges of the tarp and pulled the rope tight around the inflated innertubes! Without a passenger, the tarp and inner-tube boat floated nicely! Daan then took a wooden broom handle and fastened plywood squares on each end to make an oar. Before he left for Holland, he climbed into it and paddled across the river to demonstrate that it was seaworthy.

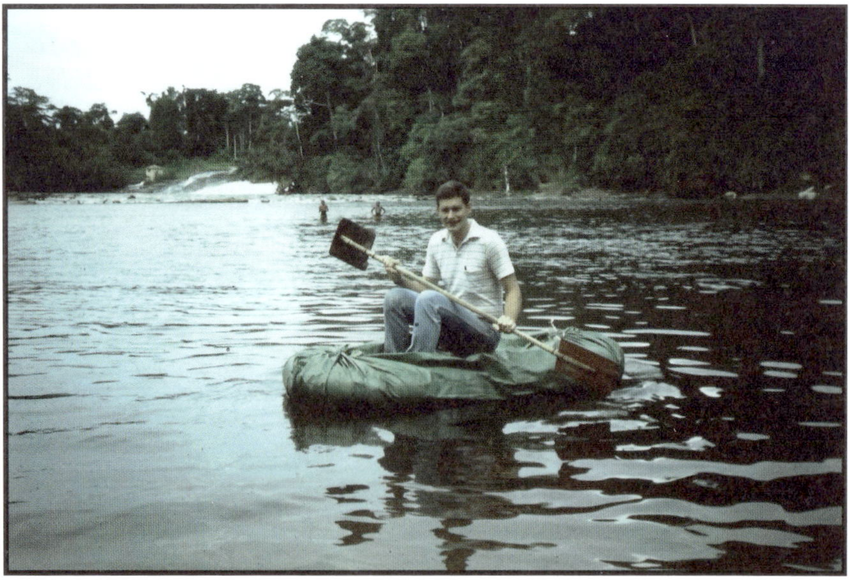

Crossing the river to the hydroelectric hut in the "Micky-Mouse" canoe!

A week after Daan left, the belt between the turbine and the generator in the hydro-electric hut broke, and I either had to cross the river to fix it or walk downriver a half mile to the ferry, cross the river, and walk back upriver a half mile to the hydro hut. I chose the innertube boat and paddled across. After I made a new belt and connected the turbine and the generator to it, we again had power. It was after days like that I struggled to understand why the Lord wouldn't let me just be a doctor!

Two weeks later the two-phase electric pump that pumped water up to a large reservoir above the falls quit working. I had seen Daan replace it before and had not paid close attention, assuming it was like wiring any other two 220 electrical outlet. Once again, I climbed into the canvas-innertube contraption, but this time I had a heavy toolbox with me that I placed between my feet inside the front innertube. Daan had left a spare pump in the hydro hut, so I didn't have to carry it too! The toolbox weighed about ten pounds, so we were lower in the water than before. I had paddled to the middle of the river when quite suddenly the tarp that held the boat together split in two! I had just enough time to grab the toolbox with my right hand. As the plywood and the oar floated away, the toolbox pulled my hand and arm down inside the front inner-tube and kept me afloat. The water was deep, and the swift current carried me downriver as I kicked and with one free arm thrashed my way toward the other side!

As soon as the Micky-Mouse canoe disintegrated, the women on the Bongolo shore who were washing clothes began shouting and wailing, but when they saw I hadn't drowned and was thrashing my way towards the far shore, they laughed and made jokes about my swimming technique! But when I arrived on the other side and held my toolbox up in triumph, they clapped and cheered!

Ten minutes later I unlocked the hydro hut and shut off the current. The burned-out water pump was six feet from the shore above the falls on a three-foot cement post in a foot of white water. I waded out to it with a screwdriver and wrench, pulled the top off of the pump to expose the wiring, and was immediately confused. Instead of two wires, there were three! As I stood there wondering what to do, one word came to mind: pray! So, I stood in the river and prayed. All of a sudden, I remembered hearing Daan talk about two-phase, 220-volt current. Since the replacement pump was exactly the same as the burned out one, I could just duplicate what I was seeing. What could be simpler?

Ten minutes later the new pump was secured on the post and rewired. Back in the hut I threw the circuit breaker on, and the pump immediately began humming! Just to be sure it was pumping water, I waded back out and felt the PVC pipe that carried water to the reservoir on top of the cliff. Oddly enough, it wasn't vibrating as it should if water was flowing through it. With a sigh, I returned to the Bongolo side, using my salvaged inner tube, drove up to the reservoir, and checked to see if water was coming into it or not. Nothing was coming out of the pipe.

About then I remembered a conversation I had with Daan after he had replaced another pump. He had said something about the pump running backwards if you didn't wire it right. That was it! I drove back down to the river, swam across with my innertube, and took the cover off the pump. This time I looked carefully to see if the motor was turning clockwise, or counterclockwise. It was turning counterclockwise! Back in the hut I shut off the power, reversed two of the wires, and turned the power back on. This time the pump slowed briefly, then picked up speed. Better yet, I could feel the pipe vibrating.

Later that evening as I was sharing with Becki what had happened with the Mickey-Mouse canoe and voiced the question that was troubling me: why was God putting me through this? Why couldn't I just be a doctor and a surgeon? Why did I have to balance caring for the sick with being the maintenance guy risking his life in Mickey-Mouse canoe? Becki didn't know the answer either, so we ended the discussion with prayer, asking God to help us.

A day or two later I read two verses in Mark 10:43-44 that I had read many times before. Jesus said to His disciples, *"But among you it will be different. Whoever wants to be a leader among you must be your servant, and whoever wants to be the first among you must be the slave of everyone else. For even the Son of Man came not to be served but to serve others and to give his life as a ransom for many."*

Far too slowly I was understanding a heavy truth: those words of Jesus were meant for me. I was called to be different. Jesus was challenging me to be more than a doctor. Not just to be the first among others, but the *slave* of others. That's why He brought us to Bongolo. And as I would soon see, He wasn't kidding about being a slave.

Are You My Servant?

The old woman paused at the top of the hill to catch her breath and to survey the hospital. She adjusted the woven bamboo strap that supported the small basket on her back Leaning on her walking stick, she shuffled forward, her swollen, toe-less feet sliding slowly over the smooth path. The veins in her neck were visible in the late afternoon sun, and several times she wiped her face with a filthy cloth. She had come more than ten miles alone and on foot. Her grandchildren had promised to follow in a day or so, but because of her leprosy. They had long since ceased to care about her. She knew they would not be coming.

In the waiting area she wearily swung her basket to the ground and rummaged in it until she found her tattered notebook. She had only enough strength to carry one cooking pot and a small amount of food in the smoke-stained basket. She placed her notebook in the wooden box outside the consultation room.

A few minutes later a nurse came out, picked up the notebook, and called her into the room. The nurse examined her and saw that she was suffering from advanced congestive heart failure and would have to be hospitalized. Of course she couldn't pay the $2 a day for hospitalization, but it didn't matter anyway, since lepers were treated free at our hospital.

I saw her a few hours later. Because there were not enough mattresses, she was lying on the bare boards of the bed. She was dirty and probably had not washed with soap for years. On examining her I learned her heart was enlarged and was beating irregularly. She had several open sores on her feet because leprosy had deprived them of sensation, and she had injured herself so many times without knowing it that most of her toes were gone. Her medical record revealed that during the past five years she had taken her medicine for leprosy faithfully. I dressed the sores on her hands and feet and wrote a prescription in her tattered notebook for heart failure. Assuming that one of her children or grandchildren had accompanied her, I failed to ask if she had come alone.

On rounds the next morning I thought she looked better. The diuretics and heart medicine appeared to be working, and she had already lost several pounds of fluid. I suggested that the family member who had accompanied her wash her clothes and told her we would give her a bar of soap. She looked down at her hands and said nothing, and I assumed she was embarrassed.

The following day she was very weak. It was only then that our nurses discovered she was not eating because she had no one to prepare her food and could not do it herself. I paid one of the nurses to get her some food, but when she brought it, the old woman wasn't hungry. That night she died.

Early in the morning the nurse on duty called me on our ham radio system with the news that the old woman and died. I asked the nurses to move the body to a private area until we could figure out what to do. I sent a message to a couple of men who had worked for the hospital before and asked them to dig a grave for her in the village cemetery. I continued seeing patients all morning, and it was noon before I realized the men had not come. I sent another message to an elder of the Bongolo Church and asked him to find two workers for us who could dig a grave. Still, nobody came.

In the late afternoon after I finished seeing patients, several male nurses helped me place the old woman's body in the back of my truck on a stretcher with some digging tools. Then I drove the half mile to the village of Dakar and stopped at the house of one of the church deacons He apologized that he couldn't help me dig a grave for the woman because of something else he had to do. When I drove to the house of another deacon and asked him for help, he declined because of a sore back. I went from house to house, asking believers that I saw in church every Sunday, and asked them to help me bury the old woman. Everyone was sympathetic but excused themselves. By the fifth or sixth stop, I was so angry that I roared out of the village towards the cemetery in a cloud of angry dust!

The cemetery was covered with l ow brush and vines, and s o I had to clear a site with a machete before digging. I slashed at the brush and vines until I had cleared a ten-foot by fifteen-foot area.

Then I attacked the ground with a pickaxe and shovel, showering dirt in all directions. My actions were a perfect reflection my rage at the hypocrites who had declined to help me! I was a doctor, a doctor, not grave digger! And I was burying my own patient, a stranger, alone! Who ever heard of such a thing? The relatives of sick and the dying patients would soon expect me to pick up their dead at their doorsteps, and after doctoring them day and night, bury them! As I flailed at the ground and all but cursed those who had refused to help, my thoughts became less and less rational.

By this time, I had popped half-a-dozen blisters on my soft, doctor hands, but I was too angry to even feel them! By then the hole I was digging was halfway done when four men from the village walked up, their faces averted with shame. Without a word, I handed them the tools and stood back to catch my breath. For the first time I noticed my hands were bleeding from torn blisters.

When the hole was ready, we lowered the old woman's body into it, covered her with a sheet, and filled in the grave. One of the men planted a stick at one end of the mound to mark the grave, but I could not bring myself to pray over it. I paid the men half the amount I usually paid workers, loaded the tools in my truck, and still smoldering, left without thanking them. As I drove home, a feeling of heaviness settled over me. *I had buried the woman, hadn't I? I had even dug half of the grave myself! Didn't I have the right to be angry?* As I justified my attitude, the Lord clearly spoke to me, His Spirit to my spirit.

"Why are you angry?" he asked.

"Since when do doctors bury their patients?" I shouted at God. "I should *never* have had to do this!" As I continued up the hill past the hospital and toward our house, the Lord asked,

"Do you think you're too good to bury this woman?" The question caught me by surprise, and I shouted and pounded the steering wheel, "It's not my job to bury people! I'm a doctor, not a gravedigger!"

By this time, I was in front of my house, so I pushed through the screen door and stomped into our bedroom, undressed, and got into the shower. But instead of feeling relieved as cold water flowed over me, I felt terrible. Then the Lord asked, "David, are you my servant, or not?" I stood under the cold water, pondering the question.

"You know I'm your servant, Lord," I replied reluctantly. God's Spirit answered me instantly: "Then don't give me this doctor stuff! My servant does whatever I tell him to do!" And that was all. As

I toweled myself dry, I realized how childish I had been. Being a doctor did not make me better than my patients, or anyone else. Whether I dug graves or repaired hernias changed nothing. I finally knelt at the edge of my bed and asked the Lord to forgive me for my anger and my pride.

When God looks at us, He does not see us as doctors, lawyers, truck drivers, migrant workers, grave diggers, or anything else. He is fully aware of the color of our skin, our sex, our intelligence, our level of education, our skills, and our weaknesses. But he doesn't define us by these things. He only sees us as willing or unwilling, proud or humble, useless or useful, disobedient or obedient… *servants.*

Whispers from God

As more and more people came to the hospital, we ran out of benches in our waiting area. I was still the only doctor, but since we needed to solve the problem, I suggested to the team that we make more benches. We had a carpenter from the Bongolo church who agreed to make them for a good price. It was up to us to purchase 20 hardwood boards from the nearest sawmill. Fortunately, it was only twenty miles away on a logging road deep in the forest. The sawmill always had hardwood boards for sale and didn't make deliveries, so customers had to drive to the mill, purchase them, then transport them. In those days we couldn't hire a local truck and driver to transport heavy loads, so I volunteered to take a day off from the hospital, drive to the sawmill in our Land Rover and do what was needed.

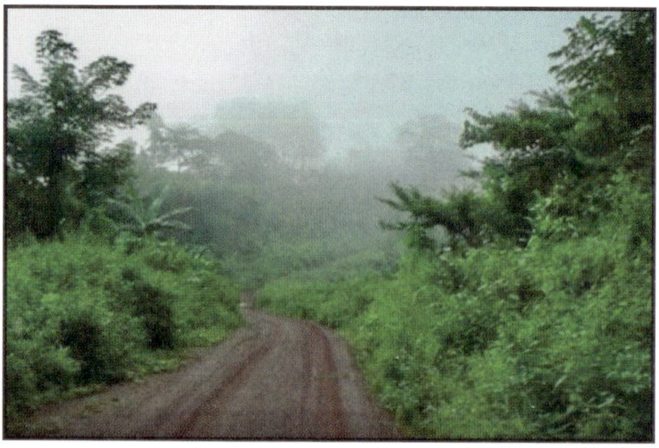

The road to the sawmill.

The logging road was unpaved but well maintained, and though it snaked for miles through dense jungle and across log bridges, it was usually an easy, 20-mile drive. The sawmill always had a good supply of freshly cut, 15-foot hardwood boards, so we didn't need to send an order in advance. The drive to the mill was uneventful, and after I picked out the boards and paid for them, the boss had one of his workmen help me load them onto my roof rack. The boards were still moist with sap and surprisingly heavy. By the time they were all loaded and securely tied down, the leaf springs on my Land Rover were flat. It was so top-heavy I would have to drive slowly and carefully.

After driving for about twenty minutes, I was on a long curve in the road with a deep ravine on the left when my Land Rover kind of wobbled. It was weird, and the moment it happened I had such a strong impression from the Lord to stop that I braked immediately. Thinking I might have a flat tire, I walked around the vehicle looking at the tires. All four were fully inflated and looked just fine, and none of the boards on the roof rack were loose. Thinking that I must have imagined the Lord's warning, I opened the door to get back into the driver's seat. For some reason that could only have come from the Lord, I glanced to the right one last time and looked at the rear tire on the driver's side. Then I froze! *There was only one lug nut on that wheel*! I quickly walked to it and squatted down to get a better look. When I touched the lug nut, *it fell to the ground*, leaving the wheel with NO lug nuts! I was so shocked that I fell backward, realizing that NOTHING was holding that rear wheel from falling off! As I picked up the lug nut my hands were shaking, but I managed to screw it on until it was finger tight. When I stood up, I was shocked to see that the distance from my wheel to the edge of gulley was less than two feet. If my wheel had fallen off while I was driving, my top-heavy Rover would have rolled down the ravine with me in it until it hit a tree 50 feet down. Still shaking, I got my lug wrench and tightened the lug nut securely. Obviously, I couldn't keep driving with just one lug nut on the wheel! The spare tire holder on the back door had long since broken the door, so I carried my spare on the floor behind the second seat. There were no lug nuts there. Then I had a silly idea: maybe if I walked back up the road, I could find my missing lug nuts! I was still shaking from the adrenaline rush, so I wasn't thinking clearly enough to take a lug nut off each of my other three wheels to make up the shortfall. Finding the lost lug nuts seemed supremely import- ant! Standing behind Rover and looking back from where I'd come, I prayed and asked God for something ridiculous: "Lord Jesus, help me find my other lug-nuts so I can get this load of lumber safely home!" Then I started walking slowly up the road, looking for my lug nuts.

What happened next was surreal. Fifteen feet up the road I found the first one, just inches from my tire track! I kept walking, and after twenty more feet I found the second one, an inch from the edge of the ravine! Fifteen more feet up the road I found the third lug nut and kept walking! At forty feet, I found the fourth one! I don't know what you would do, but I raised my hands in the air and shouted, "Thank you, Jesus!"

There were actually *three* miracles o n t he road that day. Th e first was that my top-heavy Land Rover advanced fifteen feet down that dirt road with just one, loose lug nut on the left r ear w heel. I f that wheel had fallen off, my Rover would have rolled down into the steep ravine with me inside. The second miracle was that I heard God's urgent non-vocal call for me to stop my vehicle immediately, a command He'd never given me before! The third miracle was that God made four of my lug nuts fall on the road and remain where I could find them in just minutes!

For the rest of my drive home, I sang praises to God for saving me from disaster. The next day, our carpenter started work on the new benches, some of which are still in use at Bongolo Hospital.

Psalms 37:23-24 says, "*The Lord directs the steps of the godly. He delights in every detail of their lives. Though they stumble, they will never fall, for the Lord holds them by the hand.*" Psalms 116:6 says, "*The Lord protects those of childlike faith; I was facing death, and He saved me.*" Proverbs 2:8 says, *He guards the paths of the just and protects those who are faithful to Him.* 'And finally, Psalm 23:4 promises God's people that "*Even when I walk through the darkest valley, I will not be afraid, for you are close beside me. Your rod and your staff protect and comfort me.*" The only reason I heard God's Spirit that day was because one wonderful day many years before, I believed in Jesus. He forgave me, moved into my heart, and taught me to recognize His voice!

Learning to Build

The problem, Pastor Luke our Administrative Director cxplained, was that the hospital's outhouses were full again. Couldn't we build a really deep one that wouldn't fill up in a matter of months? In the past we had always managed to find somebody with construction know-how to supervise our building projects, but at the moment we were fresh out of experienced supervisors. Neither was there anyone around we could hire who knew how to build something as complicated as a cement hut suspended over a d1e7e6p hole!

I concluded that it couldn't be all that difficult. First, you had someone dig a deep hole, then you built a stone or brick foundation around the outside edges of the hole; and finally, you poured a steel-reinforced concrete floor over temporary scaffolding, leaving a keyhole-shaped hole in the floor. Bricking up the walls and roofing the hut was something our local masons could do with minimal supervision. With these thoughts in mind, I shrugged and said to Pastor Luke, "I'm all for it! Where should we build it?"

Pastor Luke already had a spot in mind. Since I was between operations, we walked down to look at it. The site he had chosen wasn't too far away from the center of our growing hospital and not so close that you'd be reminded of its presence every time the wind blew in the wrong direction. I picked up a nearby stick and traced a four-foot square in the dirt.

"If you can find a worker who's willing to dig a hole at least 10 feet deep," I explained, "it could last several years." Pastor Luke thought the size and location were fine and went off to find a worker. That was the last I thought about it until five days later when I saw Pastor Luke again.

"How's the outhouse coming?" I asked. His eyebrows rose over the top of his glasses.

"I don't know," he said. "I thought you were in charge!" With that disturbing news, I hastened over to the worksite to see what our worker had accomplished in five unsupervised workdays. On the way there, Pastor Luke explained that the man he had found was named Nzengue Pierre. There was no sign of Nzengue until we came to the edge of the hole and looked down. To our astonishment, he was already eighteen feet down! Unfortunately, he hadn't dug straight down but had corkscrewed clockwise as he descended. To give himself more freedom with the pickax he had also enlarged the hole as he descended. In the bright sunlight, our eyes had to adjust to even see him. It was then that we realized the ground we were standing on at the hole's edge tapered away into thin air about a yard below our feet! I couldn't help wondering where Pierre might have taken the hole had we checked on him after two weeks!

Three things were immediately clear: 1) The hole was deep enough, and 2) Pierre would have to match the top of the hole with the bottom to avoid a sudden cave-in the next time it rained, and 3) Pastor Luke's unquestioned approval of all my suggestions meant that I had become the Project Supervisor.

Pierre seemed relieved that the hole was deep enough, especially since he had to climb the ladder with each bucket-load of dirt and dump it at least three feet from the hole! When Pierre finally finished matching the top of the hole with the bottom, we had a hole eighteen-feet deep and 8-feet by 8-feet wide. It seemed quite large for an outhouse, but since there was no going back, we decided to make it a double outhouse, though as I had learned with my first outhouse there could only be one hole per room!

The next step was to find a mason and have him build a foundation of rocks and cement around the top edges of the hole so that eventually the mason could pour a steel-reinforced concrete floor over the hole. Pastor Luke recommended a mason named Jean Claude for the job and thinking that his work might take a day or two, we hired him for $1 an hour, the time was the going rate.

The next morning after staff devotions I explained to Jea n Claude what I wanted him to do. I thought I made it abundantly clear that the foundation needed to be laid *closely* around the edge of the abyss, but three hours later when I came by to see how he was doing, I discovered he had laid the foundation a foot back from the edge of the hole! Now the area of air we would have to cover with concrete measured ten feet by ten! We had gone from my original plan of twenty-five square feet of outhouse floor to 120!

Seeing my furrowed brow, Jean Claude hastened to assure me that this would not be a problem, providing I had enough steel reinforcing rods and plywood to make the forms. I had thought of neither, so the project ground to a halt for several weeks while we ordered steel and plywood from Libreville. Several weeks later a truck showed up at the ferry with our steel and plywood. Daan put it in the back of his pickup and brought it to the hospital. Jean Claude then built a plywood form to put over the top of the hole and the foundation. He also made two keyholes in it with space for a wall down the middle for a double outhouse. When he was ready, he asked for ten sacks of cement. Just to be sure he wouldn't run out, I bought fifteen sacks of cement and two tons of coarse sand to mix it with. Jean Claude had a couple of his helpers bring gravel in buckets and announced he was ready to start. Everything looked fine to my inexperienced eyes, so I told him to quit dragging his feet and get on with it!

Later that afternoon I was busy in the OR when Pastor Luke stuck his head in the door. He cleared his throat politely several times before I heard him. I looked up from the operation and asked him if he had a question.

"Uh ... hello, doctor;' he said uncertainly. "The mason needs more cement."

I looked at him over my mask in surprise and asked, "He's already used fifteen sacks of cement?" Pastor Luke nodded.

"How much more does he need?" I asked. Pastor Luke said, "Another five sacks."

I couldn't stop the operation to go and see what was happening, so I told him to go ahead and buy five more sacks. An hour later I emerged from the OR and headed for the construction site. I arrived just as the masons were putting the finishing touches on their slab. It took only one glance into the keyholes to see what had happened. As Jean Claude had poured the heavy cement onto the wide plywood form, the heavy cement had made the plywood sag into the hole. His solution was to keep pouring! By some miracle the plywood hadn't collapsed into the hole entirely! When the cement eventually dried, the middle of the slab was fifteen inches thick!

The next day the floor was still there, so we breathed a prayer of thanks and called it a success. The next phase was to brick up the walls. This went smoothly, and by the end of two weeks, the outside walls and the inside wall between the two keyholes were up, and the roof was covered with a corrugated aluminum roof. I suggested to Pastor Luke that we ask Norbert, our head nurse, to check it out before we opened it to the public. Later that day Norbert called us aside and asked if we had noticed how large the keyholes were in the outhouse floor. He seemed very disturbed, so we walked over to where Jean Claude was waiting.

"First:' Norbert explained as we peered through one of the two doorways "the opening in the floor is so big a child could fall through!' At this we all crowded in to get a better look and picture for ourselves such a ghastly event.

"How would we ever get a child back out?" Norbert asked. He was right, of course. We would never succeed in breaking through the fifteen-inch steel-reinforced concrete floor to rescue a child. In my haste I had carelessly agreed to a hole size without consulting an expert!

"The second problem," Norbert continued while straddling the hole, "is that the hole is too wide, even for adults! You can't put your feet on both sides of the holes and squat without falling backwards!" Jean Claude hotly contesting Norbert's assertion, and to prove he was right he stood with his feet on the two sides of the hole and tried to squat. To our great amusement he fell backward and had to be helped up! When we all stopped laughing, Jean Claude insisted that he could make the holes smaller. We decided to sleep on it.

The next morning, Pastor Luke came up with the best solution. The hospital would buy two porcelain toilets and Jean Claude could cement over the holes in the floor. Instead of a double outhouse, the hospital would have its first two modern bathrooms!

Jean Claude and his crew spent the better part of a week cementing in the toilets and finishing up the doors. Then we locked up the two bathrooms until we could find someone who could pipe water into the bathrooms and do the plumbing.

A year later, a fourth-year American medical student named Ross McCordic came to our hospital for a six-week medical elective. The afternoons were often slow, and one day Ross asked if there was a project he could do for us. He would soon earn his

M.D. degree, but he was so handy with electricity, mechanics and plumbing that I suggested he pipe water into the bathrooms and connect up the toilets. Ross had grown up in Chad, the son of missionary parents who home-schooled him. His father had been the maintenance director at a mission hospital, and after Ross's mother died, during his teenage years he spent most of his time helping his father.

Ross suggested that as long as we were going to pipe in water for the toilets, we should add sinks. We were able to purchase sinks, faucets, and pipe in Lébamba, so he purchased for the hospital what was needed and set to work. A week later the bathrooms were finished and ready for use. At Ross' invitation,

Pastor Luke, Ross, the workers and I went down to see what a properly installed flush toilet could really do! As water swirled noisily into the abyss beneath our feet, Pastor Luc and I grinned like schoolboys and shook hands! All that remained was to organize a proper inauguration and to decide who would be allowed to use the new bathrooms. Back then, only about a third of our patients thought that porcelain toilets were impractical because they were impossibly difficult to squat on without falling off!

By this time, it was mango season, a happy time for school children every year because it was the time of year when they assumed with impunity unlimited license to throw rocks into mango trees to cause mangoes to fall. Up until then we hadn't noticed that a massive mango tree stood just ten feet from our two new bathrooms! Even before the tree's mangoes were ripe, the season opened. Caught by surprise, Pastor Luc called on me again. I had just finished rounding on all my hospitalized patients when he approached me, and I could tell by the set of his jaw that something terrible had happened. He led me down to the bathrooms, opened the doors and pointed to the tin roof. I was shocked to see a series of large, jagged holes. Apparently, some of the children had used bricks to bring knock mangoes from the tree!

From the outset of the outhouse/bathroom project, we always seemed to find ourselves at the mercy of unexpected forces! Pierre the digger, Jean Claude the mason, and a great deal of money had combined to produce two exorbitantly expensive Western bathrooms. Now mangoes, bricks, large rocks, and children were threatening to reduce our beautiful bathrooms to rubble! The solution was obvious: the children could not be allowed to throw rocks up into the tree! To enforce our decision, we hired a young man to guard the tree from sunup to sundown. But the next morning at 4 a.m. he was nowhere to be found, and even if he had been there, he would have been outnumbered 10 to 1! Later that day we came to a fateful conclusion: if we were going to save the bathrooms we had spent a year and treasure to build, the mango tree would have to go!

This was a radical decision, so when Pastor Luke suggested that we should hire Pierre, the man who had started the project, I should have known that nothing would go as planned. The three of us met at the mango tree later that day.

"If I chop down the mango tree," Pierre said, "it will fall onto the bathrooms." For once, Pierre had thought of something we hadn't!

Pastor Luke and I walked over to the toilets and looked up at the mango tree. Sure enough, if we felled the tree the heaviest branch would land directly on top of the new bathrooms. As we stared up at the tree it occurred to me that if someone were to saw off the huge lower branch first, the tree might fall the other way when chopped, thereby sparing the bathrooms. But the big branch was bigger than any of our chainsaws. But if someone could cut most of the smaller branches on that side of the tree it might unbalance the tree enough to make it fall that way. Pastor Luc and Pierre agreed that this was what should be done, but when push came to shove, Pierre refused to climb the tree and cut anything! The only thing he was willing to chop was the tree trunk.

A week later, Pastor Luke had not found another worker willing to carry out our plan. Fearing that the bricks raining down on the new bathroom roofs each morning would damage the sinks and toilets, I volunteered to climb the tree with my chain saw and cut as many of the smaller branches on the bathroom side of the tree as I could reach.

The next Saturday I climbed into the tree on a ladder, clutching my fourteen-inch McCulloch chain saw. The main tree trunk was nearly two feet in diameter, considerably more than my chainsaw could handle, but the higher branches were within my range. Over the next hour while incurring a thousand ant bites, I managed to cut enough of the higher branches to seriously off- balance the tree. One of the branches I cut grazed a corner of the outhouse, but fortunately, the damage wasn't serious.

On Monday, I brought the mission's biggest axe for Pierre to use on the main trunk, explained to him how he needed to cut the trunk so it would fall away from the toilets, and resumed being a doctor. Hours later, Pierre knocked on my office door and asked me to come and see how he was doing.

By this time a crowd of about 50 onlookers stood a respectful distance from the tree. Using a technique, I had never seen before, Pierre had chopped the trunk circumferentially, like a beaver! I almost throttled him in frustration! There was no way of anticipating in what direction the tree would fall! Pierre's explanation was that it wouldn't fall if he cut it the way I asked

him to cut it "*because the tree is perfectly balanced!*" Too late I realized he had not understood my directions. Now if a storm came up the tree could fall in any direction, and when no one expected!

Ten years before Becki and I arrived in Bongolo our missionaries salvaged an Allis-Chalmers Road grader that the government had abandoned. Daan had repaired it and used it to keep the dirt roads on the mission station drivable. Earlier that year he showed me how to use it in case the road needed grading and he wasn't around.

The grader had a large electric winch on the back end with 50-feet of steel cable wound onto a spool. I figured that if I attached the end of the cable as high in the tree as possible and used the four-wheel drive road grader to pull it downhill on the side of the tree that had most of the branches, it would fall in the direction we wanted. By now nearly 100 people had appeared to watch the great event.

When I drove the road grader onto the hospital grounds, a murmur of admiration rippled through the crowd. I parked it thirty feet from the tree, and signaling for Pierre to come, I began unwinding the cable and dragged the end to the base of the tree. Now all we needed to do was attach the end of the cable to an upper branch of the tree on the side we wanted it to fall.

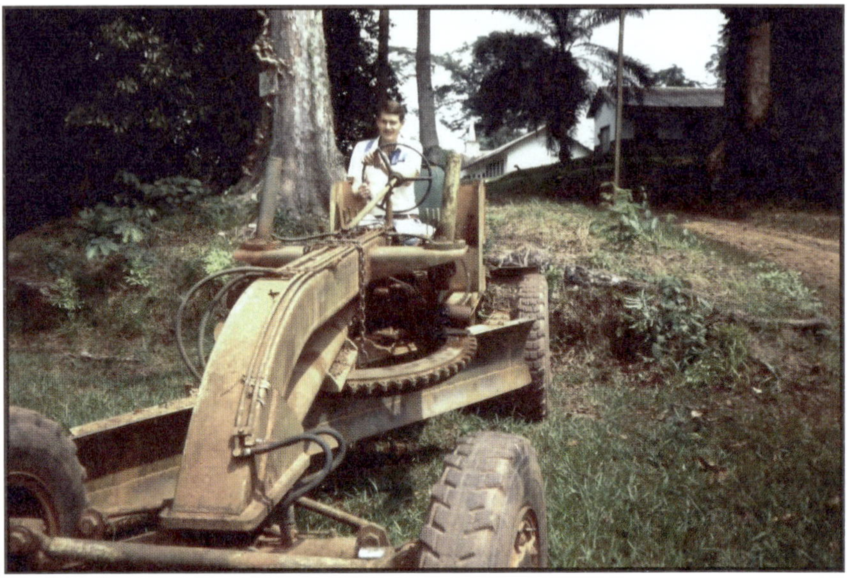

The author on Bongolo's Allis-Chalmer Road Grader

To do that I first threw the weighted end of a rope over an upper branch. When the weighted end of the rope hit the ground, I tied the rope to the hook on the road grader cable to pull the hook and cable up to the branch. The cable had a hook on the end, and I was able to hook it to itself around the branch. Then I climbed onto the road grader and drove it forward until the cable was taut and pulling on the tree branch. When I motioned for Pierre to resume chopping, he swung the ax with new vigor.

The road grader had four large, knobby tires that were connected to the drive train, and had a powerful diesel engine. I put it in low gear and pulled steadily on the cable until it was taut. Pierre continued to chop, though with less and less enthusiasm. Finally, he stopped, signaling that it was too risky to continue. I couldn't imagine what could be left, so I revved the engine and gave a tremendous jerk. As the tree swayed in my direction, a cheer went up from the crowd! I accelerated the motor even more and the knobby tires started spinning and throwing up chunks of dirt. It was unbelievable! The tree should have already come down behind me, but instead it hesitated, perfectly balanced. Then, like a giant spring, it recoiled, dragging the roaring grader and its spinning wheels backward and falling with a thunderous roar directly on top of our new bathrooms!! The stunned silence that followed lasted about five seconds, and then the crowd moaned! I couldn't believe it. I had reduced my first construction project to rubble!

Later, as we picked through the ruins I found several reasons for hope. The toilets and sinks had survived, and the plumbing still worked. Best of all, the fifteen-inch-thick cement floor withstood a direct blow by one of the tree's largest branches. Jean Claude was the first to point this out, of course, stating proudly that a lesser floor would have collapsed into the hole.

Two years after the day I traced a five-by-five-foot square in the dirt and ordered Pierre to start digging, our two bathrooms were opened to the public! Since the majority of our patients didn't know what to do with sit-down flush toilets, we ended up reserving them for our city dwellers and more educated patients.

Is there a lesson in this story? The one that comes to mind relates to perseverance. In Luke 11:5-8 we read, "*Then teaching them more about prayer, He [Jesus] used this story: "Suppose you went to a friend's house at midnight, wanting to borrow three loaves of bread. You say to him, 'A friend of mine has just arrived for a visit, and I have nothing for him to eat.' And suppose he calls out from his bedroom, 'Don't bother me. The door is locked for the night, and my family and I are all in bed. I can't help you.' But I tell you this—though he won't do if for friendship's sake, if you keep knocking long enough, he will get up and give you whatever you need because of your shameless persistence."*

In our case, we never gave up building the outhouse for our patients until we ended up with a modern, two-room bathroom and the stump of a giant mango tree!

Jeremy's Welcome

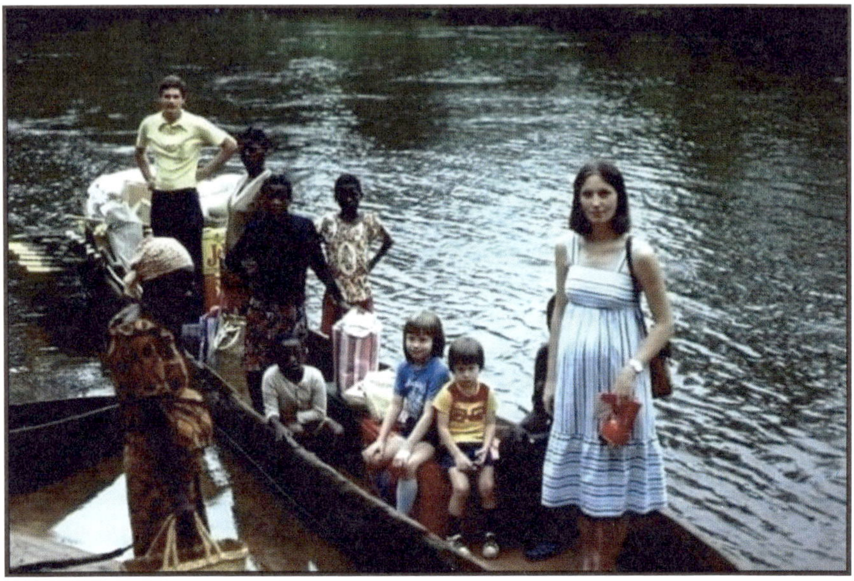

In late 1980, Becki informed me that God was going to bless us with another child! She kept busy taking care of our two older children, working in the lab, training an African to take over, and teaching in the hospital's new nursing school. We had not had a vacation for almost a year, so before she got too close to her due date we decided to travel to Gabon's beautiful southern coast and spend some time on the beach. After asking advice from veteran missionaries, we brought canvas stretchers to serve as our The ferry was out for repairs, and the back road had broken bridges, so we crossed the river in the 30-foot dugout canoe and traveled with our friends to a beach on Gabon's southern coast. That week-long vacation was without doubt the most miserable vacation we every took, thanks to unremitting heat, mosquitos, sleepless nights on the cots, and sunburned skin. Becki suffered by far the most!

Several months after the disaster on the coast, on April 18, 1981, Becki gave birth to our third child, Jeremy. By this time, we had built and equipped a surgery and maternity building that included a delivery room and an operating room, so we were ready should a C-section be necessary. Of course, it would be emotionally challenging to perform a C-section on my own wife, but at least this time I didn't have to worry about driving in a panic to Schweitzer Hospital if she ran into problems!

An hour after delivering Jeremy, Becki stepped out of the delivery room and showed our new son to the African women in the maternity ward. When she uncovered his head and face, they looked up in surprise and concern and said, "Oh! Oh! He's so pale and pink! What's the matter with him? Is he sick? And where's his hair?"

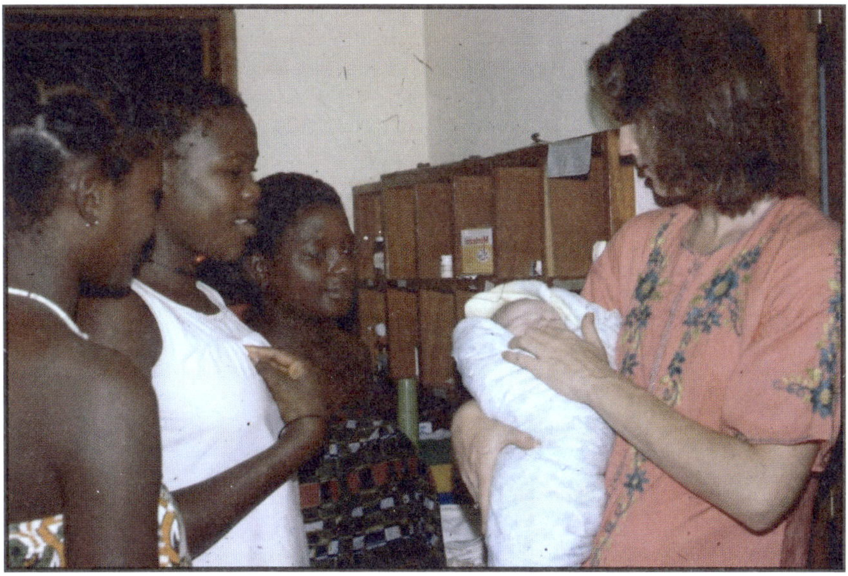

We laughed and explained that unlike their babies who were born with hair and healthy brown skin, white babies were born pink and sometimes had little or no hair! As Becki talked with the ladies, I went outside with her bag of diapers and drove our Land Rover over to the sidewalk in front of the maternity door.

A minute after I took this picture, she came out holding Jeremy in her arms. She was wearing only her red bathrobe and slippers, and when she stepped down between the sidewalk and the Land Rover, she didn't notice a dark column of army ants marching through the grass. All of a sudden, she yelped and cried, "Driver ants! Their biting me and are running up my legs! Go, David, go fast!" As I raced the half mile and up the hill to our house, she kept yelping and scooting around on her seat as she pulled the biting ants off with one hand and held onto Jeremy with the other! As soon as we pulled up to the front door she ran inside with Jeremy, dropped him on our bed, and disrobed in the bathroom! Only after she had pulled them all off and Rachael and Joshua were admiring him, could we stop and laugh at our Jeremy's frantic welcome to Bongolo!

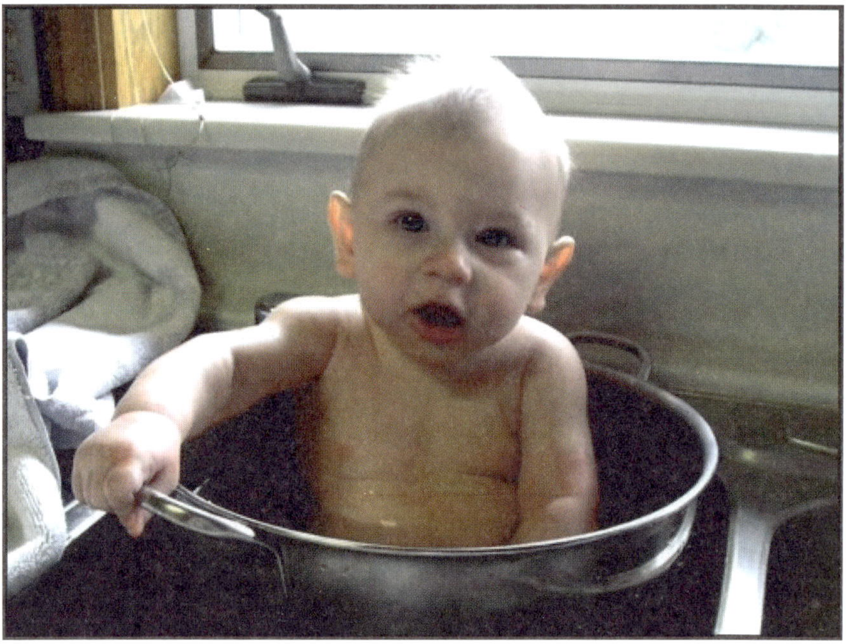

Jeremy, at 2 months

Chapter Four:

THE LOUETSI RIVER

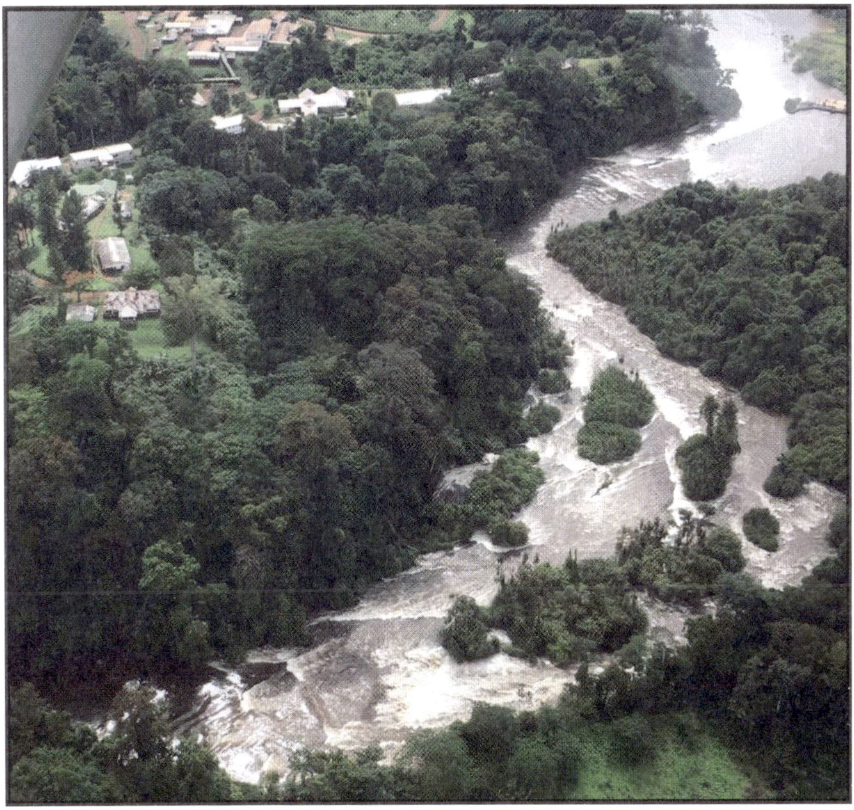

The Louetsi River, as it loops around Bongolo

The Mayor's Wife

I awoke to the sound of my name being called over the CB radio. "Yes, this is the doctor," I answered. "What is it?"

"The mayor of Lebamba is at the Louetsi River with his wife." If the mayor wanted to cross the Louetsi River in the dark at 5:00 a.m., something was seriously wrong!

I dressed hastily and started down the hill in my SUV. It had been raining steadily all night, and the road was slick. I decided to leave the truck at the top of the hill with the lights on and walk down. I could see the mayor and another woman helping his wife climb into the dugout canoe on the opposite shore. The boatman was there, too, and he pulled the canoe across the river. The mayor's wife was shaking and feverish, and the three of us helped her up the hill to my truck. As we drove to the hospital, I asked what had happened.

The mayor was angry and explained that his wife was pregnant. After running a high fever the day before, she had gone into labor. The mayor immediately took his wife to see the doctor at the government hospital. He was French and the government had sent him to replace Mr. Bayonne. The doctor admitted the mayor's wife and treated her for malaria. Her labor seemed to be progressing normally, but then her fever rose to 105 degrees! The doctor didn't seem to realize the seriousness of his wife's condition, and by the time the mayor finally convinced him to transfer his wife to Bongolo, it was the middle of the night. Rather than drive the mayor and his wife to the river himself, the doctor sent a message to the hospital's driver to pick up the mayor and his wife and drive them to Bongolo. Without confirming that the driver got the message, the French doctor went to bed. Unfortunately, nobody could find the hospital driver until 5 a.m.!

Once we arrived at the hospital, I helped carry the barely conscious woman into our delivery room and examined her. Her temperature was 105 and her blood pressure was 60/0. The baby was nearly ready to come, so as the nurses started an IV and we poured fluid into her veins to correct her severe dehydration. Somehow the mayor's wife pushed the baby out. But it was far too late. From what I could see, the baby had died from sepsis.

Minutes after delivering her baby, the mother went into shock and lost consciousness.

For the next two hours, we fought to keep her alive, giving her antibiotics and fluids. When her blood pressure dropped to so low that all seemed lost, we stopped and begged God to spare her. God answered, and hours later she regained consciousness and stabilized.

Over the next two days the mayor's wife was still septic, and her condition remained critical. We didn't have the latest broad-spectrum antibiotics, but we gave her what we had and prayed. Since at that point in time we didn't have an Intensive Care Unit yet, I felt we should transfer her to Libreville by plane, and her husband agreed. My SUV was about the most comfortable vehicle available, so we arranged for a driver to take the mayor and his wife to Mouila, the provincial capital 70 miles to the north so she could be evacuated to Libreville in a small plane the government would be sending down for her. As we prepared to leave, the mayor made an unusual request: he asked if one of our missionary nurses could accompany them in the airplane all the way to Libreville. One of our missionary nurses volunteered to drive our SUV to Mouila's airport and take care of the mayor's wife until the plane came.

Before they left, I asked the mayor if I could pray for his wife and for their trip. When he agreed, and I prayed the most direct evangelistic message I have ever prayed, and when I finished, the mayor wiped his eyes and said softly, "No one has ever treated us as kindly as you. We will never forget it."

The mayor's wife spent nearly a month convalescing in a lovely hospital in Libreville. About six months later a government car drove up to the hospital and a sharply dressed and attractive woman got out and greeted me. I think she was secretly pleased that I didn't recognize her, and she seemed happy to be back. She greeted our staff in the maternity and thanked them for saving her life. She and her husband became enthusiastic supporters of the Bongolo Hospital ministry, but regrettably, neither of them became believers. We later learned, however, that their oldest son decided to follow Christ and was baptized.

Our mayor was reassigned to another post, and the last time I saw him I gave him a Christian book in French and a tract that explained how to come to Jesus. The mayor's wife told me she remembered the morning when she nearly died, and I drove she and her husband to the hospital. Barely conscious as we drove up to the hospital, she looked out the window and saw a white light shining in the sky over the hospital, and a feeling of inexpressible peace filled her soul.

"In that moment, I believed in your God," she told me. "I could feel He was there and that He would help me."

I thought back to that dark and bitter night. I didn't see a light shining over the hospital, But I don't doubt the mayor's wife saw something supernatural. As we fought for her life, Jesus was there, guiding us and helping her. Proverbs 3:27 says, *"Do not withhold good from those who deserve it when it's in your power to help them."*

One patient at a time the curse of Bongolo Falls grew weaker, and the power of God grew mightier!

Living on the River

A major river in the African rain forest is a formidable obstacle to travelers, unless one is traveling in a canoe or a boat. Until roads and bridges came to rural Gabon, the rivers were the people's highways. Living in America where we often cross two or three bridges on the way to the supermarket, we tend not to even think about the bridges we cross. But in Africa where bridges are precious and few, the value of a sturdy bridge is immeasurable.

The simplest way to cross the Louetsi River in the 1930's was in an African dugout canoe. The locals still make dugout canoes from the trunk of an Okoumé tree because Okoumé wood takes years to rot, even when continuously wet.

Even today it is a visual delight to watch expert paddlers skim their small, two-man dugout canoes up, down and across the river! Experienced Africans who ride with them show little concern, even when the gunwale is only a half inch above the water! A careless shift of one's weight can allow water to pour in, but even water-filled canoes float, allowing passengers to hold on and kick themselves to the nearest shore.

Large dugout canoes are made out of a single, massive Okoumé tree trunk and are heavy and difficult to control with paddles. To make a large canoe practical for crossing the Louetsi River with up to 20 passengers at a time, the early missionaries rigged a cable across the river so that an operator standing on the prow could hold onto it and pull the canoe across hand-over-hand.

The cheapest way to cross large numbers of people, cars, and small trucks over a river like the Louetsi is to use a ferry made of pontoons with a platform on top that cars can drive on or pedestrians can stand on. Don Fairley built the first ferry in Bongolo by welding fifty-five-gallon steel drums together and building a wooden platform over them. Because the barrels were made with thin sheet metal and rusted quickly, it lasted about a year. In the 1960's a skilled and determined missionary named Don Dirks spent six months designing and welding together an open-hulled ferry that two SUVs could drive down into at once. He made sturdy ramps on each end and connected them to each other by cables so that when one ramp was down so a car could drive on, the other end was up. The project took so much work that it caused him a bleeding ulcer and nearly killed him. Nevertheless, when he finished his ferry was a thing of beauty. The ferry's only weakness was that after a heavy rain, water had to be pumped out before attempting to cross the river. To facilitate this, he installed a Japy hand pump.

When we arrived in 1977, this was the ferry we found. Newly arrived and still accustomed to bridges, at first, we at first looked down our noses at it and didn't appreciate it for what it was— a Cadillac among hand-pulled ferries! The Dirks ferry served as a floating bridge to Bongolo for roughly ten years. Then one day a couple of teenage boys foolishly attempted to take it across in a driving rainstorm. During the previous day, heavy rains had filled the hull with tons of water, and the hired river crosser hadn't pumped the water out. Ten feet into the river the heavy current overflowed into ferry and sank it, leaving Bongolo without a way to cross cars and trucks until a new ferry could be built!

Our efforts to retrieve the ferry proved fruitless. Six months after it sank the government finally sent a bulldozer and dragged it ashore, but by then it was a useless mess of twisted steel and rotting wood. In the interim, our team reopened an old logging road behind the village on the Bongolo side that was called "Dakar." The logging road wandered 10 miles through the forest before connecting to Gabon's main north-south highway. The town of Lébamba was fifteen kilometers south of the intersection with the logging road. By then our team and the 500 villagers who lived in Dakar were buying much of our food, fuel, and maintenance supplies in the town. Lebamba was also our primary post office. Where before it had taken us fifteen minutes to cross the ferry and drive to Lébamba, for the next six months a trip to Lébamba required an hour of driving in each direction on a jungle that required constant maintenance. Of course, the long-term solution for crossing large numbers of people between Lébamba and Bongolo would have been to build a bridge, but until 1997 the government didn't consider Bongolo important enough to merit one!

Several months after the Dirks ferry sank, friends from America provided funds to build a new one, but nobody had the time or resources to replicate Don Dirk's ferry. Our Dutch maintenance missionary came up with a simple plan that included pontoons, and ordered steel plating, welding rods, and steel cables from Libreville. Over the next four months he welded together four large steel pontoons, built ramps for each end of the ferry, and bolted a wooden platform on top of the pontoons so cars could drive onto it.

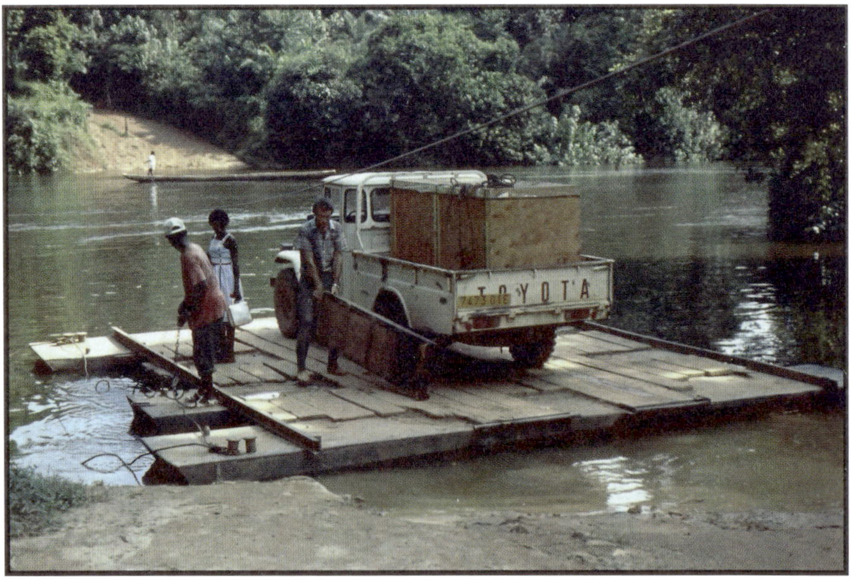

Daan crossing his truck on his "replacement ferry." Note the 30-foot long canoe on the Bongolo side.

During the six months we were between ferries, there were only two ways our patients could cross. The first was to wait in line for a place in the 30-foot dugout canoe. The second way was to pay a local fisherman and ride in his small dugout canoe for 50 cents. When crossing in the small dugout canoes passengers had to sit still to avoid capsizing. With the addition of a suitcase or two, the gunwales would sometimes be only a quarter of an inch above the water!

During those difficult days, thousands of the hospital's patients had to cross the river and either walk a mile to the hospital or wait for a car on the Bongolo side to show up. Few Africans learned to swim, so for many the small dugout canoe crossings were stressful. Adding to the congestion in the mornings and late afternoons were hundreds of high school students from Lébamba who five days a week crossed in the morning to attend Bongolo's high school, and in the late afternoon crossed back to return to their homes in Lébamba.

One day, Becki and I drove onto the ferry on our way back from an afternoon shopping trip in Lébamba. By this time the replacement ferry had been in service for a year. As I drove onto it and braked, I noticed that one of the pontoons was low in the water. I wasn't too concerned because three of the four pontoons were fine, but just as we started to pull away from the shore, a group of fifteen high school students ran up and jumped on! The ferry crosser and I shouted at them to wait, but they ignored our warnings. Seconds later the ferry moved into the current, and with the extra weight, and water-filled pontoon, water began flowing over the boards we were standing on. A minute later we were standing in water up to our knees and holding onto our SUV to keep from being swept off the ferry. the students were screaming, and we began praying for God to help us and to keep the students from drowning! As ferry continued to sink deeper, Becki and I realized we had only seconds before we and our $30,000 SUV would be floating!

At that moment the screaming students began jumping into the water and swimming to the nearest shore. Fortunately, all of them made it, though they lost all their notebooks, papers, and pens. As soon as the students jumped off, the ferry struggled back to the surface, leaving only our feet underwater.

To this day I don't understand why our SUV didn't float away, or why one of the ferry cables didn't break under the strain. Most

Africans don't know how to swim, but that day, all of the students apparently learned quickly and made it to safety! I have no doubt the Lord sent one of His angels to save the students, us, and our SUV!

While God never promises that we won't experience loss or suffering as we serve Him in hard places, Psalm 91:8-12 gives us this promise: "*If you make the Most High your shelter, no evil will conquer you; no plague will come near your home. For He will order his angels to protect you wherever you go. They will hold you up with their hands, so you won't even hurt your foot on a stone.*"

After that incident with the ferry, I realized we had to do something about the leaking pontoon. It was again a time when our Dutch maintenance man Daan was away, and if I couldn't keep the Bongolo Station and the ferry humming, our patients would suffer even more.

Bongolo and the village of Dakar were considered part of Lébamba, so it really wasn't my job to maintain the ferry and keep Lébamba's high school students from drowning. It was the mayor's! At the time, roughly a thousand people lived on the Bongolo side of the river, and up until then I had never seen our mayors do anything more to maintain the ferry than pay the two ferry crossers.

The next day I paid to cross the Louetsi in a fisherman's canoe and drove into town to visit the mayor. He must have heard an earful from the parents of the students who had jumped off the sinking ferry, because he quickly promised to send two of his workmen to fix the leaking pontoon! A few days later two of his men showed up. Before they took the ferry apart, I crossed our SUV to the Lébamba side and parked it, so we and our missionary colleagues would still have a car to drive the three miles to Lébamba. The mayor's workers came later that day, unbolted the leaking pontoon, and took it to their garage in Lébamba.

A week later I stopped by to see how the repairs were progressing. It turned out the mayor's workmen didn't have welding rods, so they had done nothing more! I immediately sent welding rods from our stock over to them. A week later I checked their progress and was pleased to learn they had finished repairing the pontoon but were stuck because they didn't have rust paint! Nobody in town sold rust paint, so I sent over a can of that!

Then, a few days later, I discovered that another pontoon on the parked ferry had sprung a leak. I notified the mayor. Eventually his workers came and took it to Lébamba. A week later they informed me that the second leaking pontoon was so rusty they couldn't repair it without replacing its bottom panel. Steel plating was only available in Libreville, so the mayor's men would have to travel to Libreville, purchase more steel plating, and bring it down-country. By then five weeks had passed on a project that our Dutch maintenance man Daan would have finished in a week!

Because the ferry was our most important means for transporting patients across the Louetsi River, I kept stopping at the mayor's office to keep the pressure on and see what was happening. The next time I checked he told me he had sent his foreman to Libreville 10 days before to purchase steel plating. A week after that—now 17 days— his worker returned with the needed steel! Two weeks later the workers finished repairing the second pontoon, painting it, and putting the ferry back together. Their repair job took seven weeks, and during all that time the taxi buses and vans that brought sick people to the hospital had to drop them off at the river's edge to cross in the dug-out canoe. We eventually set up a shuttle service on our side of the river to pick patients up when they got to the Bongolo side and bring them to the hospital. In Africa, one either learns patience, adapts, or goes crazy! But that would not be the only adventure I would have with the ferry!

On multiple occasions when I had to travel away, I arrived back at the river late at night and found both the ferry and the large dugout canoe tied up on the Bongolo side. Whenever that happened, I had little choice but to take off my shoes, shirt, and pants, l eave them in my car, and wade into the river in my underwear. Walking into the water I would hold onto the lower cable and pull myself across the river hand-over-hand. Then I would cross the ferry back to the Lébamba side, put my clothes back on, drive onto the ferry, pull it across to the Bongolo side, and drive home.

The first few times I did this my imagination went wild! What would happen if my hands slipped from the cable in the middle and I had to swim in the dark, as the current swiftly took me downstream? I could see myself swimming the river in the dark, with no light but the stars, and eventually dragging myself ashore over thorny bushes, dangling vines, and of course— poisonous snakes! Eventually I learned to focus on Isaiah 35:4: *"Say to those with fearful hearts, 'Be strong and do not fear, for your God is coming to destroy your enemies. He is coming to save you!'"* In more than ten nighttime crossings, God crossed the dark and swift current with me, and I never once lost my grip on the cable or encountered a snake!

Not long after fixing the ferry leaks Gabon scheduled national congressional elections. A local political party decided to highlight the failure of the Gabonese government to build a bridge across the Louetsi River for easy access to the hospital. What they ended up doing made the problem ten times worse!

One night in the dark of night, hired goons took down the upper cable that crossed the river. The upper cable had a pulley on it that was attached by a 20-foot cable to the ferry. As the ferry went from one side to the other, the pully ran on the high cable and followed. The connection to the high cable kept the ferry from floating downriver with the current. So, when the goons took down the upper cable, the ferry floated downriver and out of sight. The only cable they left was the lower one so people could cross in the 30-foot dugout canoe.

The next morning carloads of patients arrived at the river's edge, only to discover the ferry was gone! Their only way to cross was now on the dugout canoe, and it could only take 30 people at a time. It was hours before enough local fishermen showed up in their six-foot dugout canoes and started crossing the waiting patients and hundreds of high school students.

After setting up a shuttle service between the river and the hospital, the hospital director crossed the river, hitchhiked a ride to Lébamba, and asked the mayor for help. The mayor told him the police had no knowledge of who sent the ferry downriver and would report the incident to the President of the country. But that did not solve the problem!

At the time that these events occurred, a Canadian construction team was building a dam and a hydroelectric plant at the Bongolo Falls that included the installation of huge turbine-driven generators. Up until then, Bongolo had been the only location within 100 miles to have 24-hour electricity. The mayor suggested that our director ask the Canadians to use their heavy equipment to retrieve the ferry. At our director's request, the Canadians agreed to help and later that day located the ferry several miles downriver. They managed to drag it to shore, lift it out of the water with a crane, and load it onto one of their huge trucks. At the river's edge they used their crane and put the back in the river. Then they chained it to a tree at the river's edge until morning. But there more misdeeds were to come.

Late that night twenty thugs broke into the Canadian's camp and beat them with clubs so savagely that some of them had to be medevacked to Gabon's capital city. The thugs left a message in writing promising that if the Canadians reconnected the cables and put the ferry back in use, their attackers would come back and kill them!

When we heard what had happened and the threat against anyone who interfered with the blockade, the Bongolo Christians and our missionary team began praying that God would quickly provide a solution. But without the government's intervention, the Canadians were not willing to risk further bloodshed. Weeks dragged by, and our patients continued to suffer. The blockade became tremendously unpopular with the voters, and because it was working in the government's favor so well, the government officials chose to do nothing.

After two months of waiting and praying, I sensed that God wanted us to be bold. I called a meeting of our missionary team and suggested that we take the initiative and put the ferry back into service ourselves. We all understood that if our Gabonese brothers tried to do something the political goons would beat them without hesitation. But would they beat us up?

When I asked for volunteers, only one of my colleagues volunteered: a young missionary named Jim Timberlake. He and his wife had been with us for a year or more, and though the threats were real, my faith that God would protect us strengthened his faith. The rest of our team promised to pray for us.

The next day Jim and I loaded new cables, a new pulley, cable clamps, and all the tools and equipment we might need to put the high cable back up with its pulley and connect it to the ferry. After a brief prayer, we drove down to the ferry crossing, got out, and started unloading our equipment and tools. Two muscular young men sitting on a nearby log stood up and asked us what we were doing. I knew they were with the goons, so I said as cheerfully as I could, "Hi! We're going to reconnect the upper cable and put the ferry back in service!"

They both laughed, and the older of the two said, "Doctor, you don't want to do that. Nobody's allowed to touch the ferry, and if you try anything, remember what we did to the Canadians? Do you see these clubs? We'll do it to you too." He held up an impressive club and I nodded. In that moment, I felt the Lord's presence, so I said calmly and respectfully, "Yes, we understand, but here's what we're going to do. We'll first reconnect the higher cable that goes across the river, put the pulley on it, and connect it to the ferry so it won't go downriver when we take it across. When we're done with that, you can beat us up." Both men blinked and looked confused.

By now four or five women who had been washing clothes in the river stopped their washing to listen. Both of the hired thugs stared mutely at me, trying to understand if I was serious or trying to be funny. So, I said again, "We're going to put the upper cable back up and reconnect the ferry."

The older guy shook his head and said emphatically, "Doctor, we're not kidding. If you do that, we'll beat you with these clubs and then take apart everything you've done."

Smiling as sincerely as I could muster, I said, "Okay, we have a deal! We'll put the cable back up, and then you can beat us up!" Then I turned to Jim and said, "Let's go!" Jim was still learning French and hadn't followed the conversation entirely, so he asked, "What did they say? Did they say we can go ahead?" I nodded, said, "Sort of," and rolled my eyes. Since they weren't stopping us from loading our tools, a ladder, a new 50-foot-long cable, and other needed equipment into the big canoe, Jim shrugged and helped me load everything.

The older thug said in a louder voice, "This isn't funny, doctor! If you do this, when we're done, you'll be in the hospital, and for a long time!"

"Okay," I said, "we hear you!" Then we crossed the river in the big canoe with our stuff.

For the next eight hours, Jim and I worked non-stop. We started on the Lébamba side of the river by securing one end of our 50-foot cable around the tree where it had been tied before, fifteen feet up. Every ten minutes or so the guards would shout more threats at us, but we ignored them and kept working.

After securing the high cable around the trunk of a tree on the Lébamba side, we crossed back to the Bongolo side of the river in the canoe, dragging the cable behind us and up the bank near to where our two thugs were waiting. Acting as if they weren't there, we ran the cable through the pulley that would hang on it, secured a shorter, 20-foot cable to the pully that we would eventually secure to the ferry so it couldn't go downriver. Next, we secured the free end of the high cable that crossed the river around a tree on the Bongolo side. The high cable was now 15 feet above the river and parallel to it. Jim and I then crossed back to the Lébamba side, pulling the cable behind us that we needed to connect to the ferry itself.

When we cut the chain that had held the ferry to a nearby tree for the past two months, the goons of Bongolo stood up and started shouting again, threatening to beat us until we were bloody and even break our bones! We acted as if we couldn't hear them and made the final connection by hooking the cable from the pulley on the high cable to the ferry.

As we were throwing our tools onto the ferry, a taxibus full of patients for the hospital drove up to the river's edge. The driver leaned out his window and asked if he could drive onto the ferry and cross. Jim and I smiled and said yes! By this time the two guys on the other side were again shouting threats, cursing, and waving their clubs, but it was too late. The taxibus d rove onto the ferry, ten passengers got out and stood next to it, and we pulled up the ramps. As we pulled on the lower cable, the ferry moved out into the river. When the current pushed in slightly, the cable up to the pulley grew taught and the pully rolled nicely on the upper cable as we pulled the ferry across using the lower cable. When we landed on the Bongolo shore and dropped the ramps, the taxi bus drove off and climbed the hill past the now silent goons.

Now it was time to present ourselves to the goons so they could beat us up. Jim and I walked off the ferry and up to where they were waiting, and the Lord gave us complete peace. I said to them, "Okay, you can beat us up now!"

Neither of them moved from where they were sitting or touched the clubs beside them. The bigger man said with a sigh, "Doctor, if we so much as touch you, the people of Lébamba and Bongolo will beat us up! Go on!" We smiled, thanked them, and shook hands with them, then loaded our tools and gear into the truck. The two men picked up their clubs, crossed the river on the ferry, and walked down the road toward Lébamba. I never saw them again.

In his book *My Utmost for His Highest*, Oswald Chambers wrote, *"God will take you through a multitude of experiences that are not meant for you at all, they are meant to make you useful in His hands, and to enable you to understand what transpires in other souls so that you will never be surprised by what you come across,"* (p.310). In another passage he wrote in the same book, "*When we are in fear, we can do nothing less than pray to God, but our Lord has a right to expect that those who name His name should have an understanding confidence in Him. God expects His children to be so confident in Him that in any crisis, they are the reliable ones. It is when a crisis arises that we instantly reveal upon whom we rely. If we have been learning to worship God and trust Him, the crisis will reveal that we will go to the breaking point and not break in our confidence in Him"* (p.225). Several months later I returned from Lebamba and arrived at the Bongolo Ferry. There was a new SUV in front of me with a white man sitting on the roof. He and his driver were waiting for the ferry crosser to bring the ferry back to the Lébamba side so he could drive on and cross. I stopped my car him, walked up next to his SUV, and said, "Hello! Are you visiting Bongolo?"

He looked down at me and said, "Yes, I'm the American ambassador, and I'm here to see your hospital! You guys need a bridge!" I introduced myself and told him I couldn't agree more! We talked with one another as the ferry crosser pulled the ferry to the Bongolo side. He had many questions and asked for a tour of the hospital. That night he and his driver spent the night in a guest room at the mission. He was the first ambassador to come since we had started building the hospital in 1977! That was the beginning of a seven-year effort to find funding for the project, and in 1997, Gabon, Canada, and the United States came up with $1 million dollars for a one-lane, all steel, prefabricated "Bailey Bridge!"

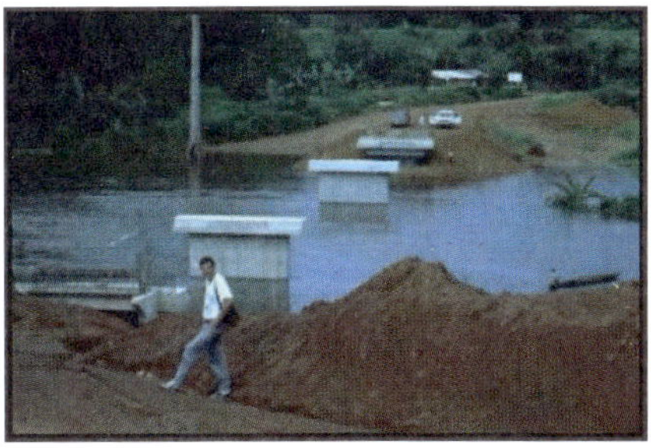 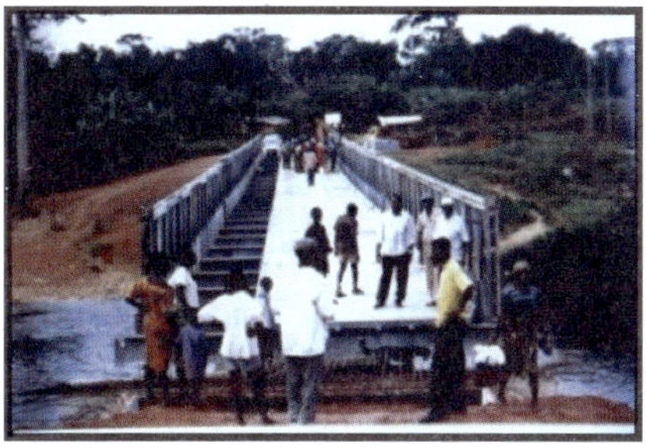

To the delight of the entire population of south Gabon and many who traveled from Libreville, the bridge was completed in 1997, ending 64 years of struggle and reducing the time to cross the river with a vehicle from 30 minutes to one!

Best of all, as a result of what he saw and heard that day and our team's witness to him about Christ over the next few years, the ambassador became a strong Christian. After he retired from the State Department, he went to seminary and became a pastor!

Lebongo's Wives

The voice calling my name over the CB radio jarred me awake. I stumbled out of bed and into our dimly lit living room to turn down the volume before the noise awakened Becki and all three kids. It was midnight, and I had been asleep for about an hour.

"Hello, this is the doctor," I answered hoarsely. "What's happening?"

"I'm sorry to call you, doctor," the nurse on the other end said, "Mister Lebongo Antoine brought his wife to the hospital tonight. She's very ill and he wants you to come down right now to see her." I was suddenly wide awake.

Lebongo Antoine's demand fanned into flame a few smoldering coals that I had nurtured in my heart for several years. Five years before I had shot and killed one of his prized goats near the hospital, and Lebongo had vowed to get his revenge by harming my children. Nothing ever came of his threat except that the church leaders sent him to work in a church school 50 miles away from Bongolo. The memory of his threat came back like a flood. It was the middle of the night, and I was not in the mood to go out of my way for either him or his wife.

"What kind of illness does she have? I asked.

"Well, her abdomen hurts very badly," he answered. "How long?"

"Since yesterday." Yesterday! And now, at midnight, Mr. Lebongo decided to bring his wife to the hospital! I thought to myself that coming in the middle of the night was probably his way of getting even. Well, I wasn't going to play his game!

How are her vital signs?" I asked suspiciously. The nurse recited them over the CB radio. Everything sounded normal. She could certainly wait until morning. The nurse was not happy with my decision to wait, especially since he would have to explain it to Lebongo.

I crawled back into bed but couldn't sleep. After twenty minutes I sat up and sighed. It was no use. I knew when the Lord was unhappy with me, and I knew he was prompting me to be charitable and go. I dressed and drove the quarter mile to the hospital.

Seeing Lebongo brought the goat incident back as though it had been yesterday. With the Lord's help I was charitable, and Lebongo responded with a smile that did not reach his eyes. His second wife's name was Brigitte, and she was not a gracious Christian woman like his first wife, Martha. Brigitte looked to be about twenty, and lay in a fetal position on the bed, moaning softly. She had been sick with continuous lower abdominal pain and nausea for two days. After examining her, I decided that she had either a pelvic infection or an extrauterine pregnancy that had ruptured. To my surprise her pregnancy test was negative, and she was not anemic, two signs that are usually positive with a ruptured ectopic pregnancy. Today I would perform an echogram of her abdomen, but at the time we didn't have one. Brigitte's vital signs were stable, so the next most likely diagnosis was a pelvic infection. I decided to start her on intravenous fluids and antibiotics and give her pain medication every four hours. I also instructed the nurses to check her vital signs hourly for the rest of the night.

When I saw Brigitte the next morning Lebongo was not around, and Brigitte looked better. Lebongo's first wife Martha was washing her rival's face, and her concern for Brigitte was touching, especially since first wives rarely want their husbands to take a second wife—unless they were lazy!

"Dr. Thompson," Martha said in a whisper, "if you have time, please talk to Brigitte about Jesus. She is not a believer, and I am very concerned about her." I could not suppress a warm smile.

"Why do you care so much about her?" I asked. "She's your rival!"

She nodded and said, "Doctor, you know I have prayed for ten years for my husband's salvation. He knows that the Jesus way is right, but he doesn't want to give up his womanizing and his drinking. When he took Brigitte as his second wife, I asked Jesus to help me win her to faith by praying for her and loving her. If I win her over and she becomes a believer, my husband will have two Christian wives praying for him!"

Her faith and logic left me speechless, but I smiled and said, "I promise to speak to Brigitte about Jesus."

Later that same afternoon, I stopped by to check on Brigitte's progress. The pain had returned, and her lower abdomen now seemed slightly distended and much more tender to examination, especially on the left. A repeat blood test showed that her blood count had dropped, which increased the likelihood she was bleeding into her abdomen. I asked her husband to donate a unit of blood, and because they had the same blood type I was able to transfuse her quickly, then take her to the operating room. Brigitte was fearful and cried as I gave her a spinal anesthetic, but once it took hold and her pain ended, she relaxed.

As was our custom, before we started the operation, I leaned over the anesthesia screen and told Brigitte I was going to pray and ask Jesus to guide and bless us as we operated. She nodded, and I prayed, "Father, please help us now as we operate on Brigitte. Give us the wisdom and the skill to deal with what we find and help Brigitte to recover completely and without complications. Above all, help Brigitte to learn to trust in you! Amen!"

When I opened Brigitte's lower abdomen, I was chagrined to find a quart and a half of fresh blood mixed with old blood clots. The bleeding was coming from a ruptured fallopian tube pregnancy, a condition that can be lethal. Brigitte was either extremely lucky, or God had protected her from a catastrophic hemorrhage. I said thatto her, and she looked thoughtful but said nothing. Martha smiled though! A few days later we discharged Martha. Somewhat to Lebongo's irritation, the illness had bound his two wives together like sisters! About six months later, Brigitte decided to follow Jesus and was publicly baptized in the town where they lived. Just as Martha had hoped, her wayward husband now had two wives working and praying that he would turn from his sinful ways and come to Jesus!

A Dream Reborn

By the time we were in our fourth year of serving in Gabon, our hospital had grown from two buildings to four. We were still using the dispensary and the mud-brick ward, but with the completion of a $50,000 surgical/maternity building complete with a delivery room and an operating room, I could conceivably start operating on hernias, perform C-sections, as well as drain abscesses, of which there many. I used spinal anesthesia for operations below the chest, including C-sections, hernias, ruptured ectopic pregnancies, and used local anesthesia for suturing lacerations.

That year, we inherited an old school building and renovated it to serve as 30-bed pediatric and medical ward. About that same time, we also started building a 10-foot by 15- foot warehouse for our medicines. Soon after, we received a 1950's M.A.S.H. X-ray machine and added a second room. Also included in the crates was an operating table for a shorter generation of surgeons! There was no way to raise or lower it!

Friends in Holland sent us a second-hand ceiling mounted operating light with bulbs we could only order from Holland. For autoclaves, we ordered two giant pressure cookers with large gas burners to sterilize our surgical instruments, drapes, and bandages.

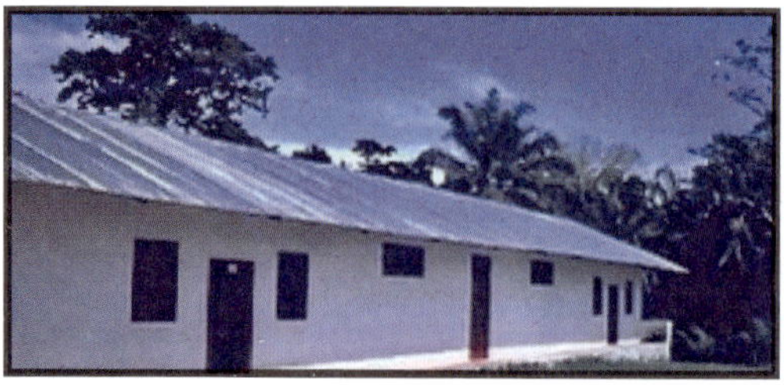

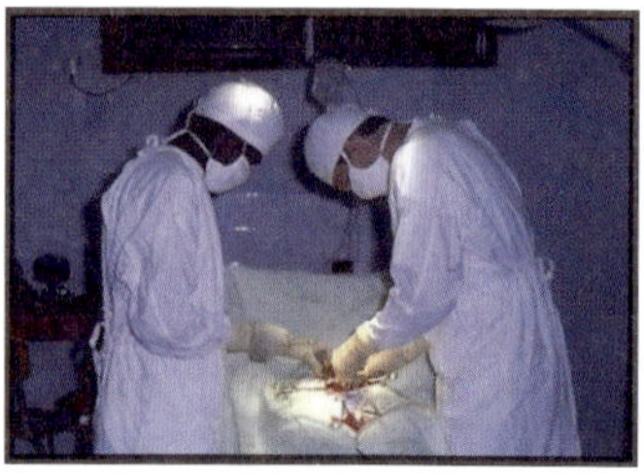

When everything was ready, I announced at the end of the Sunday-morning service of the Bongolo church that we were about to start operating on hernias and C-sections. The whole church applauded and cheered! Our first surgical patient was a church elder who had suffered from a hernia for five years. I admitted him into our eight-bed surgical ward. He later told us that all of his family and friends advised him against being our first surgical patient, because nobody knew if I was really capable or not!

That night he couldn't sleep. Around midnight a male nurse in a white uniform came into the ward and assured him that "Dr. David" was an excellent surgeon and that he had nothing to fear. Greatly comforted, the church elder slept soundly for the rest of the night. The next morning, I gave him a spinal anesthetic and performed the operation without any problems.

Several days later when we discharged him, he asked about the male nurse who had encouraged him the night before his operation. The only nurses on duty that night were women, and none of them had gone to the surgical ward that night. Neither had they seen a male nurse on duty that night, and our two male nurses didn't have white uniforms yet. Was the mystery nurse an interloper from the Lebamba Hospital who walked 3 miles to the river, crossed it in the dark, and walked the half mile to our surgical ward to talk to our patient? We never knew for certain who the nurse in white was, but our patient was certain it was an angel sent by God to comfort him!

Six months after starting to operate, we started seeing more and bigger surgical cases, many of which I wasn't trained to deal with. When these more complex cases came to us the only thing I could do was to put them in the back of my Land Rover on a mattress and take them six hours north to Schweitzer Hospital. The round trip was exhausting. After an especially trying week when I had to make two trips to Lambarene, Becki said to me, "David, you need to finish your training in surgery!"

I shook my head and said, "Sweetheart, if I couldn't find a 3rd year surgery residency position back in 1976 when I was still a 2nd year resident in training, how am I going to find a position now, after practicing bush medicine here for almost six years?" Becki looked me in the eye and said, "If God wants you to do this, He will make a way!" I couldn't argue because she was right!Her faith gave me the courage to try again and ask the Lord for another miracle, or several, since we would have to find a doctor and a nurse to take our places in Bongolo. Soon after we began praying, a missionary doctor in the Congo heard of our need. His name was Dean Kroh, and his wife Esther was a nurse. The couple contacted us and offered to fill in for us during the four years we would be gone! They had already served for three and a half decades in what today is the Democratic Republic of Congo and had built a mission hospital from scratch. We accepted their offer with amazement and joy!

By this time our daughter Rachael was in first grade, Joshua was 3, and Becki was pregnant with our third child. Even if a miracle happened and I did find a residency position, I would be on call every 2nd or 3rd day and Becki would have little help from me for the three years it would take to finish my training. Becki's reply to these challenges to our faith was, "You need to go for it, David, and God will help us!"

On April 18, 1981, our son Jeremy was born in Bongolo Hospital's new maternity ward. The only problem occurred when Becki stepped off the hospital's front step into the grass to get into our SUV, holding Jeremy in her arms. Hidden in the grass was a column of army ants that immediately ran up her legs and started biting her! The three-minute drive to our house was loud, fast, and unforgettable!

In mid-May our family flew from Gabon to Los Angeles, California. Friends of ours invited us to stay in their large home until we figured out what we would be doing. I immediately began calling surgical residency program directors in California and asking them if they would have a 3rd year residency position open, starting July 1, 1981. Every program director I called and talked with was sympathetic, but no one had an open position at the third-year level. June slid into July, and I continued to call training program after training program in many other states. Most of the program directors suggested I start over or look for a position at the first or second-year level.

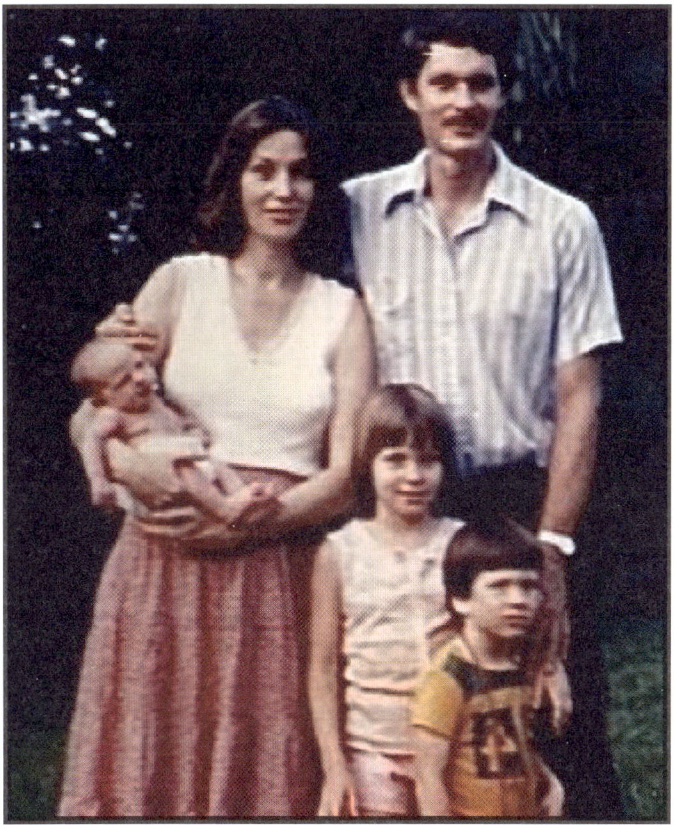

Our family in 1981

Every morning Becki and I started the day on our knees, asking the Lord for a miracle. One day, I talked with a Christian program di rector in Los Angeles. Although he was very sympathetic, he didn't have an open position, but he offered to call other program directors he knew around the country. I was delighted and said, "Thank you! I need all the help I can get!"

By mid-June I was starting to panic. Then late one day the phone rang and the Christian program director who had been calling other program directors for me asked me to come to White Memorial Medical Center in downtown Los Angeles so we could talk. I immediately accepted. The next day I drove to the hospital and found my way to his office. The professor's name was Dr. Gerald Longerbeam, and he attended a Baptist Church. He had been an academic surgeon for several decades, and the walls of his office were covered with diplomas and honors.

After we sat down, Dr. Longerbeam asked me to describe what I had been doing over the previous six years. He listened without commenting and looked at my documentation for my first two years of training at Mercy Hospital in San Diego, six years earlier. As I talked, he listened with surprising interest.

Finally, he leaned back in his chair and said, "One of my residents just quit. She was finishing up her second year of residency, which means that I'll have an opening for a third-year resident starting on July 1st. Would you be interested?"

I almost fell off my chair! When I was able to speak, I said, "Yes, I would be honored to take that position!"

He nodded and said, "I don't think you can do it, but I'm willing to give you a chance. Be here on time on July 1st, and I will introduce you to the other residents and faculty members."

For the next three years, I served as a surgical resident at White Memorial Medical Center. For two of the three years I worked there, I was on call every other night and every other weekend. Thanks to the help of a generous friend, Becki and I were able to purchase a home in Van Nuys, a 45-minute minute drive by car from the hospital. My salary was only $17,000 a year, but during those three years the dollar was stronger, and Becki pinched every penny. Despite my long hours away at the hospital she was such a great mom that our kids have only happy memories of those years!

During my last six months of residency, Dr. Longerbeam moved to Loma Linda and took over as the Chief of Surgery at the Veterans Hospital. After I graduated, he invited me to work under him for one year as a Surgical Educator, supervising the surgical residents who rotated through the VA from Loma Linda University. It was a wonderful year for our family, and the position did wonders for my salary!

In June of 1984, our family moved back to Bongolo and immediately resumed our ministries at the hospital. I had been able to ship hundreds of surgical instruments, and the extensive variety of operations I found myself performing almost covered the skin and its contents! I was soon operating six days a week and emergency cases at night. A year later, I returned to Los Angeles, took my written board exam in general surgery, and passed. Soon after, the American Board of Surgery sent me a formal invitation to take my oral board exam the following year.

As the time approached for my oral board exam, I was worried. As the only surgeon for perhaps 200,000 people in southwest Gabon, I hadn't had time to study for my oral exam. To give myself more time to prepare, I traveled to California ten days before my exam. Becki's uncle and aunt had invited me to stay with them in northern California, and during the first three days I spent hunched over surgical books. On day three, I developed a terrible headache, followed by a fever and chills. I knew right away what was happening: I had malaria. Despite taking the standard medication to prevent malaria, I had come down with a resistant strain. That morning, I prayed, "Lord, help me! I need to pass this exam, and I won't be able to take it if I'm sick with malaria! Help me find the medication I need!

At the time the standard medication for resistant malaria was Quinine, and the nearest pharmacy that had it in stock was 50 miles away, in Chico, California. By this time, I had a temperature of 104 and was shaking with chills and fever. Becki's uncle was kind enough to drive me to Chico to see a doctor friend of his. By the time we got there, my head was pounding! Fortunately, the doctor agreed to see me right away, but unfortunately, Chico didn't have a lab that could perform a rapid malaria test. However, he took my word that I had resistant malaria and prescribed Quinine! During our conversation he asked me what I was doing in Gabon and why had I come home.

When I told him that I was prepping for my oral surgery board examination he said, "Hey, I have a friend who is a surgeon who just passed his oral boards last year! Let me call him so you can meet him! Maybe he can help you prepare for the exam!

All I really wanted to do was to take two quinine pills, two aspirins, and go to bed! But the doctor wouldn't take no for an answer and telephoned his surgeon friend. The surgeon went by the unlikely name of "Pokey Cleek," though I would later discover he was one of the fastest surgeons I would ever meet! To my dismay, he told my doctor to bring me to his home! We first went to a pharmacy, and after they served me, I swallowed the quinine and laid down in the back seat in Becki's uncle's car.

Dr. and Mrs. Cleek were waiting at the door of their house and greeted me enthusiastically. "David," Dr. Cleek said, "I'm Pokey, and this here is my wife Laurel and some of my kids."

I greeted them all as cordially as I could muster. Dr. Pokey Cleek was tall, lanky and gracious. When he told his kids I was from Africa, their eyes widened, and they reverently shook my hand.

Pokey asked, "Is it true you're taking your oral boards next week?" When I mumbled that it was, he said, "Would you mind if I prepped you by asking you some of the oral questions that they asked me and my surgeon friends?"

Trying to stay focused over the pounding of my head, I mumbled, "Sure, but I'm not going to do well because I'm fighting malaria." Pokey chuckled and never having experienced malaria said cheerfully, "I'm sure you'll do fine!"

For the next hour I sat in a straight-back chair, my head pounding mercilessly. Pokey took on the role of an examiner and asked me hundreds of questions about surgical diseases and injuries, how to diagnosis them, how to treat them surgically and manage their complications—it seemed endless! As I mumbled my answers— most of them incomplete or wrong— I though my head was going to explode! All I wanted to do was crawl into the nearest dark corner and sleep!

After what seemed like 3 hours but was probably only 45 minutes, Pokey's wife Laurel urged him to relent, and he did. At the end he said, "David, I know you're tired and not feeling well, but this is what your oral exam is going to be like. Hopefully, this will help you get you ready." He would later tell me that he thought I was doomed to fail!

I thanked Pokey sincerely, said goodbye to the Cleeks, and while I slept in the back seat Becki's uncle drove us back to their home.

By the next morning, I was feeling considerably better, and later in the day flew to Seattle where my exam would take place. That evening in my hotel room I made a list of all the questions I could remember Dr. Cleek asked me. The next morning, I went to the medical library at Washington State University, pulled out four or five major new-looking surgical textbooks, and reviewed every topic on my list. At the end of the day, I had twenty pages of notes which I studied until late that night.

The next morning, I got on my knees and asked the Lord to help me remember everything Pokey had reviewed with me and that I had studied the day before. Then I drove to the hotel where the board examinations would be held.

There were perhaps seventy-five young surgeons in the large hotel lobby waiting to take the oral exam. Around 11 a.m. my name was called, and I entered a room where three middle- aged academic surgeons were waiting. After the introductions were over, the clinical questions began. Each examiner described a patient who had certain complaints and symptoms. Then the questions came: What other physical findings might I find? What other diagnostic tests would I want before making a diagnosis? What various diagnoses should I consider? What was my final diagnosis, and how would I deal with it surgically? After I finished all three professors' questions, the exam was over. It took less than 15 minutes.

As I walked out of the room, I felt like I was walking on air. To my amazement, two of the three scenarios they had asked me were among the questions Dr. Cleek had asked me at his house in Chico, and the third question I was familiar with. I also realized that God had used a painful bout of malaria to bring me to Pokey Cleek, and to prepare me for my examination. A week later I was back at Bongolo, and a month later I received in the mail my Certificate of Competency in General Surgery from the American Board of Surgery. Once again, my heavenly Father had helped me every step of the way and had prepared me so I could succeed. But that was not the last exam I would take. Every ten years after that I had to take a recertification examination to maintain my board status, and every time the Lord helped me prepare well and pass!

Deuteronomy 33:26 says it best: *There is no one like the God of Israel. He rides across the heavens to help you, across the skies in majestic splendor!"*

Freeing Hearts

As an American physician working in rural Africa, I had to either adapt with the help of Jesus or give up. I will never forget a day in 1980 when I was making rounds in our five-bed tuberculosis ward. I was the only physician on duty that day, and the 30 or so hospitalized medical patients on a separate ward were being cared for by two African nurses who didn't have time to round with me in the TB ward. When I checked on a 28-year-old woman we had been treating for several days for Tuberculosis, I was shocked to see her gasping for air! That can happen to TB patients if they suddenly start hemorrhaging inside their lungs, but she wasn't coughing up anything. The only diagnostic instruments I had that day were my eyes, a blood pressure cuff, and a stethoscope. Our X-ray machine had quit working months before, so that was not an option.

A quick assessment showed that the woman's blood pressure was 80/30 and her pulse was 120. I checked her neck and saw that both of her jugular veins were visibly distended. When I put my stethoscope to her chest, I could hardly hear her heartbeat. Knowing that in advanced tuberculosis, inflammatory fluid can fill the non-elastic sac around the heart with so much fluid that the heart can only fill partially. In an emergency like I was seeing, the solution is to remove the fluid around the heart as quickly as possible!

Trying to find the two nurses who had made rounds with me in the medical ward would take precious minutes and wouldn't solve the problem, so I ran to our medical warehouse and grabbed a 50cc syringe and a six-inch sterile needle. On my way back I ran into the medicine ward for a nurse just in case, but when I couldn't find one after looking, I realized that time was running out for my patient. I needed to get on with the procedure as quickly as possible!

By the time I showed up with my supplies, my patient was gasping for air and was paler than any African I'd ever seen. When I explained that I would need to put a needle into her chest and draw out fluid around her heart, she closed her eyes and nodded. After splashing disinfectant on her chest, I connected my 50cc syringe to the long needle I had and inserted it below her sternum, slowly advancing it towards her heart and watching to see if fluid was coming. She was so afraid she was dying that she didn't even wince as I pushed the needle towards her heart.

Seconds later I felt a slight "pop" which I hoped was the needle entering the swollen pericardial sac. Then pinkish-clear fluid rushed into the syringe. Because it wasn't bright red blood, I knew I was draining the swollen sac around her heart and not her heart. Once my syringe was full, I connected IV tubing to the needle and watched as pink fluid continued to flow into the basin on the floor. With every beat, her heart filled more with blood and pumped it to her lungs, her brain, and the rest of her body. Her breathing gradually slowed, and color gradually returned to her face. After ten minutes the last of the drainage stopped and I removed the needle. The woman's heart rate, breathing, and blood pressure were nearly normal, and for the first time she opened her eyes and smiled!

Several weeks later we discharged her to her home in another village, with enough TB meds for a month. By the end of six months, she had completed her treatment and was completely healed. But the best cure of all occurred the day she renounced her faith in the demon gods she and her family had worshipped all their lives— Bwiti and Mwiri and gave her life to Jesus. At the same time, she shared with all her family members how Jesus saved her life!

Many years later, I operated on a 10-year-old boy who was having heart failure from tuberculosis of the sac around his heart, called the "pericardium." Our pediatrician, Dr. Deborah Walker, had asked visiting cardiologist Ron Johannsen from Minneapolis to see the boy because he was having signs of heart failure. After performing a cardiac ultrasound Dr. Johannsen concluded that the tuberculosis infection in the boy's lungs had spread to the pericardium, which normally is as thin as an eyelid. The boy's pericardium had thickened to a quarter inch and in some places, half an inch thick! Dr. Johannsen suggested that we open the boy's chest under general anesthesia and remove a good portion of his pericardium. His wife had come with him, and she was an experienced cardiac nurse.

We explained all this to the boy's parents, and because their son's condition was not improving with medical treatment alone, they agreed to the procedure. On the day of the boy's operation, I had an experienced surgery resident assisting me, an anesthesiologist, cardiologist Ron Johannsen a pediatrician, and a cardiac nurse looking over the anesthesia screen! What a contrast to the day several years earlier when I had to drain fluid from the pericardium of the woman in distress by myself!

As was our custom, before starting the operation we went through a safety check, prayed together and asked the Lord to protect the boy and help us operate without any complications. Half an hour later we had the boy's chest open and were looking at the thickest pericardium I had ever seen! In places it was half an inch thick. Within minutes of cutting through it and gently dissecting it away from the heart with my finger, the boy's heart began to fill with blood and expand. Dr. Johannsen's experience was invaluable, and after half an hour of careful dissection, most of the anterior part of the boy's heart was cleared, his heart was filling well and significantly unimpeded. It was time to close and go home! A week later, the boy went home with his mother, with a return appointment to see Dr. Walker.

The world seems to be filled with the most amazing coincidences! Except they're not coincidences, are they? Romans 8:28 says, *"And we know that God causes everything to work together for the good of those who love God and are called according to His purpose for them"* (NLT). Oswald Chambers comments on this verse in his book: *My Utmost for His Highest*, *"The circumstances of a saint's life are ordained of God. In the life of the saint there is no such thing as chance. God by His providence brings you into circumstances that you cannot understand at all, but the Spirit of God understands."*

Freeing this little boy's heart from disease was one of those moments!

Chapter Five:

CHRONICLES OF GRACE

Low Tech Surgery

Not long after the drama with the mayor's wife, a young man named John came to our hospital to begin training as a nurse. As a boy he had contracted polio, and though he had survived his right leg was paralyzed and wasted. He was able to walk, but with each step he had to use his right hand to lock his right knee. This forced him to walk bent over and left him with only one hand for carrying things or working. When an orthopedic surgeon named Bob Greene came from the Congo to visit our hospital, I asked him what he thought about fusing John's knee so he could walk upright with both hands free. Bob thought it would be possible, but we would need a compression device to hold the fused knee together while it healed. We would have to innovate.

Bob came up with a simple, low-tech solution. Under spinal anesthesia he opened Jean's knee joint and sawed the lower tip of his femur, so it had a flat, horizontal plateau of bone facing downward. He then cut off the rounded the top of John's tibia, so it had a flat plateau of bone facing up. Then we put the two flat ends of John's knee together, bone on bone. To keep them compressed together until it healed, Bob drilled stainless steel nails horizontally above and below the joint, so they would be parallel to each other with their ends sticking out of the skin on both sides. To squeeze the ends of the pins together on each side of the fusion, Dr. Greene cut two-foot-long strips of rubber from a bicycle inner tube and wrapped them around nails that stuck out above and below the knee joint. The rubber strips held the pins tightly together, allowing the knee joint firmly together and his leg permanently straight.

After t wo w eeks, D r. Greene encouraged John t o s tart putting weight on the operated knee as he walked with the help of crutches. A month later we took the rubber straps off and removed the pins. John's knee had firmly fused, allowing him to walk upright and get around with one normal leg and one stiff leg. Th is left both hands free to for his work as a student nurse.

John's new confidence impacted his commitment to Christ, and after he graduated, he got a job working in a rural government dispensary. We saw him about five years later at a refresher course for nurses. John told us that he had married, and God gave him and his wife three beautiful children. Tragically, all three of them died in one year from resistant malaria. Though John and his wife were crushed with grief, they continued to serve God and others.

John not only overcame his handicap, learned to serve God and others, as well as overcome tragedy, but exemplified the lesson of Proverbs 24:16: "*The godly may trip seven times, but they will get up again. But one disaster is enough to overthrow the wicked.*"

One morning when I came to the hospital, I learned that during the night a car had brought a forty-year-old logger to the emergency room. The man had apparently broken a leg and was in severe pain. Surprised that the nurses hadn't called me during the night, I went to the emergency room where I found him lying on a gurney. His vital signs were stable, but even without removing his trousers I could see that his right leg was almost six inches shorter than his left leg! If he had a fracture, it was a really serious one!

The injured man's name was Mouloungui, and he worked for a logging company that was clearing a path for high-voltage power lines through the rain forest. His job was to fell trees with a chain saw and trim off the branches so a bulldozer could push the branches and the tree trunks away and eventually be loaded on logging trucks. Several days earlier while he was cutting a large branch with a chain saw, the large branch suddenly flipped and smashed into his right knee. Since then, he had been in severe pain and hadn't been able to stand. It had taken three days for his employer to get him out to a main road and to our hospital.

An X-ray of Moulongui's leg revealed that he didn't have a fracture but a seriously dislocated knee! The head of his tibia— which is the larger of the two bones in the lower leg below the knee — was at least six inches north of his knee joint! I was amazed that he still had pulses in his foot! I didn't want to frighten him unnecessarily about the seriousness of his injury, but I had never even seen a dislocation of the knee before and had no experience in putting one back in place! That being the case, the first thing I did was go to my office to look up what our orthopedic textbooks said about the problem!

I found several descriptions of dislocations, including some as serious as Moulongui's. The books used words like "serious," "difficult," "nerve damage" and "arterial compromise," all somber enough to inform me that he was in trouble. The textbooks also stated that if we failed to relocate his knee non-operatively, the only alternative would be surgery.

The thought of evacuating him to Libreville worked its way through my mind, but because his knee had already been dislocated for three days, further delay could be catastrophic. At the time there were three orthopedic surgeons in the country, all working in Libreville, 250 miles away on a dirt road. None of Moulingui's family members had come with him, and if I drove him to Libreville, they might not catch up to him for another two or three days. Once he arrived in Libreville, he could be one of ten or twenty other patients evacuated from around the country with serious orthopedic injuries. In light of these realities, I decided to make a cautious effort to reduce Moulingui's knee dislocation so I could save his leg.

I explained what I planned to do and asked Moulingui's permission to take him to the operating room, give him a spinal anesthetic, and reduce his dislocation non-surgically. He grunted "yes," and closed his eyes.

My OR assistant, Etienne expertly started an IV and administered a spinal anesthetic, and for the first time in a week Mouloungui was pain-free and able to sleep.

"Here's what we're going to do," I explained to Etienne with far more confidence than I felt. "We're going to pull his knee back into place slowly and carefully. It won't be easy, but God will help us."

Etienne and I bowed and prayed and asked God for his help and wisdom, then began.

Because of the spinal anesthetic, Mouloungui could feel nothing below his hips, so I planted both feet on the base of the operating table, grasped his calf and ankle and pulled with all my might. All I succeeded in doing was to drag his entire body a few inches toward my end of the OR table. It was going to take something greater than my strength to overcome an already three-day-old knee dislocation.

Then God gave me an idea. My mind's eye pictured the hand-operated come-along in my truck. That was it! If I could figure out a way to use the come-along I had up at my house and gradually pull Moulingui's lower leg down to where it belonged, the come- along would give us the power to reduce the dislocation.

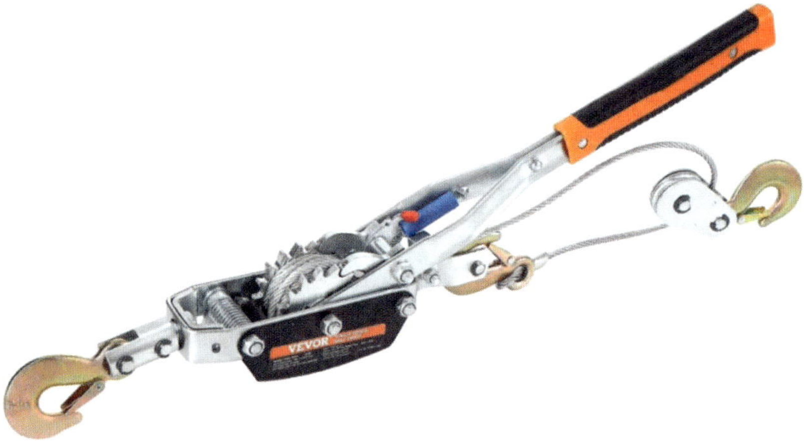

A Come-along

The end of the OR table was about six feet from a door leading to another operating room, so I nailed a 2x4 to the outside of the door frame, tied one end of a towing strap to Moulingui's foot, and hooked one end of the come-along to the 2x4 outside the door. When every- thing was ready, we locked the wheels of the OR table, and I began to ratchet the come-along. The strap tied to Moulingui's foot quickly grew taut, and Moulingui's foot began to move! Sensing victory, I continued ratcheting. His foot moved an inch, four inches, six inches!

But when we stopped to check our progress, I realized that we had only succeeded in dragging Mouloungui down the OR table!

After pulling Mouloungui back up to the top of the table, I placed a small, padded post between Moulingui's legs and into a slot in the OR table, taking care to protect his privates. This time when I cranked the come-along, the post between his legs kept him from sliding. As I resumed ratcheting the come-along, Moulingui's foot began to move towards the door! But a moment later we realized we were dragging the entire 350 pound OR table and its locked wheels towards the door, leaving Moulingui's knee *still* dislocated!

Mercifully, during all this time, Mouloungui continued to sleep. Dismayed but not defeated, we released the come-along, unlocked the wheels of the OR table, rolled it back into place, and again locked the wheels. To keep the OR table from sliding across the floor again we carried in two sturdy tables and placed them end to end between the foot of the OR table and the door frame. Once again, we ratcheted the come-along, but as the tow strap tightened, the ends of the two tables buckled up! This development led to my final epiphany, which was to seat grown male nurses on top of the two wooden tables!

When everyone was ready, I ratcheted the come-along again. The strap tied to Moulingui's ankle tightened until his foot was blue, and I began praying that the ligaments in his foot would stand up to the strain! Inch by inch, as I ratcheted the come-along Moulingui's foot began to move. I continued cranking until his left foot was parallel with his right foot. When I gently manipulated his knee the upper end of his tibia slid back into the knee joint with an audible click. We cheered as if we had scored a goal, waking Mouloungui from his nap!

After making sure he had good pulses in his foot, I applied a cylinder cast to his leg and knee, released the traction, and sent him back to his room with his leg elevated. When the anesthesia wore off, he complained about a bruise in his groin and pain in his knee, but otherwise he recovered extraordinarily well!

That evening, I stopped in to see Mouloungui and talk to him about the Lord's mercy in helping us reduce his severe dislocation without any evident complications. He expressed his thanks to us but showed no interest in thanking God. I said to him, "Mouloungui,

God did something remarkable for you today. You could have had terrible complications from your dislocation, and from what we had to do to reduce it. God protected you and helped us! Do you know that God cares about you, and sent his son Jesus to die on a cross for your sins? God says that if you believe in His Jesus, He will forgive your sins and welcome you into His family."

Mouloungui looked away, embarrassed by all the attention. "Thanks, doctor," he mumbled. "I really appreciate what you did for me today. But I have my own religion."

I nodded sadly and gave him a friendly pat on his good leg. "I'm glad we were able to help you."

A week later, I removed Moulingui's cast and started him walking with crutches. A few days later I discharged him with a letter asking an orthopedic surgeon in Libreville to check him out. Mouloungui re- turned to our hospital several weeks later and told me he never wants to see any other doctors in Libreville. Six months later, he stopped me as I was walking between buildings. I didn't recognize him until he greeted me. Incredibly, his lower leg and foot weren't even swollen!

"I suppose you know," I reminded him, "that God made our efforts succeed that day when we put your knee back in place because we prayed to Him on your behalf and asked Him to help. If He had not helped us, we might not have succeeded and was God who kept you from any complications!" He nodded and smiled politely but clearly did not want me to continue. The last I heard he was living the way he had lived before the accident, as though God had never done anything for him at all. Sometimes the best success stories turn out to be quite sad.

James 4:13-17 says it all: "*Look here, you who say, 'Today or tomorrow we are going to a certain town and will stay there a year. We will do business there and make a profit.' How do you know what your life will be like tomorrow? Your life is like the morning fog—it's here a little while, then it's gone. What you ought to say is, 'If the Lord wants us to, we will live and do this or that.' Otherwise, you are boasting about your own pretentious plans, and all such boasting is evil.*"

Not *My* Child, Lord!

One of my most difficult moments came when I had to operate on my son, Jeremy. When he was five years old, Becki noticed he had a small inguinal hernia. I confirmed her diagnosis, and during the following three months we kept checking as it enlarged. Since we were not due to return to the United States for two or three more years, we decided to take care of it in Gabon.

We had two choices: drive 300 miles to the Schweitzer Hospital in Lambaréné to have it fixed by a European general surgeon or do it myself. I was operating on Gabonese children and infants almost every week for the same condition, so I felt confident that I could do as good a job on my own child.

In our operating room we put Jeremy to sleep and thirty minutes later, the operation was over. The next day he was up and running around more than he was supposed to! On the fourth day, he began to complain of pain in his abdomen, and that evening he ran a low-grade fever. He didn't want to eat supper. and by morning the pain had localized to the area of his appendix. The operative incision looked healthy, but I began to wonder if I had done something wrong. Again, we were faced with a choice: treat him ourselves, including possible surgery for acute appendicitis, or go to Schweitzer Hospital in Lambaréné. Although it was the week before Christmas, we decided to go to Lambaréné, in part because the Schweitzer Hospital had a more sophisticated laboratory than ours and could perform tests that might prove helpful. Besides, I was not enthusiastic about operating a second time on my own son!

We left Bongolo around noon. Jeremy was uncomfortable during the six-hour ride over rough, dirt roads, but his condition didn't worsen. We arrived in Lambaréné around 6:00 p.m. A short time later, a pediatrician came to examine him. Her husband was the hospital surgeon, and he examined Jeremy as well. To our relief, they both agreed that Jeremy's condition did not warrant surgery. As a special courtesy they let us stay in one of their fully furnished guest houses.

The next morning Jeremy was hungry, and his blood tests were normal. The two doctors reexamined him and concluded that he did not have appendicitis and was improving. They thought he might have been suffering from a virus and agreed with me that it was safe for us to return to Bongolo. We arrived home on Christmas eve and had one of the happiest celebrations ever!

Not all missionary stories involving sick children turn out this well. On January 17, 1938, missionaries Louis and Carol Klein's identical twin daughters were born prematurely at Schweitzer Hospital. Baby Beth weighed 4 pounds and baby Alice weighed 3. In those days, breastfeeding was considered to be inferior to powdered milk, so from birth, the twins were fed powdered milk. Both babies vomited their feedings frequently, slowing their growth considerably. Dr. Schweitzer checked on them daily, but when they were a few days shy of being a month old, Alice died unexpectedly in the middle of the night. Her small gravestone still marks the spot where in 1938, the Kleins laid her to rest.

To this day, Alice Klein is the only child of missionaries who died in south Gabon. Before Dr. Schweitzer built his hospital in Lambaréné In the 1800's, missionary children under five died frequently from malaria and dysentery. Even in the early decades of the 1900's, an astonishing number of missionary women died in labor. Eventually, the missionaries built a beautiful New England style chapel near the hospital. Many American and French Protestant missionaries who died at the hospital were buried between the chapel the nearby Ogoué River. The church has long since collapsed into rubble, but when the grass is cut, the graves of many of the forgotten missionaries and their children can still be seen.

In 1974, Carol Klein looked ahead to the last visit she would make to that cemetery to see her daughter Alice's grave. Before her visit she wrote, *"We will proceed downriver a few miles to a steepled church on the riverbank and a cemetery where Alice, flesh of our flesh and bone of our bones, awaits the resurrection. And as I gaze at that little grave, I shall think of the hundreds of Massangou people who are being instructed today by Scripture they can read, who praise God through hymns in their own language, who have been brought to Christ through the testimony of faithful workers. And I shall thank God for giving us grace in bereavement, and for allowing us a long and fruitful ministry in Equatorial Africa. And in that moment as I hold it all within my grasp—the blue sky, the broad Ogoué River, the earthly fragrance of the rain forest, the memory of wonderful people who wrapped themselves around our hearts—I shall stand extra tall and extra firm, and I shall thank God once again for sending us as His missionaries to Gabon.*[4]

A Mustard Seed of Faith

The room was darkened, but there was enough light coming through the window of the mud-brick hospital room to see the young Gabonese nursing student lying comatose. Fluid dripped into a vein in his arm from a bottle above his bed. In the tropical heat, his face was shiny with perspiration. From time to time, a young woman sitting next to him wiped his sweaty face with a towel.

There were other family members in the room too, and they watched his steady breathing in silence, hopelessness written on their faces. His older brother, also a nurse, stood by his bed for long hours, silently praying.

Frederic was in a deep coma, and the outlook for him was grim. Three days earlier I had started him on a treatment for filaria, the hair worm that's transmitted by the bite of a small fly. It then multiplies a hundred times. Frederic's body was filled with thousands of the tiny hairlike worms we call filaria. They live the lymphatics of the skin and cause constant, intense itching. Frederic had begged me for the treatment to eradicate the pests, and I had refused. Filaria were not life-threatening, but the dangers of a lethal reaction to the treatment could be fatal. Frederic knew my warning was true, but he still wanted the treatment. After holding him off for several months, I finally agreed, on the condition that his older brother would supervise the careful process of taking the medication, and that at the first sign of a headache he would stop taking the medication.

During the first and second days he took the minuscule doses I prescribed and experienced the usual symptoms of fatigue and heaviness. On the third day, he began having severe, unrelenting headaches. Instead of stopping the treatment as I had instructed him, he took the third dose and went to bed. In the morning, he didn't wake up.

Frederic's fellow students brought him to the hospital as soon as they saw what happened, and I immediately and regretfully began

4 *We Went to Gabon*, by Carol Klein (p.180-81)

a course of drugs to decrease the swelling of his brain and other organs. In spite of my treatment, he ran a high fever and worsened by the hour.

As we went about our work that day, a black cloud hovered over our staff. Instead of the usual smiles there was heaviness. Uppermost in our minds was a similar case we had seen a year before when a pastor's daughter who was taking the same medication went into a coma that lasted for weeks. When the elders of the church anointed her with oil and prayed for her, she came out of the coma but remained partially paralyzed and unable to talk. Realizing that she would probably not improve, she gave up the will to live. A month later she died.

I had promised myself after her death that I would never prescribe the treatment again, and now it had happened once more. Every day on rounds that week as I looked down at Frederic's swollen and feverish body, I asked God to heal him and to spare him from what had happened to the pastor's daughter.

Standing by his bed on the fourth day of his coma, God spoke to me and said, "If all of you pray and believe, I will heal him! If you don't all pray, I will do nothing. This has happened to show My power."

A moment later I was filled with self-doubt. Perhaps I didn't really hear God and was just thinking what I wanted to believe! Maybe I imagined it! But what I did know was that God wanted me to step out in faith. After all, if we didn't pray God wouldn't heal!

I looked around the room at the students, all of them young and immature Christians. Most had never even attended a prayer meeting, so how could I get them to come together to pray and really believe? None of them had ever seen a person healed, and neither had any of our Gabonese nurses. Meanwhile, despite the best treatment I could devise, Frederic's condition was not improving.

As I looked into the faces of the students the Lord affirmed what he had said to me before: "I want everyone to see My power and believe in Me." I invited everyone to a prayer meeting that night at the church, which just 30 yards from the hospital.

By 8:00 p.m. about twenty of us were gathered. I opened my Bible to Mark 9:23 and read aloud the words of Jesus: *"Everything is possible for him who believes."* I looked around at the young faces. They seemed to be saying, "Really? Everything?" Or was it the questioning of my own heart?

I then turned to Matthew 9:29 and read: *"According to your faith will it be done to you."* If only it could be true for Frederic! One by one we began to pray. Some prayed with hesitancy, others with great fervor. For the next hour we sang choruses and hymns in Yinzebi and French.

After some time, I stood and read again the words of Jesus, this time from Matthew 17:20 and 21: *"I tell you the truth, if you have faith as small as a mustard seed, you can say to this mountain, 'Move from here to there' and it will move. Nothing will be impossible for you."*

That verse seemed to instill true hope in our hearts. There was a longing to believe and not doubt that God would heal Frederic. In my own heart there came the conviction that because we were praying and believing, God would bring healing. Now many began to entreat the Lord for faith to believe for Frederic's healing. As it grew late some left, but many stayed, alternately praying, singing and sharing Scriptures. At midnight, weary from the day's work, we said our good night's and went home to bed, trusting God would do what we asked.

In the morning as we started our hospital rounds, there was an air of expectancy; but when we entered Frederic's room, it vanished. His condition had not visibly changed. His mother sat weeping in a corner of the room, her tears falling silently onto the floor. As I tried to take refuge in studying Frederic's chart, the Lord once again spoke to me. This time He brought to my mind one of the verses I had read the night before: *"According to your faith will it be done to you"* (Mat- thew 9:29). The Lord wanted us to believe in spite of what we saw.

I encouraged those in the room, "Let's not stop believing that God will heal Frederic! God wants all of us to believe—not just me and our missionary nurses, but all of us who prayed! This is not the time to wonder if maybe it isn't God's will! This is the time to insist before the Lord that we are trusting Him to heal Frederic!"

At 2 p.m. that afternoon, Frederic regained consciousness! Those who had nurtured in their hearts the mustard seed of faith were not surprised and rejoiced! "God heard us and healed him!" one student exulted. But the healing was only partial. He was awake, yes, but he could not talk, and he could only walk with two people holding him up. We had asked God for total healing, so we continued to pray for him.

Three days later, I brought a very shaky Frederic to the Bible study we held in our home every Friday night for our male nurses and nursing students. After the Bible study, we laid hands on Frederic and prayed for his complete recovery. His improvement during the following week was dramatic. He began to talk and soon was able to walk unassisted. But because his eyes could not focus, he still couldn't read or write.

The following Friday night Frederic asked us to l ay hands on him again and pray, this time for his eyes and hands so that he could read and write and resume his classes. The students prayed boldly for their classmate.

Over the next six weeks Frederic recovered completely, caught up on his studies, and resumed working at the hospital. For all of us, he was living, walking proof of the power of God, and when we ask Him to do the impossible, the importance of unified and persistent faith. Would we have learned the power of perseverance in prayer if God had healed Frederic immediately? We would certainly have celebrated and rejoiced, but we would not have learned the importance of perseverance in prayer.

Makaya

The little man sitting in front of me was upset. His name was Makaya, and the dusty fan wobbling in the comer did little to move the sticky air in my office. I waited for him to decide whether or not he was going to follow my advice to remain in the hospital until we got his irregular heartbeat controlled or reject my advice and risk dying on the four-hour trip home.

"Doctor, I did not come here prepared to stay. The car that brought my wife and I for this checkup is waiting. We didn't come with money to pay for a stay in the hospital or buy food for a long stay."

"Makaya," I said firmly, "your heart has a very dangerous rhythm. It could stop suddenly while you're on your way home." I could picture him bouncing around in the back of an open pickup truck for three hours over the rough dirt roads. "You must stay here until your heart is regulated."

He sighed heavily. "Very well, I'll stay. But if I'm to eat, I'll need some money. Will you lend me $75?"

Surprised, I grappled with the implications of his request! Did it make sense for me, the doctor, to start loaning patients money so they could pay their bills? If I made it a habit, I'd soon be a pauper! Besides, I didn't have $75 in Gabonese money. Just then the Lord brought to mind what He said to His disciples in Matthew 5:43, *"Give to those who ask, and don't turn away from those who want to borrow."* They were words from Jesus's Sermon on the Mount, and they weren't just a suggestion. I paused to take a deep breath, smiled, and said "yes." I would give him the money in the morning so he could pay his hospital bill and buy food. Relief and gratitude spread across his face.

Most of our beds were taken, so I instructed the ward nurse to find a bed for Makaya in one of our few private rooms. The next morning when I walked into his room, I was shocked! The nurses had put him in a room with a woman named Brigitte! She was recovering from a hysterectomy, and I had promised her that she and her daughter would have the room to themselves! Worse yet, the mother and daughter were sharing one the beds in the room, and Makaya and his wife were sleeping in the other one! I couldn't believe the nurses had not informed me of the problem! I quickly apologized to all four of them for the embarrassing situation and immediately set out to find another room. Unfortunately, there weren't any other free rooms or beds! When I explained the situation to the four roommates, Brigitte smiled and shrugged.

Makaya had retired from the civil service several years before. He and his wife lived in the town of Tchibanga, a four- hour drive to the west. I didn't know it at the time, but for years missionaries working in Tchibanga to him about the Lord. His job was delivering messages between different government officials in town, so he was always in a hurry running here or there and never had time to talk to them. Besides, as a devout Catholic he wasn't interested in the

Protestant religion. From my brief contact with him, he really didn't seem to know the Lord. Brigitte, however, was a faithful and enthusiastic believer. She had come from eastern Gabon and a distance of 800 kilometers to have her surgery done at Bongolo Hospital. Our African nurses had been impressed by her quiet and gentle spirit.

Several days later I made rounds again, and as I entered Makaya and Brigitte's room, I could see that the two families had become friends. I asked if either of them would like to move to another room, since we now had a private room available. Much to my surprise, both couples declined! Seeing the look of surprise on my face, Makaya explained that he and his wife had prayed with the hospital chaplain the night before and had invited Jesus into their hearts! Now that they had found the Lord, they wanted to take every opportunity to learn more!

Several days later, both couples were ready to go home. Makaya's heart arrythmia had been controlled with medication, and Brigitte and her husband were ready to return to eastern Gabon. I prayed with all four of them, committing them to the Lord Jesus. A month later, I drove my family to the coast for a week. The trip took us through Tchibanga, and we stopped at the church to deliver some books to the local pastor, and he seemed very happy to see us. "How are things going?" I asked.

"Well," he said, his face beaming, "the church is overflowing every Sunday. We don't have enough room for all the people who are coming to the Lord!" This was wonderful news indeed. "You know," he added thoughtfully, "there's a fellow who's attending the church now who found the Lord at Bongolo Hospital. He and his wife attend every meeting, and they have brought many others into the faith in Jesus too."

"Is his name Makaya?" I asked.

"Why, yes!" he exclaimed, slapping his hands together. "That's him! What a blessing he has been to me and to this church!"

When I saw Makaya again for his three-month checkup, his heart was ticking along smoothly. He thanked me and praised the Lord for restoring his health. Then, he took out $75 in Gabonese bills and handed it to me. Somewhat confused, I asked him what the money was for. A look of amusement crossed his face.

"Doctor, I'm repaying you the money you loaned me. Don't you remember?" Embarrassed at my lapse of memory, I laughed and took the bills. He became serious as he stood up to leave.

"You know, doctor, you're one of the reasons I found Jesus. When you loaned me that money, I knew God was at your hospital, and that you knew and loved God. You hardly knew me, and you had no way of getting the money back if I didn't bring it. When Brigitte began talking to me about Jesus, I had already decided I wanted to follow Jesus."

I could barely choke out a goodbye as he left. It had never entered my mind that by loaning Makaya $75—a stranger at the time, God would use my gift to lead Makaya and his wife to faith.

Makaya believed in Jesus because of sacrifices—not just my miniscule sacrifice, but the even greater sacrifice that Brigitte and her daughter made by sharing their hospital room with complete strangers and then leading to faith in Jesus! But there were other, even greater sacrifices made by the thousands of believers who sent us to Gabon and helped to sustain and extend the ministries of Bongolo Hospital. It takes sacrifices to free people who previously were under the curse of demon gods and live in God's forgiveness and light. It is the sacrifices of God's people that sends the light of Jesus to places where previously there was only darkness. It's a light so bright that it dispels the curse of demon gods and brings in its place God's forgiveness, life eternal, and joy to those who were perishing.

Panga

As the years rolled by, Bongolo Hospital grew larger and busier, and so did our three children. At first, we tried taking a vacation with them in Libreville, the capital city. Our mission had a small guest house where we could stay when in the city when there was room. Libreville's beaches were lovely, but sometimes French ladies would walk down the beach topless. There were private beaches farther up the coast, but they were privately owned and climbing over fences and past "no trespassing" signs was nerve-wracking! We knew there were lovely beaches on God's southern coast just six hours west of Bongolo, near a small town called Mayumba. A couple of times we tried staying in a rented house, but it had rats, unscreened windows, and sleeping under mosquito nets in a closed-up house that had no screens was unbearably hot!

Eventually, we bought a tent and a 30 x 40-foot tarpaulin that we set up on a beach south of Mayumba. Our kids loved it but setting up the camp entailed digging an outhouse, hauling water from town every other day, and cooking over a fire. At least twice a week and sometimes in the middle of the night a thunderstorm came that would roar down on our lovely camp, blow down our tarp and tents and leave us and everything we owned soaked. Everything! One memorable night, the storm broke the ridgepole on our family's tent at 2 a.m. in the morning. I was able to keep the tent intact by holding he two ends of the broken ridge pole together, but it was a very long night of standing like Atlas to keep our tent from collapsing while the family slept!

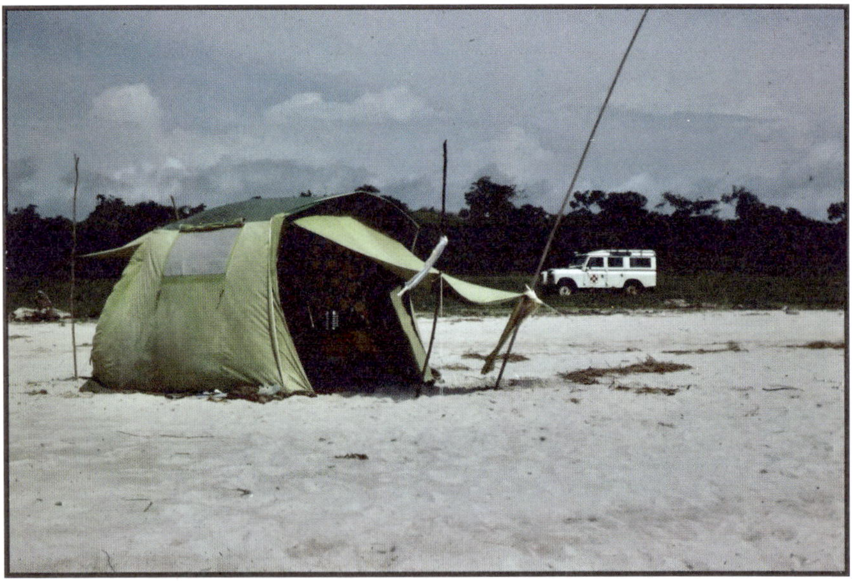

The next year, a French businessman named Bernard invited us to stay in his cabin near a village called Panga. His cabin was on a grassy hill overlooking the beach, and just 100 yards from the beach. The village of Panga was twenty miles north of Mayumba, and the cabin was a mile from the village. The cabin had a living room, three bedrooms, a kitchen with a gas stove, and a bathroom!

A 55-gallon drum collected water off the roof, and the cabin was fully furnished. We were delighted and accepted Bernard's offer.

A week before our planned trip, I drove to Bernard's house and got the key to his cabin. The drive to Panga took 4 hours, and the final five miles through the jungle to the village was so rough we could only advance in 4-wheel drive and low gear. Bernard's cabin was a mile from the village on a grassy hill that overlooked the ocean and a pristine beach. The view was so beautiful we were ecstatic! The cabin looked like it had been thrown together by a bunch of high school students, but it was far better than a tent and tarps! After moving our stuff into the cabin, we hiked 100 yards down to the beach in our bathing suits. The surf was perfect for body surfing, and Becki found hundreds of seashells, some of them spectacular. After an hour of exploring and swimming in the surf, we climbed back up the hill to the cabin, ate a hearty supper, and after putting sheets and pillows on the beds, went to sleep. The sound of the ocean soon lulled us to sleep.

Around 1 a.m., Becki and I heard what at we thought at first were mice in the wall just six inches from our heads. The inside walls of the bedrooms had been adorned with split bamboo, leaving a one-inch space between the outside walls of rough boards and the bamboo slats. Eventually we realized the squeaking noises were bats that had moved in, and for the rest of the night they squeaked and scratched the bamboo just inches from our pillows! The next morning, we awakened bleary-eyed and tired. But with such a lovely beach all to ourselves, we decided to chase the bats away later, eat a hearty breakfast, and spend the morning at the beach!

Around noon we climbed the hill and were sitting down to a simple lunch when a pick-up truck drove up and a white- haired Frenchman stepped out, accompanied by his 20- year-old Gabonese girlfriend. I stood out on the porch as they drove up, and as the Frenchman got out of his car he said, "What the %&!!$ are you doing in my cabin?"

I said, "*Your* cabin? This is Bernard's cabin, and he told us we could spend a week here! He gave me the key last week!"

The Frenchman pointed his finger at me and shouted, "Bernard is not the owner of this house, I am! I built it, not him, and I'm his father!"

Astonished, I said, "Bernard told us it was his cabin! I'm sorry if Bernard didn't tell you, but he didn't tell us anything about you being the owner. Don't you and your son talk to each other?"

That was too much for the Frenchman and he shouted back, "I don't have to talk to my son about my house! He's supposed to talk to me! And I say you need to leave!"

We were not in a position to refuse, and by now the kids had appeared and were huddled behind us. Seeing them, the Frenchman turned to his girlfriend and said to her, "This is crazy!"

She shrugged and said, "Let them stay! We can sleep in the bedroom they're not using."

Becki and I sighed and took a deep breath. It was too late to drive home, and the kids wanted to spend more time at the beach. So, we cleared our belongings out of the living room and kitchen and spent the rest of the afternoon at the beach. Sharing the kitchen to cook supper that evening was awkward, so we ate supper on the porch and went to bed early. The kids wanted to spend the morning at the beach, so we decided to go down in the morning, then pack up and go home after lunch.

That afternoon while the kids played on the beach, Becki and I drove over to a hill half a mile away that was higher than the hill the Frenchman's house was on. It had an even more spectacular view of the beach and the ocean.

I said to Becki, "Wouldn't this be a beautiful place to build a cabin for our team?"

Becki laughed, and said, "In your dreams, David! Who would give money for a beach cabin? Who would build it? And with everything you're doing you certainly couldn't do it!"

The grass was about eight feet high, and we had to get up onto our roof rack of our SUV to really see the view. As I was looking at the waves and the beautiful beaches below, the Lord said to me very clearly, "David, I will build it!"

I was so surprised I turned to Becki and said, "Honey, the Lord just said to me, 'I will build it!' He's going to build us a cabin here on this hill, so we and our teammates will have a place to go and rest and play with their children!"

Becki laughed again and said, "Well, I didn't hear anything, so don't get your hopes up!" But my hopes were up, and though I knew it would take a miracle, I also knew that we served a God who loved us and was always doing miracles!

The next year, we returned to the U.S. to speak in Alliance churches, raise our support for the next four years, and raise money for the hospital's most urgent building needs. Several months later a builder in our church named Marvin Root came to me and asked if there was a way he could help us in our ministry. A light bulb flashed in my head, and I said, "Yes, Marvin! Our missionaries have nowhere to go during their vacations, and God showed us a beautiful spot on the southern coast of Gabon. Could you help me design a cabin that could house two families at a time, and that we could build?"

His eyes widened in excitement, and he said, "I would love to do that for you! Tell me what you're thinking about!" After we talked for an hour Marvin went to work and I went back home, praying for God's blessing on the project. A few weeks later Marvin showed me a beautiful plan for a cabin that would be up on 4-foot hardwood stilts. This would provide a better view of the ocean and beaches and better protection from termites. It would have two large bedrooms, each with two bunkbeds and a queen bed, a living-room sized front porch with a view of the ocean, and a roomy kitchen. Each bedroom would have a bathroom that included a shower. Water would be collected from the roof and stored in a tank below the house, then pumped to a water tower.

Then Marvin said something that took my breath away: "If God provides for the project, I will come with my wife Sherrie and our four children, and together we'll build your vacation cabin!" One piece at a time, God was putting the project together!

But how would He provide the money? Thinking ahead, I wrote a one-page explanation of what it would cost to build a cabin in Panga, which at the time was $20,000. I entitled it, "A Vacation Cabin for Gabon's Missionaries." That year, Becki and I spoke in 20 or more churches in the United States to raise our support with the Christian & Missionary Alliance. In every church, we put up a display of Bongolo Hospital that included photos and explanations of the needs. I also included a one-page proposal to build a vacation house in Panga. But at the end of the year, not a single person had taken the Panga flyer! I was so disappointed that I asked the Lord, "Father, did I misunderstand you? Next week we'll be on a plane back to Gabon, and nobody has given us a dime for the cabin!" But the Lord didn't answer.

A week before we were scheduled to get on a plane back to Gabon, my surgeon friend Pokey Cleek asked me to assist him with an operation he had scheduled. As we were scrubbing at the sink outside the operating room Dr. Cleek said, "Uh…David, do you have a project for the hospital that I could help you with? Something that would benefit or encourage the whole team, or…whatever?" Trying to sound calm I told Pokey about the beach house we wanted to build so our missionaries had a place to go with their families for vacation. At the end of my explanation he said, "Great! We'll send you a check of $10,000 for that!" I humbly thanked him, and as I finished scrubbing, he stepped into the operating room.

Before I went into the operating room I said, "Thank you, Lord! This wonderful! But we can't build this cabin for $10,000, we need $20,000!" I sighed and joined Dr. Cleek in the O.R. As we prepared to start, he said, "By the way, David, I didn't ask you what the vacation cabin is going to cost to build. What's it going to cost?"

As calmly as I could, I said over the pounding of my heart, "$20,000."

"You got it!" Pokey said. As I thanked him and started the operation, I said to Jesus in my heart, "You're amazing, Lord! Just amazing!"

A few months later and back in Gabon again, I went to Panga to meet with the village chief and ask her permission to build our vacation cabin on the hill we had picked out. The chief was an elderly woman, and when I asked her, she looked at me and said, "Doctor, you've forgotten me already! How could I refuse your request? You operated on me five years ago when I was bleeding to death from fibroid tumors of the uterus!" It had been ten years since then, and I hadn't recognized her!

Later, the provincial government gave us a deed for the entire hill we hoped to build on. Six months later, Marvin Root arrived in Bongolo with his family. Before he came, he had sent me a list of hardwood lumber we would need to purchase from a local sawmill and truck to Panga, as well as plywood and roofing tins from Libreville. I hired a truck to deliver the hardwood needed for the posts the house would sit on, the 2"x10" hardwood beams that would be under the floors, and hardwood for framing the roof. Later, we sent another truckload of aluminum roofing tin and cement to pour footings for the posts the house would sit on.

During the Root family's first two weeks in Bongolo, Marvin prefabricated the walls, using hardwood two-by-fours and treated plywood. We then hired an additional 5-ton truck to take the prefab walls to the building site.

To house the Roots while they were building the cabin, Becki and I rented the best house we could find in the village of Panga for the Root's family of six. It American terms, it was "a shack," though at the time it was one of the better shacks in the village! The walls were made of rough boards and there was no ceiling. The shack had three tiny bedrooms, each with a double bed frame, worn mattresses, and mosquito nets. Though the house had cement floors it had no ceilings. The living room was 8-foot by 10-foot and had just one window. Of course, none of the windows were screened, there was no running water, no electricity and an outhouse for a toilet! They would have to cook over a small, gas stove and wash their dishes outside the kitchen in a simple aluminum basin.

The only car we had for them was a small Suzuki Samurai. That meant that every morning, all six of the Root family would have to pile into the five seat Suzuki for the 1-mile drive to the work site! Since their only lights were kerosine lanterns, they had to get home every evening well before sundown!

On the Roots first trip to Panga, Becki and I drove out with them, carrying their bags, a kerosine refrigerator, food supplies, and several of their kids. When we were within a half a mile of Panga the skies opened in a violent rainstorm. Our 4WD SUV promptly got stuck in a mud hole. As rain poured down in buckets, I dragged my winch cable 50 yards to the nearest tree and wrapped the cable around it. But when the winch started pulling, our SUV stayed in the mudhole while the tree fell down! We tried again on a second tree and brought it down too! The third tree held, and this time our winch dragged us out of the mudhole. By then I was totally soaked and covered with mud!

That afternoon after the rain stopped, we moved into their shack, then drove up to the building site and set up our ten. We tried to join them every weekend to help with the building and to bring additional food and supplies. On one of those occasions, I was walking on the beams that would hold up the plywood floors when my foot slipped and I fell, breaking several of my ribs! After that I stayed out of their way! One of our enduring memories was watching the two youngest girls paint the cabin's plywood floors, hanging upside down from the rafters!

One day when the family arrived back in their shack there was a chair with three legs sitting in front of their door. That night, Marvin made a new leg for it and left it outside their door the next morning. The next night and many nights after, another three-legged chair would be waiting for them. Though he never told us how many chairs he fixed, Marvin fixed every chair the people brought to him.

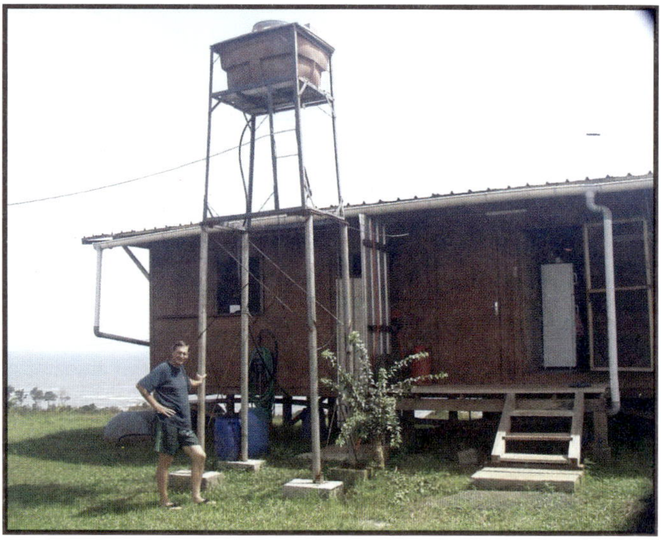

The Completed Panga Cabin!

That was the beginning of a church in Panga. It eventually grew to around 20 believers who met every Sunday in the chief 's house. A decade later, Becki and I helped the Christians build a 20-foot x 30-foot church building. The chief 's son eventually became the l ay pastor, and he led the church for years.

The sacrifices of Dr. Cleek, Dr. Cleek's family, and the Root family for the missionaries and for the people of Panga caused God's name to be exalted to the highest heavens and His glory to shine in Gabon!

Psalm 112:1-6 says it best: "*Praise the Lord! Blessed are those who fear the Lord, who find great delight in His commands. Their children will be mighty in the land; the generation of the upright will be blessed. Wealth and riches are in their houses, and their righteousness endures forever. Even in darkness light dawns for the upright, for those who are gracious and compassionate and righteous. God will come to those who are generous and lend freely, who conduct their affairs with justice. Surely the righteous will never be shaken; they will be remembered forever.*"

Forgiven

The young woman was feverish, crying and holding her abdomen in severe pain as I examined her in the emergency room. I concluded that Anne Marie had an abscess in one of her fallopian tubes. Since I was afraid it might rupture, I took her straight to the operating room. It was a Saturday morning during a national holiday, so most of the experienced OR staff were across the river for the celebrations. Only one of the two nurses who were on call for the operating room showed up when I sent a message for her to come. Unfortunately, she had worked in the operating room only once before! Four of our five missionary nurses were on vacation, leaving me with no alternative but to ask the inexperienced nurse to circulate. For those who don't know what that means, it's the circulating nurse who makes sure the surgeon, his assistants, and the anesthetist have everything they need as the operation progresses.

We were short-staffed everywhere, but I finally drafted a first-year nursing student to be my surgical assistant. She had never been in the operating room before and was terrified. However, after seeing Anne Marie crying in pain and hearing my assurances that I would show her what to do, she agreed to help.

I made a conscious effort to relax as I explained to my two rookie assistants what they needed to do. We rolled Anne Marie into the OR on the gurney, slid her onto the table and positioned her for a spinal anesthetic. The circulating nurse didn't know where the blood pressure cuff or stethoscope was, so I found them for her. I set my OR assistant to scrubbing her hands and arms at the scrub sink while I opened the surgery packs and washed the patient's back with disinfectant for the spinal anesthetic. The circulating nurse looked dazed when I explained how the table controls worked, so to keep my gloves sterile I manipulated the controls with my right knee and foot to raise and lower the table the way I wanted it.

Anne Marie was writhing in pain and would not lay still for the spinal. Eventually, the circulating nurse understood how to hold her on her side in the fetal position, so I could get the spinal needle in the right place in Anne Marie's back and administer the anesthetic. As it began to work, our patient's pain disappeared, and she slept.

By this time, my surgical assistant had scrubbed her brown hands and arms nearly pink. She didn't know how to dry her hands or put on a gown or gloves without contaminating herself, so I made her stand in the middle of the floor with her hands and arms in the air until I could do it for her. Eventually I got us both gowned and gloved and on opposite sides of the OR table.

Nobody had remembered to shave the patient, so we waited another five minutes while the circulating nurse located a razor blade and shaved Anne Marie's abdomen to my satisfaction. While she was doing this, the IV ran out. She hunted around for another bottle but couldn't find one in the OR, so told her to go to the pharmacy for more IV bottles. When she came back, I used an instrument to scrub the patient's abdomen with disinfectant and draped her with sterile towels and drapes for surgery.

About that time Anne Marie started looking pale and clammy, the blood pressure alarm went off, and the oxygen alarm clipped to her finger began chirping. I worked the controls to the OR table with my knee and foot and lowered the head of the table so that her head was lower than her feet, which brought her blood pressure back up. I was counting to ten for the third time and was on the verge of ripping my gown and gloves off to do things myself when the circulating nurse triumphantly returned with three full IV bottles. They had no hooks on them, so we waited another three minutes while she rigged up a halter out of rolled bandages and hung one of the bottles on the IV pole.

Just then, the blood pressure alarm again sounded again. My patient was going into shock! Contaminating my gloves and robe, I quickly inserted a large IV needle into a vein in the girl's other arm. Once I got the IV going, I let saline pour into her vein rapidly until her blood pressure stabilized and *my* heart rate returned to normal! Then I changed into another sterile gown and put on a fresh pair of gloves.

The spinal anesthetic did not work as well as I had hoped, providing adequate anesthesia to only the lower half of my patient's abdomen. Because of that, I made a low transverse incision well be- low her navel. My rookie assistant clutched the drapes and swayed a bit at the sight of blood spurting here and there, but she managed to stay upright and hang onto the retractors we used to keep the incision open.

The pelvic abscess in Anne's lower abdomen had ruptured, and things were a bit messy. I had to pack a large abdominal compress into the upper abdomen to hold the intestines away from the uterus, ovaries and fallopian tubes, but because the anesthesia level was low, our patient reacted to my pushing her intestines around and vomited. The circulating nurse got an emesis basin to Anne's mouth thirty seconds too late, but at least the girl didn't inhale what she threw up and aspirate!

To clean out the mess in her abdomen, I had to suction, pull, clamp, cut and tie. All this activity served to aggravate Anne Marie's discomfort, and she began to moan and squirm on the table. When several loops of intestine popped out of the wound, my young assistant nearly fainted. I could have instructed an experienced circulating nurse to give an additional anesthetic intravenously, but the nursing student helping us didn't know where anything was. Somehow, we managed to keep going. When the only thing left to do was to close the abdomen, we were almost home!

I placed a drain into the cleaned-out abscess cavity and suctioned out the last bit of pus while Anne Marie groggily fought to get off the table. Somehow, I managed to sew the abdominal cavity closed. After that, Anne Marie quieted down, and my assistant regained her usual color. I felt badly that Anne Marie had experienced so much pain, but we had gotten her through the operation, and she would live.

For the first three days, Anne Marie did well. Her fever disappeared, her pain diminished, she got out of bed and walked around, and she drank some liquids. I treated her with intravenous antibiotics and checked on her every day. But on the third day her temperature spiked to 105 degrees, and she complained of bloating. Her lower abdomen was again tender and swollen.

I got an X-ray and when I saw it, I felt sick. The X ray revealed a ribbon-like irregular white streak in her lower pelvis that confirmed my worst fears: she would need a second operation. Several hours later in the operating room, this time with an experienced OR crew, I removed the abdominal compress I had left in her abdomen during the first operation. Afterward I showed Anne Marie's husband the compress I had just removed, now wrapped in a plastic bag.

"I left this compress in your wife's abdomen during her first operation," I explained. "That's why she didn't get better." Her husband looked at the bag in horror.

"Will she get better now?" he asked faintly. I assured him that she would. The relief on his face was wonderful.

"Thank you, doctor," he breathed, "thank you!"

He obviously didn't understand what had happened, so the next day I explained it to him again, this time adding that we would not be charging him for his wife's second operation and that we would be refunding their money for the first one. At that he blinked in surprise.

"Doctor, I can't take your money back!" he said earnestly. I assured him he could, and that I wanted him to because my mistake had caused his wife a serious complication. Thinking he needed some time to think about it. I told him I'd see him the next day.

The next morning, I instructed the hospital cashier to refund the money the couple had paid for the first operation. About midway through the morning, the circulating nurse brought a message from the cashier—Anne Marie and her husband were very upset and wanted to see me as soon as possible. I was not surprised. They were finally understanding the seriousness of my error. With a heavy heart, I headed to their room. Anne-Marie was sitting up on the bed talking to her husband when I entered. Her welcoming smile caught me off guard.

"Doctor!" she said happily when I entered her room, "I feel so much better today!"

I smiled nervously and glanced at her husband. He looked troubled. Then her smile faded.

"Please, doctor," she said, "we don't understand. The cashier came and tried to give our money back to, but we refused." She paused and looked at her husband. "We don't understand why you don't want to be our doctor anymore."

I took a deep breath and started in again, explaining that was not the issue. We couldn't accept their money after the blunder I had made in leaving a sponge in her abdomen that had put her life in danger. At that, her husband interrupted.

"If you had not operated on my wife she would have died!"

"I should have done better," I insisted. And then Anne Marie spoke words that took my breath away.

"Doctor," she said gently, reaching out and touching my arm, "why are you so hard on yourself? Nobody's perfect!"

I couldn't think of anything to reply to that!

"The important thing is that she got better, doctor," her husband added. "That's all we care about."

I could have told them that in my country a similar blunder would have cost me my reputation and my insurance company a million dollars, but I didn't. We weren't in my country, we were in theirs, where women with her condition died often, without every seeing a doctor. When I finally found my voice, I thanked them for forgiving me and assured them that I would be their doctor as long as they wanted. To make them happy, I also agreed that the hospital would keep the money they had paid for the first operation! Anne Marie went on to recover completely and went home a few days later.

Undeserved kindness somehow seems more precious than any other kind. God calls it "grace."

Chapter Six:

The Enemy Counters!

Faith Trials

In 1993, I accepted an invitation from the Christian Blind Mission to spend six weeks at the Ebolowa Presbyterian Hospital in south- ern Cameroon to learn how to better care for the many patients we encountered with eye injuries and glaucoma. I had had a month of similar training in Zaire in 1981, but I wanted to upgrade my knowledge so I could effectively treat glaucoma and operate on eyelids scarred from leprosy.

The Ebolowa Presbyterian Hospital was built between the years of 1920 and 1950. At the peak of its glory, it had a staff of five or six missionary doctors, a dentist, a nursing school and 200 hospital beds. The hospital buildings were made of brick and mortar with lovely glass windows that patients could open or close, running water, electricity and linoleum floors. The operating rooms were spacious and well-lit, but their operating tables and lights belonged in museums! Though they only had one surgeon, they had the capacity to accommodate four surgical teams at a time. In its heyday, one or two missionary surgeons supervised three to four teams of African nurse-surgeons operating simultaneously at the four tables. In the 1960s, the Presbyterian Church of Cameroon took over, and the American Presbyterian Church withdrew its missionaries. It was not a happy transition.

When I visited the hospital in 1987, it was ably directed by a dedicated Camerounese general surgeon named Dr. Daniel Ety'ala. A short-term Belgian ophthalmologist who ran the clinic and was supported by the Christian Blind Mission. It was the Belgian ophthalmologist's job to teach me to competently diagnose glaucoma, cataracts, and treat injuries to the cornea.

I quickly adapted to the routine of the eye clinic, spending most of my time assisting the ophthalmologist. African nurses in the clinic performed the initial eye examinations before sending the patients on to the doctors for further evaluation. Three or four afternoons a week, the eye team operated on patients who had surgically correctable diseases. In the evenings I studied ophthalmology textbooks for three to four hours before going to bed.

My first inkling that my faith in Christ was different from the staff of the hospital came on a Sunday morning when I attended the local Camerounese Presbyterian church. The church building had been built by the early missionaries and was well maintained. It comfortably seated two-hundred and fifty people, and a had a large stage for choirs. The service proceeded smoothly with hymn singing, accompanied by a competent pianist and several guitarists. After the offering was taken, a choir of about twenty young women took the stage. They sang in French, and I was familiar with the songs. The second song was lively and accompanied by a drummer who at certain times during the song would beat the drum in a brief staccato rhythm. Whenever he did this, the women in the choir pulled their elbows back, pushed out their chests, and shook their shoulders in unison! The effect was startling and brought laughter from the men and cheers from the women in the congregation!

I was sitting with a male nurse from the eye clinic, and when he saw the look of surprise on my face, he laughed and asked, "What do you think, doctor? Aren't the ladies great?" Since I knew he approved, I gave him a withering look and kept my thoughts to myself. In any other setting what the women did in concert with the drummer was sexually suggestive, but we were sitting in a church ostensibly to worship God! Even more disturbing to me was that the pastor smiled when it happened. I also knew it was not an African custom, because I had been in many African church services in numerous countries, and I had never seen anything like this.

After the service was over, my young friend asked what I thought, and I told him it was something one might expect to see in a bar or dance hall, never in God's house during a worship service!

Keeping a grip on my emotions I asked him why he thought it was funny? He laughed and said I was too serious.

From that moment on the nurses in the ophthalmology department—some of whom were choir members jokingly called me "Father Thompson." The next Sunday I debated if I would attend or stay home, but since I didn't know if it was a thoughtless and momentary prank, I decided to attend. I was again disappointed and did not attend again.

During the third week of my month-long immersion in ophthalmology, the ophthalmologist had the team pack up our equipment and instruments and load everything into the hospital van. The next day we headed north to a small, crumbling mission hospital for a three-day mobile clinic. During the trip, I sat in the front seat of the van and talked with the thirty-something driver whose name was Joseph. He wanted to know why I was in Gabon and why I came to their hospital. After a while, we got onto the subject of my beliefs, and I told him that I loved God, was a follower of Jesus, and did my best to obey all that God teaches in the Bible. When I asked him if he believed in Jesus, he laughed and said, "Oh yes! I'm a Presbyterian."

But the more we talked about faith in Jesus, the more irritated he seemed to get. It bothered him that I did not drink alcohol because I didn't want to get drunk, dishonor God or cause others to stumble. In response to his question about extramarital sex, I told him that the Bible clearly taught that sex outside of marriage displeases God and is harmful to those who practice it. When I told him that I'd rather please God than be rich, he laughed outright. He seemed to think I was putting on an act.

Initially Joseph's questions were couched in respectful tones, but he soon let me know that anyone who took the Bible seriously was naïve. God created the body for pleasure. To refuse to indulge was to contradict God's real intent for humans. As Joseph talked, I was struck by his complete lack of fear of God. I told him that I loved God, wanted to please him by the way I lived, and feared His anger. He just shook his head, ending the conversation.

A few hours later, we arrived at an old mission hospital. Its condition surprised and saddened me, because it had obviously been a beautiful place. The ancient hospital buildings were dilapidated and, in some cases, falling down. Years of heavy rains had washed away so much dirt around the foundations that the buildings sat up on islands of dirt a foot higher than the rest of the grounds. The pitted and uneven cement floors in the wards were swept, but the overall appearance was that of decay. The weary metal beds wore mottled from multiple coats of paint and chipped. In the wards only a few beds had mattresses, and they were deeply stained. There were few patients to be seen in either the wards or the outpatient clinic. The whole place seemed to be falling apart.

A tired-looking Camerounese doctor appeared and introduced himself as the hospital director. He gave the driver a key to the house where our team would be staying and hurried off to take care of a problem in the operating room. Joseph drove the van up to the house we were to stay in. It was an old mission house and was fifty yards from the hospital, across a main road. Grass and weeds grew two feet high on all sides. Bougainvillea had nearly taken over one half of the house! My sense of gloom deepened. Was this what Bongolo would look like in another thirty years?

We entered the front door and found the furniture and floors covered with a fine layer of dust. The once-polished hardwood was now scratched and dull with grime. Carved, hardwood living room chairs sat in a room bare of any cushions, curtains, pictures, or color. It was apparent that the house had once been a missionary family's home; now it looked more like a multi-room storeroom!

Sweeping aside cobwebs we threw open the windows and carried our bags into the bedrooms. There was no water, so Joseph went off to look for the doctor. An hour later, he returned with the news that the water would be turned on for one hour. Because electricity was so expensive, the hospital could only afford to pump water two hours a day. We took turns in the bathroom, standing in a rusting porcelain tub and pouring cold water over ourselves with a pitcher. I was grateful that I had brought my own soap and toilet paper, but I had forgotten to bring a towel. I finally used my dirty shirt to dry off and changed into clean clothes.

By the time everyone was ready for dinner, it was 8 p.m. We were hungry and ready to see the town, so we climbed back into the van and headed down a mile-long collection of dust-covered houses facing each other across a rutted, unpaved street. The hulks of abandoned and stripped cars lay every twenty feet or so on both sides of the road, shrouded in red dust. In the eerie light of the headlights, the thick dust and wrecked autos made the town look like it had taken a direct hit from an atomic bomb. We stopped at several restaurants, but every restaurant we stopped at had already closed. It looked like we would have to go to bed hungry.

Joseph, however, had hidden resources. Winding deep into the town's labyrinth of back streets, he stopped pedestrians and asked for directions. The third man he stopped apparently told him what he wanted to know, because he pulled away with a wave and drove directly to a modest, cement-block house. As we waited in the van, he talked to a middle-aged woman standing in the front door. A moment later, he motioned for us to join him.

We were pleased that Joseph had found an open restaurant and entered what seemed to be a private home. Two well-dressed young women greeted us at the door and ushered us into a spacious and well-furnished living room. There did not appear to be any tables in this restaurant, so we sat on comfortable over-stuffed chairs and sofas and watched an old French movie on a color TV that sat against the opposite wall.

The young ladies asked us what we would like to drink, and we all ordered Cokes, except for Joseph who ordered a beer. The hostesses served us peanuts and refilled our glasses as soon as we emptied them. I couldn't help thinking that the service was extraordinarily good.

About thirty minutes after we sat in what we thought was the living room, the meal arrived, and we were served where we sat. It smelled delicious and appeared to be chicken in a gravy sauce mixed with tomatoes and onions, served over rice. I know my chicken anatomy well, but as I gnawed on an odd-looking leg, I looked over at my ophthalmologist friend. He was looking hard at a lump of meat graced with several long whiskers. One of the African nurses with us noticed our perplexity.

"It's bush rat," she explained with a smile, as though she was describing spaghetti. After that, the ophthalmologist left his piece of meat alone and ate his rice. I managed to finish the meat and all my rice. As much as I hated to admit it, the bush rat was quite tasty!

About the time we were scraping the last forkful of rice off our plates, two middle-aged Cameroonese men entered the room. The young women greeted them so warmly that I assumed they were family. Our hosts escorted them to seats next to us in the living room, and the men greeted us casually. The young ladies served them glasses of wine, chatted with them for a few minutes and then turned to leave. Then, the gentleman sitting next to me grabbed one of the girls by the hand and pulled her onto his lap. She giggled in a very unsisterly way and kissed him warmly on the mouth. The other man did exactly the same thing with the other girl.

I chanced a sidelong glance at my ophthalmologist friend. He was more a man of the world than I, but when I noticed a pink flush spreading up his neck, confirming my worst fears. We were eating in a brothel!

I glanced furtively at our four African nurses, but they were watching the television as though they had never seen one before. Eventually, the men with the girls on their laps realized that the ophthalmologist and I were looking at them and looked over at us. We swung our gaze toward Joseph, who smiled and shrugged.

It was time to go, so we stood, thanked our hosts for the meal, and paid the bill. As we drove back to the hospital, it was very quiet in the van. I finally asked Joseph why he had taken us to a brothel.

"What difference does it make?" he asked defensively. "We ate, didn't we?" He was right, of course, but it didn't make me feel any better.

The next day, our team set up in two examining rooms in the dilapidated outpatient clinic and examined about sixty people for various eye problems. We found six who needed surgery and scheduled them for the next day. Lunch was served at the hospital doctor's house.

He and his wife were Dutch citizens and looked to be about twenty-five years old. Despite their youth, they had a look of desperation and impending exhaustion. I asked the doctor how it was that he was working there alone, and he explained that they had been recruited in Holland by the Cameroun Presbyterian and an adventure. The church paid their airfare and promised to pay them a monthly living allowance, but after nine months they were just surviving. Despite their best efforts, the hospital was not making enough money to pay their salaries, so during the last six months, their parents had been supporting them from Holland. I asked several leading questions but was unable to discern from their answers any evidence of faith in God. Their idea of what a missionary was and did was quite different from mine.

That afternoon, we finished up in the eye clinic around 3 p.m., so I went back to the house to rest while the others took care of the paperwork and visited old friends. There was a single sheet on my bed, so I lay down for a nap. I had just begun to doze when I heard a knock at the front door. When I opened it, I was surprised to see an attractive young woman.

"Can I help you?" I asked. She smiled as though she knew me, looked away without saying anything for a few moments, then gave me a look that only an idiot could misunderstand.

"Joseph sent me here for you," she finally explained. I was shocked but collected my wits enough to say that I was not interested. She looked disappointed and went off pouting. I was too angry to sleep, so I went for a walk.

An hour later, when I got back to the house the girl was just emerging from Joseph's bedroom. She walked by me and out the door without a word. A moment later, Joseph emerged and followed her out.

Two days later, we finished operating on our six patients and drove back to the main hospital. During the first hour of the trip, Joseph was very quiet, but halfway home he suddenly asked me, "How can someone who is used to doing wrong things stop doing them?"

Unlike our conversation during the ride up, this time he seemed sincere. So, for the remainder of our trip, I explained as clearly as I could how someone can become a child of God through repentance, faith, and obedience to Jesus Christ. To my delight, everyone in the car listened and asked questions.

A few weeks later my month was up, and we went our separate ways. I never found out what Joseph eventually decided to do about Jesus. What I did learn was that God tests us about the things we publicly say we believe—not to tempt us, but to test us and show us what's in our hearts.

Oswald Chambers wrote, *"Do not forecast where the temptation will come, it is the least likely thing that is the peril. You have remained true to God under great and intense trials, now beware of the undercurrent. Unguarded strength is double weakness. The Bible characters fell on their strong points, never on their weak ones. 'Kept by the power of God,' that is the only safety."*[5]

An Angel from the Dark Side

Christian appeared at the hospital one day complaining of terrible pain just about everywhere! He was a muscular, healthy-looking twenty-year-old, but he moaned and groaned so effectively during his examination that I finally admitted him to the hospital. During the following week he never ran a fever and seemed remarkably active for someone with such severe complaints. When, after two weeks of various creative medical therapies we proposed to discharge him, he came up with a new list of symptoms. We began to suspect he was a shirker.

Finally, one day we needed his bed for someone who was very ill, so we discharged Christian and told him to come back to the outpatient clinic when he needed treatment for something we could actually document! He nearly wept, begging to be allowed to stay anywhere on the hospital grounds. For the first time I realized Christian was afraid to leave. But why? We finally decided to let him stay in an empty storage room.

During the following weeks, we saw him often in church services and around the hospital. The chaplain talked with him for many hours, and Christian confessed to him that he had come to the hospital to escape spirits that were haunting him. For years, he said, spirits had talked to him at night, telling him to do certain things. He had tried to ignore them, but they became increasingly insistent and finally began threatening him. When someone told him that our hospital was a place where God was, he decided to visit and the moment he stepped onto the hospital grounds, the spirits that had been troubling him were subdued! After the hospital chaplain related this to me, we

5 *My Utmost for His Highest*, by Oswald Chambers, p.110

concluded he was either demonized or a budding schizophrenic. A week later, he prayed with the chaplain to receive Jesus as his Savior.

Christian was very intelligent and told us that he had completed two years at the university in Libreville, Gabon's capital city. While a student, he consulted several Ngangas to enhance his ability to learn. This was not unusual in Gabon. The Nganga sold him a sacred object called a fetish to give Christian special intelligence. Soon after, Christian began hearing voices at night, but he never associated them with the fetish. In fact, when he went back to the sorcerer to try to obtain protection and relief from the voices, the sorcerer gave him more fetishes! This only made his problems worse until he couldn't sleep at night. He finally dropped out of school. He had been unable to find relief until coming to Bongolo Hospital.

The hospital needed a new burn pit for medical trash, so we hired Christian to dig it for us. He worked so well that the hospital administrator gave him another job. When there was no more work at the hospital, we hired him to help mow the grass around the mission houses.

Christian was a member of the Bapounou tribe, and it just so happened that a retired missionary who had served among the Bapounou in Gabon came back to Bongolo for one year on special assignment. His name was Pastor Raymond Cook, and he and his wife had joined the Piersons in the 1950's to preach the gospel and plant churches among the Bapounou people. Our hospital chaplain asked Pastor Cook to disciple Christian and teach him the Bible. Every 2d5a3y after work, Christian spent an hour with Pastor Cook as they read and discussed the Bible. He showed a remarkable ability to understand the Bible, and his spiritual growth was exciting to watch. Three months after his conversion, h e w as baptized a s a public indication o f h is desire to follow Jesus.

On several occasions, Ray Cook and I asked Christian about his family, but he was curiously reluctant to talk about them. When pressed, he explained that his parents had died, and that his closet living relative was an uncle. He was terrified of his uncle and believed that it was his uncle who had sent evil spirits to torment him at the university. Before he was baptized Christian assured the pastor of the Bongolo Church that he had burned all his fetishes. All of us felt he should declare his new faith in Christ to his family before he was baptized, but he convinced us it would be better to tell them after he was baptized, not before. On Christmas day, Christian was baptized in the Louetsi River, along with ten other new believers.

Christian was one of the most exuberant Christians I ever encountered. From the day of his conversion, all he wanted to do was talk or sing about Jesus and about his deliverance from the spirits. As he mowed the lawns around the mission houses, you could hear his strong, baritone voice singing songs of praise. Except for his great fear of his uncle, he gave no evidence of mental or emotional imbalance. When asked why he was so happy, he would smile and say, "Because Jesus has set me free!" To this day I do not doubt that his conversion was genuine, though later events would leave many of us wondering.

A year later, Christian announced that he wanted to go to Bible school and become a pastor. This generated considerable discussion among the pastors and missionaries at Bongolo. Some felt it was too soon after his conversion, while others wondered about his complete isolation from his family. No one doubted his love for the Lord, or his sincerity as a follower of Jesus. He argued convincingly that his decision to follow Jesus was what separated him from his family.

A special bond developed between Ray Cook and Christian. Ray's counsel and encouragement seemed to influence Christian the most. Eventually, Ray and the church leaders decided that if Christian wanted to go to Bible School, he would have to reestablish contact with his family and inform them of his decision.

It was almost a month before Christian felt ready to go. During this time many of us counseled him and prayed with him. Although he expressed fear that his uncle might somehow strip him of his faith, he refused to let anyone accompany him. He was gone for two weeks, and during that time we prayed for him often. When he returned, we welcomed him warmly and asked him what happened. His answers were disturbingly vague. Apparently, his family had accepted his decision to follow Christ, and his uncle had not been a problem.

I felt that for some reason, Christian was hiding something from us. But in response to my questioning, he assured me he had told us everything. Something did not ring true. Several weeks later he was accepted as a first-year student at the Bible school, and moved to Moanda, 300 miles away in eastern Gabon.

It was two months before we heard from him again. He wrote in a letter that although his studies were progressing well, he was again experiencing abdominal pain. And there was something else in his letter than disturbed me—he wanted me to pray that he would "resist." My question was, "Resist what?"

About that time his fellow students at the Bible school noticed he was eating strangely. First, he stopped eating meat. For a Bible school student that was not unreasonable, since meat was expensive. But then, he stopped eating anything prepared from palm nuts. Since palm oil is about the only cooking oil available in the interior of Gabon, this posed a real problem. He began to lose weight and became increasingly eccentric, fasting first one meal a day, then one day a week, then several days or a week. At night, he sang aloud for hours, and the other students didn't recognize his songs. Then he began taking long walks in the forest. At first, he went for an hour or two, but then one day disappeared for an entire afternoon, missing some of his classes. Then one night he didn't return.

The Gabonese are afraid to be out alone at night because they believe that the night belongs to the spirits. Even on hot, humid nights, they will close every window in the house. It does not matter if the windows are screened or if the family is sleeping under mosquito nets, the windows must be closed! If asked why, they may tell you that it's to keep out thieves, but even if the windows have security bars most will be uneasy until the windows are shuttered. So, when Christian stayed out in the forest all night it could only mean that he wanted to be there and was either going mad or consorting with spirits! When he returned to school the next morning, the Pastor Moukingui, who was the Bible school dean, had a talk with him. Christian told him he had been talking with an angel. It was the angel who told him to stop eating the products of the palm tree, and to stop eating meat. It was also the angel that taught him the songs he sang at night. Eventually he admitted to Pastor Moukingui that it was the angel who led him to the forest and communed with him all night!

When Pastor Moukingui asked Christian to describe the angel, he said it was a being of great beauty, very bright and glowing like a white-hot coal. He was certain that the angel was sent by God to help him, and Pastor Moukingui was unable to convince him otherwise. On a hunch, he asked Christian if he had kept any of the fetishes from his pagan life. Christian would not admit to having them, but he refused to break off his relationship with the angel. In the end, Pastor Moukingui decided to take Christian back to Bongolo, hoping that perhaps those who had led him to Christ would be able to counsel him. Christian thought returning to Bongolo would be a good idea.

I was in my office at the hospital when Pastor Moukingui arrived. After the customary greetings and friendly banter, we got down to the subject of Christian. Moukingui recounted everything that had happened at the school. We prayed together and agreed that the local pastors should be the first to talk with Christian. Ray Cook had returned to the United States, but I promised to see Christian and talk with him after he talked with the church pastors.

The meeting between Christian and the pastors did not go well. They later said Christian was evasive and seemed distracted. He was like a closed book that nobody could open. The pastors finally told him that I wanted to see him around 7 p.m. He agreed to come if I was alone.

At 8 o'clock he appeared suddenly on my front porch. I greeted him warmly and we sat down in chairs, next to each other. He asked me to turn out the porch light, which I reluctantly did. Then I asked him how he was doing. For the next five minutes, he said nothing, and we sat in absolute silence. I prayed for wisdom and discernment, wondering if he was psychotic, spiritually troubled, or both.

Finally, Christian said, "I have learned many wonderful things since I left here."

"In the Bible, you mean?" I asked, trying to get the conversation going.

"Well," he said, "in the Bible, but from other places as well."
"What other places?" I asked.

"From an angel of God," he replied, starting to warm up. "What's this angel like?" I asked.

"He's very beautiful and very wise. He glows like a white light."
"What does he tell you?" I persisted.

"If I am obedient to God he will do miracles through me," Christian replied.

"How do you know the angel is from God?" I asked.

"Believe me," Christian answered forcefully, "I know! I can tell the difference between and evil spirit and an angel of God!"

"How?" I asked quietly.

"By what he says. He says that the Bible is true and that I am on the right path. God has sent him to lead me on that path!"

"What does he say about Jesus?" I asked.

"He says he's Jesus's messenger and spokesman," he explained. "Is it true that you haven't thrown away all your old fetishes?" I asked. His friendly mood changed immediately.

"Who told you that I have kept fetishes?" There was anger in his voice now, and I sensed the presence of great evil.

"Do you still have your old fetishes?" I asked again. "If you've kept even one, it gives Satan the right to oppress you and delude you." A minute of heavy silence passed.

"The angel told me to keep them, so I did!"

"But Christian, the Bible says that Christians must have nothing to do with the things that belong to Satan. Why would an angel of God contradict God?"

"It is an angel of God, I tell you!" he almost shouted, leaning forward in his chair. "Do you want to see him for yourself?"

A feeling of apprehension passed over me. There was indeed something terribly evil with us on that porch. I could feel the hair stand up on the back of my neck, and my arms were covered with goosebumps!

I continued, "I don't need to see your angel friend to know that he doesn't come from God and that he's deluding you, Christian. An angel of God would never permit you to keep a fetish! He's taking you off to hell, Christian. If you want to follow Jesus, you must renounce this evil angel. Otherwise, he will have you in his power forever!"

With that Christian leaped to his feet and stood over me, his hands clenching and unclenching, his breathing heavy. I sat motionless, praying for God to protect me. After a long minute, Christian relaxed and leaned against the porch wall. But he would not look at me.

Finally, I said, "Christian, you are being deceived by an angel of light. It is Satan's oldest tactic. It's what he did to Eve in the garden, when the world was new. He may look like an angel of God, but he is evil, and when he has finished with you, he will destroy you. I beg you, Christian, let me help you get free of this thing!"

Without another word Christian turned and walked off the porch into the opaque darkness. His bare feet made his departure noiseless, and the black night seemed to swallow him whole. I prayed silently for him, then got up and went into the house.

The next morning, I told Pastor Moukingui and the Bongolo Pastor what had happened. During the day, someone saw him leaving with his machete and a small shoulder bag. Without saying a word to anyone, he walked into the forest. We never saw Christian or heard from him again. Eventually, we found his uncle. He told us that he had not seen Christian since he had gone to the university in Libreville two years before. The family had thought that Christian was dead and of course knew nothing about his time as a Bible school student.

Christian's whereabouts remain a mystery. Perhaps he wandered into the nearby Republic of Congo, to Libreville, the capital city. What is important to remember, however, is that when he was questioned by all of us about fetishes (the sacred objects that give demons power over humans) Christian never answered the question. The lesson to us in James 4:7 is clear: "*So, humble yourselves before God. Resist the devil, and he will flee from you.*"

In Karl Payne's excellent book, *Spiritual Warfare*, he writes, "*When I fail to deal with my sin, I provide Satan, or more likely his helpers, the opportunity to start chipping out hand and footholds in my life. What starts as a fingertip grip will end up a firm handhold attempting to control and strangle me. I can stop the process when I choose to confess my sin rather than ignore it. But as long as I choose to play the game, I am going to pay the dues. And the longer the games go on, the more severe the consequence will become.*" [6]

"But what about the person playing games? My consistent experience is that demons will not voluntarily leave individuals who are unwilling to fully submit every area of their lives to God."[7]

6 *Spiritual Warfare, Christians, Demonization, and Deliverance*, by Dr. Karl I. Payne M.D., Republic Book Publishers, 2020, p.129

7 Ibid.

The Sting of the Curse

The young woman writhing in pain on the examining table held her hand over her left ear. She was fifteen years old, and her older sister had accompanied her to the hospital. I managed to get her to sit still long enough to look inside her ear with an otoscope. Everything looked perfectly normal. She was running a fever of about 102 degrees, but she had no other physical findings. Baffled, I gave her an antibiotic and pain medicine. The next day, her fever was gone, but the pain in her ear was worse! I examined her ear once again and everything appeared normal. She denied any history of trauma to her face, head or ear, and was able to open her mouth and close it without difficulty. Because she was in agony and the oral pain medication had not helped, I gave her an injection of Demerol. It worked for an hour, but during the night her pain came back. I increased the dose and combined it with a tranquilizer, but even that didn't help!

On morning rounds I suggested to her that God could heal her if she was willing for us to pray for her. Instead, she told us she preferred returning to her village so she could consult the Nganga.

Somewhat taken aback, I asked how she thought that would help. She was in too much pain to offer much of an explanation, but her sister explained that the girl's spirit had left her body "in vampire."

The sister's explanation sounded so bizarre I decided to ask my good friend Pastor Philippe about it. Pastor Philippe didn't seem surprised by the story. The girl was from the Mitsogo tribe, and he explained they believe that every person has a friendly spirit that inhabits their own spirit. If this friendly spirit becomes offended by something it has done it supposedly leaves and wanders around outside of the owner's body. When this happens the Mitsogo say the friendly spirit is "in vampire." When that happens, the person it has left can experience any number of violently unpleasant symptoms. For these reasons, a spirit "in vampire" is a matter of grave concern to everyone in the village. According to the Ngangas, whenever a friendly spirit leaves its host in anger, it can cause illnesses, accidents, family fights and even death in the community. The only solution, of course, is to call in the Nganga to placate the spirit and call it back into the person it left.

When the people in the girl's community learned that we were not able to help the girl, the chief and the Nganga ordered her to return to the village or face serious consequences. The pastor had counseled her and offered to help her escape from the spirit that was torturing her, but she refused.

Pastor Phillipe could see that I was skeptical, so he suggested that I take her to the village and talk to the sorcerer myself. He felt I needed to understand that the power of the spirits was not imagined or just superstition, but real. He accompanied me as we drove the girl the ten miles to her village on a back road. During the trip, the girl cried and held her head in her hands. Because of the pain, she had not been able to eat for three days and had lost weight.

The village elders were relieved to see her, and as soon as she got out of the car, they hustled her over to the Nganga's house. The pastor asked a bystander to tell the Nganga that I wanted to talk with him. A few minutes later, the Nganga emerged from his house. To my surprise he looked very ordinary and was dressed in simple clothes. There was nothing to distinguish him from any other man in the village. He greeted me with a friendly handshake and to my chagrin thanked me for bringing the girl back to her village. I asked him to explain what he thought the problem was, and not surprisingly, his explanation was almost identical to the pastor's.

The Nganga explained he planned to call the wandering spirit back into the girl that same evening, and that afterward he would send her back so that I could see for myself she was healed. As we drove back to the hospital, I expressed my skepticism.

"You will learn, doctor," my pastor friend said gently, "that evil spirits can perform miracles, too."

The next afternoon the girl reappeared at the hospital, having walked all morning from her village. She was smiling, showed no signs of illness, and related that when her "friendly spirit" come back into her body, the pain in her ear immediately ceased.

A great sadness filled me as I watched her walk away. Unwilling to place her faith in Christ, she had received a cure from Christ's defeated enemy. If she continued down the road she was on, her decision would come at the price of her soul. Her story was clear evidence that in villages more than 10 miles outside of Bongolo, the curse of the Ngangas was still very much alive.

Marie was fifteen years old and unmarried when she became pregnant. This was not unusual, since most girls in Gabon get pregnant at a young age before marrying "to prove they can have children." Sterility due to venereal disease had become so serious a problem that in proving themselves, young women almost invariably contract one or more venereal diseases. This was not Marie's concern, however.

After a long and very difficult labor at a nearby government hospital, she gave birth to a normal baby. Two days later, she suddenly went blind!

Postpartum blindness is typically referred to in developed countries as "cortical blindness." It occurs from injury to the brain's occipital cortex, with either unilateral or bilateral posterior cerebral artery blockage, making it a kind of "stroke." Fortunately, in most cases the condition is not permanent.

Marie's family brought her to our hospital the next day, expressing hope that I would be able to cure her. Though I had heard of post-partum cortical blindness, I had never seen one and was unable to find much about it in our limited medical library. When I examined Marie's eyes with an ophthalmoscope, they looked completely normal. I told the family that there was a good possibility her blindness was temporary, but I also encouraged them to pray and ask God to heal her. In any case, I thought it best to wait and see.

Unfortunately, the family thought that praying and waiting was the equivalent of doing nothing, so they took Marie to a Nganga. Most of the people in Gabon are spirit-worshippers and believe there are good spirits and evil spirits, though the "good spirits" are not totally good. If angered, they, too, can do serious harm! The Ngangas believe they can manipulate the spirits to serve them, reveal secrets, and punish their enemies through illnesses or accidents.

Revelation 12:9 says, "This great dragon—the ancient serpent called the devil, or Satan, the one deceiving the whole world—was thrown to the earth with all his angels." That means that these fallen angels are the very spirits many Africans have worshipped and feared for centuries. All spiritual beings are invisible to us, and according to the Bible, Satan and his demons are in a constant battle for the souls of men. Demons will do anything to deceive, enslave and destroy humans, even convincing them that they are really good and willing to offer their services to us for free! But what demons and Satan carefully hide is their malicious intent to deceive, dominate, and control humans so they will suffer the same fate that awaits them.

Demons were once beautiful angels, but sometime after the creation of the universe the most beautiful and powerful angel in heaven tried to overthrow God, who created him! His name was Lucifer, and when a third of the angels joined him, a great battle ensued in heaven that the rebels lost. As we read in Revelation 12:9, God threw the rebels out of heaven and down to Earth, and one day soon will throw them all into hell, a place God made specifically for them. Humans who reject God's salvation through faith in His son Jesus will suffer the same punishment.

God's obedient angels are holy and powerful and are in a constant fight against Satan and his evil spirits to save those deceived by Satan and protect Christ's followers on the earth. What the demons fear more than anything else is "The Great White Throne Judgment" that will occur at the end of time when God judges all the angels and humans who reject him.

We did not hear anything more from Marie for a month. Then one day she reappeared. Her eyesight had returned, and her family wanted me to know that it was the Nganga who cured her! While it's remotely possible that an evil spirit was responsible for Marie's restored sight, it is more likely that she suffered a known complication of childbirth that most of the time resolves after a few weeks as the body heals itself. Regrettably, the Nganga and his demons received great credit for this supposed miracle.

The last time I saw Marie I was impressed by her sadness. Instead of joy that her sight had been restored, she was listless and disinterested in life. In asking the spirits to help her, Marie enslaved herself to ruthless spiritual beings who's power she will not escape unless she comes to Jesus.

African Justice

In many ways, my medical practice in Africa was delightful, com- pared to the practice of medicine in America today. I didn't have to worry about malpractice insurance because nobody in their right mind would sue the only board-certified surgeon within 200 miles. Medical services are paid for in either cash, goats or cutting grass with a machete. This seemingly stress-free arrangement might tempt physicians and nurses in North America to consider serving short term or long term in Africa! Before making any hasty decisions about serving there, you should probably know how the law works in most, though not all African settings.

Compared to Europe and the United States, police departments have fewer cars. For that reason, policemen generally enforce the law using check points on key intersections where at their leisure they can minutely inspect passports, drivers' licenses, and make snap decisions about fines. The police have little need to refer to written laws because there are few lawyers outside of Africa's biggest cities, and the police have the authority to stop, hold, question, and legislate laws on the spot, should there be a need! This is tolerated by governments because the police also nab criminals on the run, identify illegal immigrants, make sure tourists don't take photographs willy-nilly (especially at airports and around presidential palaces) without written permission. The police are generally encouraged to collect enough in fines from travelers to make up any shortfall in their pay.

On average, a drive between Libreville and Bongolo, a distance of 350 miles, is punctuated by between five to ten police stops. This pattern holds true for travel on most major routes throughout Central and West Africa, although Gabon's police are relatively well-paid, making them tend to be less demanding.

In 1998 I flew from Libreville to Douala, Cameroun and took a series of buses and minibuses to Banso Baptist Hospital in northwest Cameroun. After a tour of the hospital, I held fruitful talks with the hospital director and a missionary surgeon about opening a PAA-CS program at their hospital. When it was time to return home, I decided to save money on my return and use public transportation. From Banso I rode in a series of minivans, pickup trucks, and buses to the capital city Yaoundé and spent the night at a mission guest house. At 6 a.m. the next morning, I took a taxi to where minibuses congregated and bought a ticket to a town near Cameroun's border with Gabon. I had to pay extra to get a seat in the middle row, then waited for an hour until enough customers had bought tickets for all eleven seats. Only then did the driver tie our bags onto the roof rack and start down the road.

We got as far as the edge of town before encountering our first police stop. All of us presented our IDs to a policeman, and I was told to get out of the van and sit in one of five chairs arranged in a circle under a tree by the road. Minutes later, three or four others from the bus joined me. A few minutes later, a policeman came along with a small pad of forms. When I asked him why I was being detained, he explained that because I was a foreigner I could not leave town without paying a "departure permit, "which for me was $5. Arguing was pointless, since if you refused your bags would come off the roof and you would be left! Once I paid the policeman gave me a small receipt let me get back in the van.

After an hour of driving, the pavement ended, and soon after the drive stopped next to three women who waved is down. I was surprised that he took their money, and shocked when he indicated they could sit in "my" row, which already held four passengers! Since there was no possibility of squeezing another person onto the seat, the ladies sat on our laps! At first, I adamantly refused, but when the driver said he would leave me on the side of the road if I didn't comply, I gave in. Fortunately, the woman who sat on my lap was on the lean side. I learned somewhat belatedly that if you paid for *two* seats, you could refuse, unless it was an "emergency," in which case the driver could "confiscate" any unused lap space without giving you a refund!

An hour later we reached the outskirts of a town. A half mile later the driver informed me that my ride was over, and I would have to change to another taxi-bus to get to the border. But instead of driving to the marketplace where the taxi-buses loaded and unloaded their passengers, we drove a half mile out of the way to the town's police station. After we stopped, the driver explained that all foreign tourists were required by law to report to the police upon arrival. As the van drove away, I carried my bags into the police station and stood in a dingy hallway just inside the door, wondering what to do next. Eventually, a young policeman came out of a doorway and asked to see my passport. After looking at every page, he asked why I hadn't purchased a permit to travel through their province! I was momentarily speechless but then explained that I had gotten a visa to his country that permitted me to travel anywhere in the country. I then produced the permit I had purchased when leaving the capital city.

With a serious look on his face, the young policeman shook his head and said, "I'm afraid you're mistaken, Monsieur. You will not be allowed to proceed to the next town until you have purchased a permit for this province. The permits are not expensive— only $20! The permit you purchased when you left Yaoundé only allowed you to leave the city, not travel through our province!" He said this with a straight face, and it was so ludicrous I nearly started laughing!

After I got a grip on myself, I said, "Sir, I'm not paying for any permit to travel through this province. I have a legal visa in my passport that authorizes me to travel from town to town and province to province in your country without any permit." The gendarme frowned briefly, then shrugged and walked off with my passport.

There was a bench in the hallway, so I dragged my suitcase over to it and sat down. An hour later I was beginning to wonder if I hadn't made a tactical blunder when the young gendarme returned—with my passport.

"Come with me," he said. "I've explained your situation to the chief of police, and he wants to question you." Then he added, you smoke?" He was hoping I would give him a cigarette. I shook my head, and then so did he.

Ordering me to see the chief of police sounded alarming, and I briefly wondered if I should tell them I was doctor, or that I was a surgeon. Of course, that might backfire and motivate the chief of police to ask for money. Instead, I prayed for wisdom, stayed calm, and followed the young policeman. At the end of the hall, he opened a door and ushered me into a small room full of smoke and talking policemen. A large man sat behind a desk in the center of the room, smoke curling upward from the cigarette between his lips. Four African men stood in front of him, their passports on his desk next to mine. They had all been arguing with the big guy when we entered, but when I walked in, the room went silent.

The young policeman switched to a t rial language and said something that made the police chief scowl at me. For at least thirty seconds he silently scowled, as though trying to communicate the frailty of my position. Then, without a word, he picked up my passport and handed it to me. I started to take it, but for another five seconds he held on to it, as if to underline the power he had over me! Then the bossman let go of my passport, and the young gendarme hustled me out of the room.

"You may go now," he said almost breathless with relief, "You've been granted an exemption!"

It took me 45 minutes to walk with my heavy suitcase to the marketplace. Eventually I found another ride, this time sharing a front seat designed for one with a fourteen-year-old boy! The border with Gabon was a 30-foot-wide river, and we arrived around 3 p.m. There was a hand-pulled ferry tied up on the opposite shore, but since I was alone, I had to negotiate a price with a man standing in his canoe on the other side of the river. His starting price was $100, but over the next 30 minutes of testy bargaining and silent waiting, I got the price down to $10. Once I was on the other side, I paid for a ride to the nearest town in the back of a compact pick-up truck and found a hotel to spend the night. That was the very last time I made a road trip between Gabon and Cameroun using public transportation!

A later time when I traveled to Cameroon, this time by air, the immigration officer at the Douala airport studied my passport for more than a minute.

"This visa is not valid," he said, looking at me suspiciously. I had gotten it only two days earlier at Cameroun's embassy in Libreville, so I knew it was valid. I asked him what was wrong with it.

"It's dated last year!" he exclaimed. Sure enough, the embassy official had written the wrong year on my visa! I suddenly remembered that I still had the wrinkled receipt in my wallet. I had never kept a receipt for a visa before, but for some reason that could only have been the Lord, I tucked this one away! When I pulled it out and showed the officer that it was properly dated, he studied it for a minute and told me to follow him. We walked for five minutes through dimly lit hallways until we came to a small waiting room outside the Director's office. The officer pointed me to a rickety metal chair next to about twenty African men who on were sitting quietly on the floor. As I sat down, my eye caught a glimmer of steel on their wrists. They were all chained together! A few minutes later a customs officer came out of the Director's office and stood looking at me.

Finally, I asked him, "Why are these men here?" He looked at them with disdain.

"They're here because they had counterfeit visas when they got off the plane! They're illegal immigrants from Mali!" My heart sank to my toes. Did they think my visa was counterfeit too?

Ten minutes later I was called into the office where the chief of police sat. He compared the visa in my passport with the receipt I had produced. After a moment he smiled and said, "This is not your fault. You may go." He must have seen the relief on my face because he laughed and waved me out the door. As I walked past the chained Malians and down the hall to freedom, I wondered what would have happened if the Lord had not prompted me to keep my receipt!

On another occasion, Becki and I were driving in our Toyota Landcruiser from Bongolo to Gabon's capital city with our fourteen-year-old son Jeremy. He was asleep in the backseat when we came around a corner and saw three battered 55-gallon drums in the middle of the road, indicating police stop. Two policemen were sitting on chairs in the shade of a tree next to the road. When we stopped, one of the men stood and came over to the car.

I had my driver's license, vehicle papers and visa in hand. He looked them over carefully to see if they were all in order. When he finished, he handed them back to me, then looked through my window at the back seat, where our fifteen-year-old son Jeremy was sleeping.

"Wake him up!" he shouted. Surprised, I explained that Jeremy was my son and was only a teenager.

"I said wake him up! Everyone must be awake and sitting up respectfully when there's police stop!" I turned and told my son we were at a police check and that they wanted to see him awake. He sat up and looked at the glaring policeman in complete bewilderment. Apparently satisfied that he was not a terrorist, the policeman grumpily waved us through!

Several years later, I drove to Libreville to buy a set of wicker living room furniture for an apartment we had built to house our African surgery residents. The set included four armchairs, a sofa and a matching coffee table. Because without the cushions the entire set of furniture didn't weigh more than 100 pounds, I had tied the entire set on our large roof rack. When I finished, the effect of all that furniture looming four to five feet above the roof rack was rather impressive. I had traveled about fifty miles down the road south when I came to the first police stop. Both gendarmes stood to their feet as I came into view, not a good sign. The older one blew his whistle vigorously. I knew I was trouble, though I wasn't sure what law I had broken. When I walked around the front of the truck and cheerfully greeted them, they were staring at the pile of furniture and rope.

The man with the whistle regarded me soberly and without trace of humor said, "You can't do this, sir. This is vehicle abuse!" I almost burst out laughing but managed to look surprised.

I respectfully explained that I had read the code for a driver's licenses and had not seen "vehicle abuse." Shaking his head, the heavier policeman motioned to follow him back to his table and chair. He sat down and pulled out his receipt book.

"You can't load your vehicle with that much stuff," he explained.

"But it's not heavy," I protested. "You know how wicker furniture is. It doesn't even weigh 100 pounds. Besides, it's for one of our new doctors at Bongolo Hospital."

"I don't care who it's for, it's too high," he replied.

"But officer," I pleaded, "It's lower than the rail overpass 50 miles south of here, and it's not as high as the logging trucks! And it doesn't endanger or impede other vehicles. My roof rack is designed to carry 500 pounds!"

He shook his head and gave me a look that indicated he was growing weary of the discussion.

"It's vehicle abuse," he said firmly. It seemed best to concede, so I asked him how much the fine was for vehicle abuse.

"Three thousand francs," he said, looking as though he had made a huge concession to me. That was the equivalent of $5, so I handed him the money as he filled out a small receipt, signed it and gave it to me. I was walking back to the truck when I thought of something.

"What's going to happen at the next police stop?" I asked. "Am I going to have to pay at every stop?"

The gendarme shook his head. "No, of course not. That's why I gave you a receipt. If you're stopped again, just show the gendarme the receipt, and he'll let you go on without paying again." Reassured, I waved and drove on.

Two hours later I came to another police check. The police had stopped several cars and trucks on the opposite side of the road in the oncoming lane, and another car was parked in front of me. A young man rolled one of the 55-gallon drums on the road out of the way as I approached. Thinking I was getting the green light to proceed, I slowly drove through the opening. That idea evaporated with the shrilling of a police whistle to my left. I stopped and looked across the road where a crowd of drivers stood in front of a small shack. A lone gendarme stood behind a table, holding a whistle to his lips and pointing right at me.

He must have said something funny to the drivers in front of him, because as I approached everyone started laughing. A well-dressed man got out of a car behind me and laughing, said to the gendarme, "Hey, this ought to be good!" The gendarme laughed and said something unintelligible. By the time I reached the policeman's desk, twenty drivers and their passengers were smirking, chuckling or covering their mouths. I gritted my teeth and turned red. "Please help me to stay calm, Lord!" I prayed.

As I approached the big gendarme remained standing and scowled as I stepped up to his table. "Monsieur," he said, waving at the car with one hand, "you are not permitted to do that with your vehicle." Several in the crowd snickered. I answered as calmly as I could, knowing I had the receipt from the last police stop in my pocket.

"Monsieur le Gendarme," I responded, "all that furniture weighs less than 100 pounds. It looks like a great deal of weight, but it is very light."

"Did you weigh it?" he asked sarcastically. This produced an explosion of guffaws from the onlookers.

"No, I didn't weigh it, but you know how light wicker furniture is. My car rack is designed to carry 500 pounds, and I'm sure that furniture weighs far less than that."

"But you didn't weigh it, did you?" "No sir," I answered reluctantly.

"Well, there you are. You'll pay me a $20 fine!"

Pulling the receipt out of my pocket, I said, "I've already paid a fine. Here's my receipt."

The policeman looked at me with mock astonishment, then burst out laughing. "Was I there? Did you see me there?" He turned to the crowd for effect, and even the kids giggled. I was seething inside and prayed the Lord would help me stay calm.

"I should not have to pay this fine twice," I said.

"Oh, we have a smart one here," the policeman said sarcastically. Then placing both hands palm down on the table in front of him he locked eyes with me and said, "If you think you're going to continue down this road without paying me a fine, you're dreaming. This is my country not yours. You can either pay me or turn your car around and go back to Libreville."

I should have remained quiet and paid him, or shrugged, or done something else—anything but what I did. Angry and humiliated, and resenting the fact that the policeman was breaking the law by making me pay twice, I held my wrists in front of me and said, "OK, sir, why don't you just arrest me and put me in jail?"

Everybody along that road knew about our hospital, everybody knew who I was and what my truck looked like. There was even a sign on the door that said "Bongolo Hospital."

For about five seconds it was so quiet you could have heard a leaf drop to the ground. Then the gendarme sort of swelled, as if he had inhaled too much air, his eyes bulged slightly, and he placed himself directly in front of me.

"White man," the big policeman said softly, "you can sit here all night if you want, but you're not going past me until you pay me." Then he turned and stomped over to the other cars on the road. I sat down next to his table and asked the Lord to give me a break!

Twenty minutes later my pride had crawled off somewhere and lay near death. When the policeman had finished making ten other drivers pay their fines for whatever sins they had committed, I paid him the $20 he asked for and walked back to my truck. But as I drove away, my fatally wounded pride miraculously revived and bounded back into the truck!

If God doesn't humiliate surgeons from time to time, could anyone stand them? Proverbs 11:2 says it all: "*Pride leads to disgrace, but with humility comes wisdom.*"

Chapter Seven:

LIVING GOD'S CALL

Courage and Its Blessings

In the wild, machines only work for a while, and replacement parts are so limited that one has to improvise constantly. In the tropics the humidity causes everything to rust. Early on, much of our equipment came from the basements of the hospitals I worked in, and nine times out of ten, they came with no accompanying instructions.

I remember one occasion when our portable and only X-ray machine quit working. Since many patients came with fractures, tuberculosis, fluid around their lungs, or bowel obstructions, X-rays often made the difference between a clinical guess and a correct diagnosis and effective treatment. A visiting doctor had previously donated his satellite phone to us, so I decided to use it to call the company that manufactured our X-ray machine and see if he could help us figure out the problem.

During the first phone call with the company's biomedical engineer, I described the problem. The engineer thought it was probably a fuse that had blown, and since there were some capabilities of the machine we weren't using, he suggested we take out a fuse our machine wasn't using and use it to replace the blown fuse. We set up a time for a call the next day so I would have time to remove the outside panels and bring a headlamp. The satellite phone wouldn't work within the X-ray department, so I dragged the portable machine outside while keeping it plugged in. At the appointed time I got the engineer on the line and told him I was ready.

The first thing he said was, "Be very careful, doc! If you touch the wrong thing you could die! Are you sure you want to do this?"

I was a bit surprised by the news, but I decided to go ahead anyway and said, "I'm ready! Just tell me what you want me to do!"

The engineer told me to look for a group of fuses that w ere several different colors. When I found it, he directed me to the red

fuse, and said, "Now pull that fuse out, just like you would for a car fuse." It was a piece of cake to pull out the red fuse and exchange it for the burned-out yellow fuse. Once I swapped them, he asked me to turn on the X-ray machine. As soon as I hit the "on" button the X- ray machine turned on and worked! He sounded just as relieved as I did.

I love donated equipment because it's free, or *almost* free. I say "almost free" because we still had to ship used and donated equipment from America to Africa, then truck it inland more than 200 miles over atrocious roads to Bongolo. What I didn't love about used donated equipment was its unpredictability and its tendency to quit working when you needed it the most!

Take, for example, our first X-ray machine, a twenty- milliamp M.A.S.H. unit that arrived in an unbelievably heavy, lead-lined crate that weighed close to 500 pounds. The steel box for it could have survived a hand-grenade, was seven-feet long, four-feet wide and two-feet high. The three-piece unit had been sitting in a U.S. military warehouse for more than thirty years without ever being opened. Since we didn't own an X-ray unit, when someone offered it, we didn't hesitate.

Six months later, the X-ray unit and roughly eight tons of other donated M.A.S.H. equipment and supplies arrived in the port of Libreville. It was then loaded onto a truck and driven to Bongolo, picking up a generous coating of dust along the way. After it arrived at the Bongolo ferry the truck was too big to cross on the ferry, so a crew of ten Gabonese workers who were hired for the day slid the X-ray crates and boxes out of the truck and loaded it into the back of a pick-up truck. It took several trips for the smaller pick-up to transport everything to our newly completed X ray room. It was at this point that I decided to help set it up.

Because little of what happened next was anticipated, it's difficult to describe. Two missionaries and ten Gabonese men dragged the heaviest box out of the truck and let the end drop it to the ground. Then the pick-up pulled away, letting the other end drop with a bang!

Two teams were then chosen and assigned to opposite sides of it. At my signal, the struggle to get it through the X-ray door began. One team lifted its end before the other team was ready. When the team on the other end was ready and lifted, the first team gave out and dropped its end, barely missing numerous bare toes. This happened several times, pinching fingers, eliciting spirited dialogue and firmly compacting the earth beneath the box!

On the fourth try, thanks to a chorus of coordinated shouts and grunts by the workers and me, the two opposing teams managed to lift both ends simultaneously. The stronger team forced the weaker team toward the x-ray door, where its members wedged solidly, unable either to lower their end or retreat. The shouts and grunts increased in volume as the stronger team fought to push the box into the X-ray room and the weaker team screamed alternative directions! When the pitch of the shouting had climbed one or two octaves higher than at the beginning, the impasse was broken and the unfortunate players who were holding onto the sides of the box were scraped off by the door frame, leaving me and one other workman—a sixty-four-year-old man with bilateral hernias and toothpick legs—holding up our end of the box! In the agony of defeat, I must have lost consciousness, because to this day I have no recollection of how the box ended up in the middle of the floor!

Sometime later, we discovered that the box was upside down. When we finally got it right side up and opened it, we found a cleverly folded X-ray table and a telescoping arm to hold the X-ray tube. The telescoping arm slid on greased runners in two directions, which we unfortunately discovered at the expense of several bruised fingers. The entire unit had been designed to be opened and assembled in just minutes, but that was not our experience. Two hours after we started, we figured out the directions and got the unit set up.

It was several more days before I learned how to take X- rays, something I failed to pick up in medical school and residency. The U.S. army had cleverly coated the inside of the trunk with lead, so that it could serve as a shield for those who took the X-rays. Unfortunately, the trunk was only four feet high when opened and stood on its end, so whoever pushed the button for an X-ray had to crouch behind the trunk, and while instructing the patient not to breathe or move, shoot the X-ray blindly. After that, one had to remove the film and develop it in tall, narrow tanks filled with toxic chemicals.

It took several weeks of experimenting to discover that a twenty-milliamps X-ray is great for taking pictures of safety pins and fingers, but to X-ray things like arms, legs, torsos and heads, long time exposures are required. For example, to X-ray an adult's leg required an exposure lasting at least four seconds, and to X-ray a patient's chest one had to hold down the button for five or six seconds. Since few patients will hold their breath that long and at the same time remain immobile, we often ended up taking time exposures that included several excursions of the diaphragm, chest walls, and heart. Not surprisingly, our blurred films could identify only the gravest of abnormalities. A clear and focused X-ray of the chest would probably be classified as a miracle!

I tried only once or twice to X-ray an adult's abdomen. The exposure lasted eleven seconds, enough time for several breaths to take place and for contracting intestines to produce triple images.

Mercifully, our twenty-milliamps X-ray tube burned out after three years, saving everybody hours of mostly fruitless effort. Some years later, someone bought us a new, 100 milliamp X-ray machine designed for use in the tropics that served us wonderfully for three years, before dying after a lightning strike.

The unpredictability of older military equipment could also be dangerous. In 1996, the U.S. military donated us a forty-foot container of surplus medical equipment. Among the many useful items were four, six-foot-long steam autoclaves. Steam autoclaves sterilize whatever is put into them by using heat and steam under pressure. The heat for them can be provided by either electricity or burners, but because of our hydroelectric plant, we had fairly reliable electricity. I set up one of the autoclaves in a shed behind the operating rooms and asked our missionary maintenance man if he would hook it up to electricity.

The autoclave worked beautifully for six months. Then, just two weeks after our wonderful Dutch maintenance man returned to Holland for a six-month furlough, a bolt of lightning during a thunderstorm burned out two of the autoclave's three heating coils. The U.S. army had thought of that possibility and had provided extra coils. Changing the coils looked like a straightforward procedure, so I explained it to the hospital's African maintenance crew and went off to take care of several medical emergencies.

When I came out of the operating room around 5 p.m. to see how they were doing, I could tell by the litter of parts, twisted coils and tools strewn about that my crew had not succeeded in changing the coils. It turned out that the replacement coils were for another model! The next morning, I had the workmen clean up the mess while I figured out what to do. Perhaps, I thought, it would be easier to use the backup gasoline burners that came with the autoclaves rather than waste more time messing with the electric coils.

I had always been taught that fire and gasoline are not just dangerous but *really* dangerous, so I approached the gas burner for the autoclave with skepticism. According to the manual, lighting it was not difficult. Once I figured out from the instructions how to safely light the gas burner under the autoclave, I tried to teach the women who worked in the sterilization room to do it. For some reason, they would have nothing to do with it!

Faced with a possible mutiny, I decided to look for one- eyed Bernard, the second-most experienced African on our hospital maintenance crew. Ever since Bernard had risked his life to kill a black mamba snake in the attic of the outpatient clinic, I had been his protector. He needed one because he worked in spurts of about two hours, after which he simply disappeared for the rest of the day. Toward the end of the day, he would magically reappear, holding a hammer or some other tool and looking suspiciously well-rested, but always able to explain what he had been doing for the previous two to four hours.

On the day that Bernard killed the black mamba, a crowd of about 100 people were calmly sitting in the outside waiting area waiting to be consulted. Suddenly a shiny, black snake poked its head out from under the eaves of the tin roof. The patients, who up until then had felt weak and sickly, suddenly found hidden reserves and stampeded in a screaming mob to a safe distance. I emerged from the operating room in an adjacent building at about 10 a.m. and found the area in front of the outpatient building surrounded by a crowd of patients and staff. Our Administrator, Pastor Luc was there too, and he had already called for the hospital maintenance crew to come and take care of the problem. Three of them eventually showed up, one of them being one-eyed Bernard, holding a hammer as usual. I explained what they already knew: one or several of them would have to climb up into the attic and kill the snake.

Two realities made this an extremely dangerous idea. The first was that the ceiling was made up of three-eighths-inch plywood that was nailed to two-by-fours spaced every three feet. The only way to walk around in the low space above the ceiling was to balance on the two-by-fours that were infested with wood bores. The second and more important reality is that the black mamba is one of the fastest and deadliest snakes in the world, if not THE deadliest. Its venom paralyzes its victims rapidly, and if it sinks its hollow fangs into a person's head or neck and injects its venom, the victim will die in minutes, not hours. We had a small supply of antivenom at the hospital, but if one of the volunteers got bitten, we would have to inject antivenom within less than a minute, and who would do that?

I was surprised when Bernard stepped forward and said with a toothy grin, "I'll kill it!"

After choosing as his weapons a pointed machete and a five-foot-long steel rod, Bernard climbed a ladder into the small opening that led into the attic. Several of us armed ourselves with machetes and took up positions on different sides of the building, in case the snake should try to escape.

For several minutes, we heard only the sound of Bernard grunting and sliding around on the weakened two-by-fours. He seemed to be having some trouble locating the snake. Five minutes passed, and our attention started to lag. The crowd began to relax and talk about other things.

Suddenly, we heard a shout, followed by the sound of a machete flailing against rafters. I realized too late that we had not cut the electrical power to the building, and there were 220-volt electrical wires running on the attic rafters. The banging continued and moved towards the front of the roof. Bernard was apparently in hot pursuit of the snake. The clattering moved to a corner where the roof came down to meet the wall. Then there was silence.

One of Bernard's colleagues ran into the building and asked Bernard if the snake had gotten away. Bernard shouted back that the snake had retreated beyond the reach of his machete. He was preparing to go after it with his steel rod. His voice sounded about an octave higher than normal.

The battle resumed abruptly with the crashing of steel against roofing tins. The snake must have counterattacked, because the steel rod popped quickly through the thin roofing tins and back in several places. Then it ripped through the roof twice more, then a third time. Since it did not seem to be the right time to admonish Bernard for putting so many holes in the roof, I bit my tongue, said a prayer for his safety, and gripped my machete tighter. The other spectators were not so thoughtful, however. Though not one of them ventured closer than twenty feet, they showered Bernard with a chorus of advice.

"Go for his head, you dummy!" a muscular, two-eyed, twenty-five-year-old shouted from my right. I could just picture Bernard hearing his advice and deciding to stop pounding the snake's tail! The sounds of battle resumed, finally reaching a crescendo. Then there was silence, and we held our breath. A moment later, Bernard threw down the body of a dead, eight-foot black mamba. He had reduced its head to a pulpy, red mass.

As he climbed down from the attic, we acclaimed him as a hero! He received my genuine thanks with a lop-sided grin and a shrug before going back to pushing the lawn mower around for an hour and then disappearing with his hammer. We should have given him a bonus, or a medal, or held a special ceremony to honor his courage, but to this day I'm ashamed to admit that we didn't even buy him a Coke. Anyway, whenever I needed someone fearless for a task like lighting the pressurized gasoline burner for the steam autoclave, I naturally thought of Bernard!

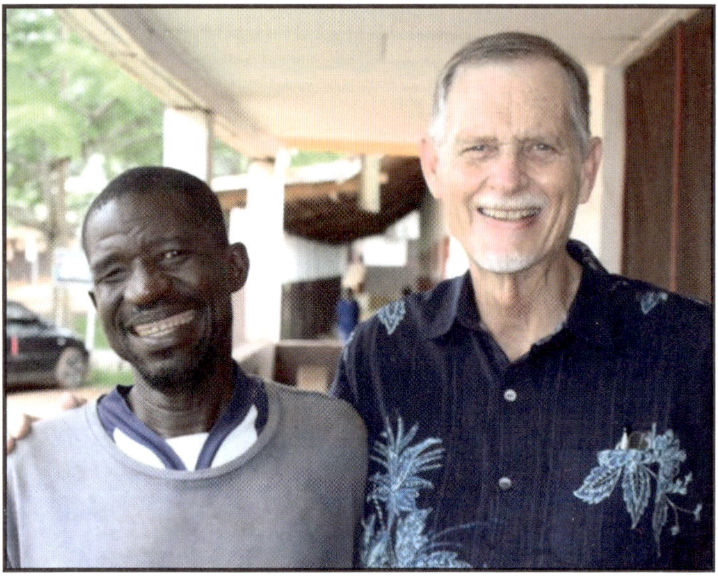

The author and Bernard, the Black Mamba killer, decades later!

The instructions for the burner gave not the slightest warning that the device was a potential bomb. Step one instructed one to pour gasoline into the five-liter tank. Step two was to use a handy, attached pump to pressurize the tank. Step three involved opening a valve and lighting a pre-burner, presumably to turn the liquid gas to a vapor for the long burner under the autoclave. Step four required nerves of steel, because the operator had to open the valve to the long burner so gasoline vapor would catch fire and heat the autoclave! Bernard quickly got the hang of it and agreed to light the autoclave for the ladies who made up our surgical packs and put them in the autoclave whenever he was needed.

The tenth day of using the M.A.S.H. gasoline autoclave dawned like any other day in Gabon-misty and humid. Our staff met together that morning at 7:30 for a Bible study and prayer as we did every morning and dispersed to begin work at 8 a.m. I made rounds on my patients and went to the operating room to fix someone's hernia. I had just finished the operation and was stripping off my gloves when the OR circulating nurse ran gray-faced into the OR.

"Corne quickly, doctor!" he cried. "The autoclave is on fire!"

I ran the twenty feet to the sterilization room and was stunned by what I saw. The gas heater was lit and burning as usual, but flaming gasoline was leaking from around the control valve below the flame. Tongues of orange and yellow flame shot out from under the autoclave, and liquid fire dripped down onto the floor to join an enlarging pool of burning gasoline. The women from the sterilization room had fled and stood crying outside the back door of the building. Bernard was frozen in the doorway, unsure of what to do.

In that millisecond, a hundred thoughts flashed through my mind. If we did nothing but protect ourselves, the entire surgical building with our three operating rooms, our anesthesia machines, our patient monitors, and all of our precious instruments would burn. In the months or years, it would take to rebuild and re-equip our operating rooms, we would have no way to deal with the hundreds of surgical emergencies that ambulances brought to our hospital. People would die. On the other hand, if I ordered Bernard into the autoclave room to try to control the fire, it might explode and burn him horribly, perhaps even blinding his remaining eye. If I tried to control the flames, the same thing could happen to me.

An empty bucket sat on the floor two feet from me. Shouting at Bernard to bring a bucket of sand, I rushed to the sink and filled the bucket with water. The only way to keep the burner from exploding was to cool it down and shut it off. As I ran with the half- filled bucket into the autoclave room, I prayed a desperate prayer: "Whatever You decide for me, Father, I put my trust in You. Only help me put out this fire!" In that instant, a picture of myself burned from head to toe flashed through my mind. Then the water from my bucket hit the fire, and the burner gave off a roar of steam and flame.

The flames did not go out but instead overflowed into rivers on the floor. One of the women met me at the door with another bucket of water, and I heard the OR nurse shouting for Bernard to hurry with the sand. Before I threw the second bucket of water I grabbed a towel, wrapped it around my hands, and reaching through the flames grabbed the burner and slid it halfway out from under the autoclave. A third bucket of water nearly extinguished the flames. Seconds later Bernard arrived with the sand, threw it over everything, and I shut off the control valve. We gave thanks to God that the fire was out, and no one was burned.

On one other occasion, we had a major hospital fire, this time in our medical warehouse where we had more than $150,000 of medicines and medical supplies in storage. It was late in the afternoon on a day when the temperature was in the high 90's. One of the nurses suddenly noticed smoke pouring out the upper window of our medical warehouse and called the alarm. We didn't have any smoke sensors in the building, so it was by the grace of God that she saw it soon after it started. As we shouted for help, people came running from every direction. I don't remember where I was, but when we unlocked the steel door of the warehouse, smoke had filled the 40-foot building. Dr. Keir Thelander, a young surgeon who had joined our team recently, showed up seconds after I arrived with his mom and dad in tow!

As we entered the building, we could see flames and hear crackling and popping coming from two large refrigerators that were on fire. We quickly identified the source of the popping noise which turned out to be burning hemorrhoid suppositories! Next to the burning refrigerator were at least twenty boxes of various medical supplies on fire. The building had a sink, but it was too near the fire to be of use. Fortunately, within twenty yards of the building there were several outdoor faucets, and nurses and other volunteers who came from a service in the nearby church building filled buckets with water for Keir me and others to throw on the fire. Someone noticed a sand pile next to the building and brought buckets of sand inside that we used to put out the burning suppositories.

Other volunteers courageously grabbed the burning boxes and dragged them out of the building where they could be extinguished with water. At the height of the fire, the flames reached up to the plywood ceiling and caught some of the rafters on fire. Using buckets to throw water to the ceiling and the rafters, we gradually brought the fire under control.

Within fifteen or twenty minutes, those of us who were fighting the fire could see we were winning. Had we noticed the fire just five minutes later, the whole building would have gone up in flames. A year later Dr. Keir's parents shipped a refurbished fire truck to Bongolo that fifteen years later is still in service!

Does courage give birth to courage? That day we all witnessed it. Does God protect us when we take great personal risks to save others? I've seen Him do it many more times than I can remember!

Psalms 46:1-3 & 7 describes the source of our courage: *"God is our refuge and strength, always ready to help in times of trouble. So, we will not fear when earthquakes come and the mountains crumble into the sea. Let the oceans roar and foam. Let the mountains tremble as the waters surge! (6-7) The nations are in chaos, and their kingdoms crumble! God's voice thunders, and the earth melts! The Lord of Heaven's armies is here among us; the God of Israel is our fortress."*

God's Paratrooper

In the 1990's, Pastor Luke retired, and a Gabonese pastor named Serge Batouboko agreed to serve as the administrative director of Bongolo Hospital. After graduating from high school at the age of 17, Serge joined the army. He was intelligent, athletic, and a natural leader, and was soon promoted. A few years later he was assigned to serve in the nation's capital at the presidential palace and was soon purchasing groceries for the officer's mess (cafeteria). Like others working in the presidential palace, Serge was able to divert funds to his own account without being discovered. After he had been doing this for several years, he heard that the French army was opening a program to train paratroopers. For every jump the trainees made, they would earn $100. Serge was not afraid of parachuting, and because of the money and the chance for further advancement, he signed up.

Serge excelled in the paratrooper training program, and by their last training jump he was looking forward to receiving another promotion. He was one of 10 officers who went on one last jump off the coast of Gabon. It was to be an easy exercise from about 10,000 feet, over a large, treeless area of sand on the coast, and south of the capital city. As they had been taught, the men hooked their parachute pull cords onto a cable down the middle of the plane before jumping. The cord would ensure that their parachutes opened immediately after they jumped from the plane. Just before the first man jumped, a stiff breeze suddenly began blowing.

Serge was the tenth man to jump, and as soon as he jumped, the 10-foot strap connected to the cable inside jammed and wouldn't disengage. Serge found himself being violently dragged behind the plane, just feet from the tail! His parachute only partially deployed, and as plane dragged him through the air, he fought to get free. By then his parachute had turned into a tangled mess. In that moment, Serge knew he was going to die, and his life instantly flashed before his eyes. An instant later, his trainer succeeded in cutting the strap holding Serge inside the plane, and he fell away from the plane. He had the presence of mind to pull the cord for his secondary parachute, but as soon as it deployed it tangled with his main parachute. As Serge plummeted to the ground, he cried out, "God, if you save me, I promise to serve you!"

Serge had never been a religious man, and seconds later he landed in five feet of water, ten feet from the beach. That was the last thing he remembered. Hours later a helicopter found him lying on his back halfway in the water. He had fractured both legs and was unconscious, but he was alive!

A day later, Serge woke up in the hospital and was surprised that he was alive. His superior officer came to see him and congratulated him for...well, surviving! But when Serge asked about the others who had jumped before him, he was told all of them were fine. A week later, however, his commanding officer told him the truth: the stiff breeze that had started blowing just before Serge and his friends jumped, blew all of the other parachutists out to sea, where they drowned. Only Serge survived. It was a terrible blow, and Serge struggled to understand why.

A week later, Christians from a local church came to visit. They brought clean towels and snacks and asked him if he was willing to share his story. At first, he refused, but after he learned they were Christians, he told them of his promise to God. When the visitors shared the gospel with Serge, he repented and put his faith and trust in Jesus. His new friends gave him a New Testament in French and encouraged him to start reading the book of John. For the next two weeks, Serge read through the New Testament his friends had given him, asked questions, and prayed with them whenever they visited.

Soon after his confession of faith, Serge's commanding officer came and told him that because he was up on crutches, he would be going back to the barracks. When Serge refused, his commander was surprised, especially when Serge explained that when he was about to die after parachuting from the airplane, he made a promise to God that if He saved him, he would serve Him—not as a soldier, but as a pastor! Serge's commander was not impressed, and he told Serge he couldn't resign because he had signed up for 10 years! If he refused to go back to the barracks, he would have to go to the military jail.

Serge shrugged and said, "Okay, Sir, put me in jail. But I'm going to keep my promise to God."

Two weeks later, Serge's commander came back and asked him if he was ready yet to obey. Without hesitating, Serge replied, "No sir. I have to obey God first!"

Two weeks later his commander sent a French psychiatrist to talk to Serge. After their meeting, the psychiatrist advised Serge's commander that because Serge had lost all of his friends to drowning and felt guilty for surviving, he should be allowed to take a two-year leave of absence. The commander and his superiors agreed. After Serge was released, he quietly returned all the money he had stolen while working in the presidential palace. When he was able to travel, he took the train to the Alliance seminary in eastern Gabon and applied. The seminary had a three-year pastoral training program, and after hearing Serge's story, his remarkable testimony, and his call to become a pastor, the school accepted him.

Over the next two years, Serge's faith and Bible knowledge grew rapidly. He became a soul-winner to some of his former friends and did well in his studies. Then at the end of two years, Serge's commanding officer called him in and told him that his two years of grace were up, and he needed to return to the army. Serge respectfully declined, stating that he had another year of Bible school to complete so he could qualify to be a pastor. Shocked, his commander threatened to throw him in jail for the duration of his contract, which was eight more years!

But Serge would not budge and told his commander he was not afraid to go back to jail! Amazed by his faith, his commanding officer finally threw up his hands in frustration and said, "I fear God too, and if I make the devil angry, God will still help me. But if I make God angry, who can help me?" He then signed a paper freeing Serge from all of his military obligations.

Serge went on to finish his third year of Bible school and was assigned by the Alliance Church to serve as the pastor of a small church in eastern Gabon. Five years later the national church leadership decided to send him to a Christian university in France to learn accounting. After he finished the course, Serge returned to Gabon and soon after was asked by the church president to serve as the Treasurer of the Gabon Alliance Church.

Five years later, Pastor Luke Mambela who had served as Bongolo Hospital's administrative director for ten years decided to retire. Bongolo Hospital needed a capable and godly Administrative Director, and we had heard Serge's story. After meeting him and getting to know him, our medical team asked him if he would be willing to serve as Bongolo Hospital's administrative director. He accepted, and soon after, the church gave its blessing.

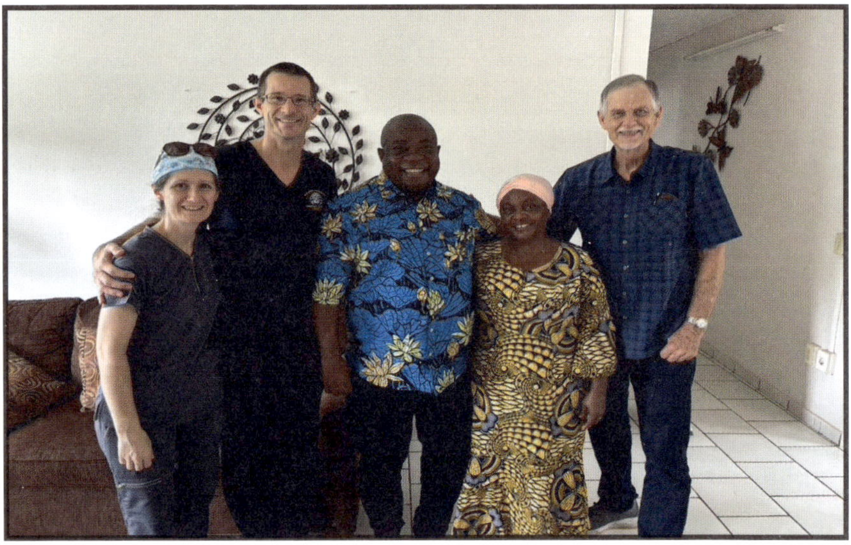

Right to left: the author, Jackie and Serge Batouboko, Dr. Zack O'Connor, at the time of this writing, is the PAACS program director at Bongolo Hospital), and his wife Dr. Jen O'Connor is also a faculty surgeon.

Pastor Serge's service was one of God's greatest blessings that God could have given Bongolo Hospital. As the only survivor of one of Gabon's worst military disasters, he was revered by both the government and the Gabonese military. In addition, his steadfast determination to serve God impressed even the atheists in the government!

The Strike

Sunday, January 31. I was writing a report on my computer in the afternoon when a battered, white pickup truck pulled up in front of our house. Four young men climbed out, came to our front door and introduced themselves as "representatives from the Lebamba Strike Committee." I invited them in and seated them in the living room. As I filled their glasses with chilled Coke, they gazed at the African paintings on the walls, the pictures of our kids, and the small African fish zooming around my twenty- gallon aquarium. After we had sipped our Cokes for a few minutes, they got down to business.

"Tomorrow morning the town will be shut down by a general strike," the oldest of them explained somberly. "All roads leading into and out of Lebamba will be barricaded. This has nothing to do with you. It's a community demonstration against the government's failure to keep its promises. We are angry that our leaders have diverted funds and have not kept their promises to build our town a water system, put up streetlights, and add enough electrical poles so everyone in town can have access to electricity."

Several years earlier, a Canadian company had completed the construction of a dam with three large turbines that the government had strung high tension lines on to connect to Bongolo, Lebamba, and three other towns in the south of Gabon. To complete the project, they had to demolish our small hydroelectric plant that Don Fairley built in 1945, but because the dam and the turbines were all was built on mission property, our electricity was free.

Becki was in Libreville and was due to fly into an airport two hours north of Bongolo on Monday and I knew she would be bringing American visitors with her. When I expressed my concern that they would not be allowed back into town during the men assured me there would be no problem. They would leave instructions at the barricades to let any of our missionaries or guests through. They also assured me that people needing urgent medical care would be allowed to cross the barricades and reach the hospital.

After they left, I shared the news with the rest of the missionaries on our station. Except for those who were planning to drive two hours north to Mouila to meet the plane on Monday, everyone agreed to remain at the mission and hospital compound until the strike was over.

Monday, February 1: The next morning, I spent a bit more time than usual in prayer, sensing that I could not afford to miss any of the Father's cues that day. When I came down to the hospital, I found about half of the usual number of patients. Instead of ten or twenty cars and taxis parked in the hospital parking lot, there were none.

Later that day, I was in the middle of a major operation when the electricity suddenly went off. It was not unusual for the power to go off for five or ten minutes, so we continued working with the aid of a flashlight. Fifteen minutes later, however, the electricity was still off, the temperature in the operating room was already in the 90's because the air conditioner quit, and the flashlight was growing dim.

The maintenance crew had been working on installing a new backup generator the day before. When I called for backup power, they came to the OR door and explained that they had disconnected the old generator before discovering that the new one lacked a key part! Worse, our missionary mechanic and one of our doctors had gone to Mouila to meet the plane! We managed to complete the operation moments before the flashlight went completely dead.

When I emerged from the operating room, I was steaming, and not just because my scrubs were drenched with sweat. Everyone outside the OR seemed to know that our town's new masters had forced their way into the large government-owned hydroelectric plant across the river and had turned the power off. Pastor Serge, our administrator, had already gone to talk to the strike leaders, so I asked two of the hospital maintenance workers and another missionary on our station to help me reconnect the old generator. The relic weighed more than a ton and was coated with a mixture of dirt and old diesel fuel. We filled it with fuel and were trying to figure out how to connect it up when the city power came back on.

A few minutes later, the hospital administrator drove up to the garage to tell us that the strikers had agreed to maintain power to the hospital. Still upset that they had shown complete disregard for our patients, I showered, changed into clean scrubs and returned to the operating room. Around 5 p.m., I got a call on the radio from Bob, our maintenance man. He and the doctor who had gone with him to Mouila had arrived at the barricade with Becki and our American visitors, but the young men at the barricade were refusing to let them through! Pastor Serge and I drove down to the edge of town where they were being held.

The barricade was made of five small logs and some old oil drums. It would take very little effort to move the barricade out of the way. The three or four young men strutting defiantly in front of the cars were half drunk and looking for a fight. About ten or fifteen adolescent boys stood by admiring them. I let Pastor Serge do the talking, and he greeted the young men and reminded them that we had been promised the right to come and go freely. They scoffed at that and replied that no one would be allowed to cross their barricade. If they persisted until dark, Bob, our doctor, Becki, and our visitors would have to turn around, drive the two hours back to Mouila and stay there until the strike was over.

While the leader of the group was talking, five middle-aged women carrying heavily loaded baskets of bananas and manioc (cassava) from their gardens walked past the cars and approached the barricade. The young men tried to stop them from crossing, but the muscular ladies shoved them aside and scolded them like children. Who did they think was going to feed them if they stopped their mamas from bringing food from the plantations? Were they planning to eat dirt? It was hard to keep a straight face as the women chewed them out and pushed through them! The women continued on their way, wondering aloud how any Gabonese woman could have produced such stupid offspring!

Serge and I thought it was wonderful, though we managed to stifle our smiles. Unfortunately, the exchange did little to serve our cause. When Serge again asked the young men what they wanted, they replied even more offensively than before. It was infuriating, but I managed to keep stay calm and let Serge do the talking. He somehow managed to stay calm and would not let their words, or their bad manners offend him.

Eventually, the young men offered to let the cars pass if Serge paid them $30. We could easily have overpowered them, but it did not seem to be God's way of solving the problem. For the sake of peace, we paid the money. As the cars drove through the barricade, Serge, and I walked back to our car, wondering how long the provincial governor was going to do nothing.

Tuesday, February 2: During the night a group of young men felled a tree across the road between Bongolo and the center of town. This made it impossible for anyone from town or even farther away to drive a vehicle to or from Bongolo. After felling the tree, the young men refused to allow even pedestrians to continue on to the hospital. That day, none of our scheduled elective surgery patients showed up. What was especially troubling was that the strikers were not willing to tell us what the strike was about!

There were patients already in the hospital who needed surgery, so that morning we did a diverting colostomy for a woman with rectal cancer, put a chest tube in a young boy with fluid around his lungs, and cleaned out an infected hip fracture. The stores in town all remained closed for a second day, and the only cars allowed on the roads were those used by the strike leaders. Nobody seemed to know what the strike was about, and the young men manning the blockades were not authorized by their leaders to explain!

During the night, a fourteen-year-old boy died in the pediatric ward. The next morning, Serge crossed the river and walked the three miles to the center of Lebamba to get a message to the boy's father on the police radio, since he lived in a town eighty-five miles away. Serge waited for three hours before the police inexplicably decided him the use their radio. Undeterred, Serge walked back to the hydroelectric plant and got permission to use their radio. After he called, he learned that the boy's father was on a remote road repairing a road grader and would not be home for another day.

By evening, the boy's body was beginning to decompose in the heat. The strikers would not allow us to drive to the town cemetery, so, we buried him next to the church. After the funeral, the young men at the barricade would not permit the boy's distraught mother to leave town, so she remained at the hospital with her two small children, mourning her son's death alone.

That afternoon, a group of the strikers drove up to the hospital in a battered white truck and demanded to see me. I came out of the operating room and found them waiting at the door. The leader asked me to give them either diesel fuel for their cars or motor oil for their chain saw. I wanted very much to give him a piece of my mind for all of the trouble the strike was causing our patients, but the still, small voice of the Lord prompted me to keep silent and give them what they asked for, even though it might enable them to make things worse!

I asked them to drive me up to my house where I had some motor oil in storage. As we drove away from the hospital the young men in the back of the pickup shouted to the patients standing around, "We're kidnapping the doctor! We're kidnapping the doctor!" They howled and slapped their knees in hilarity at the cries of alarm from our staff. All I could manage in response to their sick joke was to shake my head.

On the way up the hill, the leader of the group explained that they needed the fuel and the oil for the chain saws to remove some of the barricades. The local population had grumbled so much about the roadblocks that they had decided to remove some of them and allow the stores to reopen. The head of the strikers added that they also wanted to make additional roadblocks on the roads leading out of town to frustrate anyone trying to forcibly reopen the roads in and out of town. Then he shared they were planning to cut the electrical power that evening to Mouila, the provincial capital eighty-five miles away, as well as to the town of Ndende, a smaller town twenty-five miles to the north. When we got to the house, I told the young men that I didn't have any gasoline, only motor oil. They seemed satisfied with my explanation and produced a two-liter container for me to fill.

That night, the strikers were as good as their word and cut the electrical power to the towns of Ndende and Mouila. It made us wonder if their issue was with the governor in Mouila.

February 3, Wednesday. The day began calmly enough, but I again felt the need to get up before sunrise and pray that God would bring the conflict—whatever it was about—to a peaceful end. It seemed that more than anything else, God was teaching us to trust Him and wait for Him to act on our behalf, something exceedingly difficult for me!

For the first time since the beginning of the strike, a small number of patients arrived at the hospital in taxis and cars. We performed two operations and were preparing to do a C-section on a woman who had been in obstructed labor for twelve hours when the battered white pickup truck roared up the hospital driveway and screeched to a halt in front of Pastor Serge's office. In contrast to the previous visit, the strikers now seemed angry and pushed their way into Serge's office without knocking. A few minutes later, they stormed out and drove off. After they left, Pastor Serge came over and explained that they had informed him they were going to cut the electrical power to the hospital. Evidently, a crowd of about 200 angry people from Lebamba had demonstrated in front of the strike headquarters that morning. They were angry that they were the only ones in town deprived of electricity, while Bongolo and the hospital still had power. To pacify the town, the strike leaders decided to shut of the electricity for the town *and* Bongolo!

Serge asked the doctors to come and explain to the strike leaders how a prolonged electrical blackout would affect our patients, including several premature babies that were on oxygen concentrators. In the surgery ward, a small boy needed continuous chest suction from a continuous pump to keep his chest from filling up with fluid. We had only four hours of diesel fuel in our aging backup generator, and if we used it up the rest of our diesel fuel now, we would not be able to take X rays, order laboratory tests or operate. Furthermore, if the hospital ran out of diesel fuel and had no power for more than six hours, we would lose our entire stock of vaccines. The strike leaders were unmoved.

While we hurried up to complete another C-section, Serge crossed the river to talk with the hydroelectric plant's director. After we got the baby out it didn't start breathing and had to be resuscitated with suction and oxygen. Eventually it improved, though on oxygen. Ten minutes later the power went off.

The hospital had a smaller, fuel-efficient backup generator to run an oxygen concentrator for the premature baby ward, so the newborn baby was able to stay on oxygen. However, we could not put the boy with the draining chest tube in with the premature babies. We finally decided to watch the boy closely and leave him where he was. If he began to fail, we would start up our back-up generator and run it until we were out of fuel.

The director of the hydroelectric plant was a devout Christian, so when Serge explained to him that we only had enough fuel for six hours, and that after that, several children might die he was aghast!

He immediately went into town and begged the strike leaders to allow his men to climb one of the main pylons and disconnect the high-tension power lines leading to Lebamba. That way he could shut off the town's electricity without disturbing the hospital. Then he asked the strike leaders to consider what would happen if children died at the hospital as a result of their actions. Would the relatives seek revenge? Might the government hold them responsible for the deaths? And what if the army or police showed up the next day and some of the strikers were injured? If the operating rooms or emergency room were without power, how could the hospital help them? The more he talked, the more the strikers listened. In the end, they allowed him to disconnect the wires to Lebamba and without cutting the power to the hospital!

That night, our hospital and housing compound was the only place with electricity in an area the size of Vermont! So that we wouldn't irritate our suffering neighbors in the village and across the river, we blacked out the windows in our houses and turned off our outside lights.

Earlier that same day we had managed to call the American embassy on our satellite phone and explain our situation. The ambassador wanted to know what, if anything, the U.S. government could do to help. I assured him that we were not in any danger and did not want anyone to attempt a rescue. But if the Gabonese government could send someone with clout to talk to the strikers, the uprising could probably be resolved peacefully. I also informed the ambassador that the strike was in its third day and not a single regional or federal government official had come to talk with the strikers and see what they wanted! We didn't even know what they wanted!

That evening, Serge attended a meeting in town and learned that the government was ready to respond to the demands of the strikers, but only if they cleared the streets and turned the electricity on to all three southern towns. Later that night, the town leaders sent a representative to Mouila and invited the governor to come back for talks.

February 4, Thursday. Our hospital staff met for prayer at the hospital at 7:30 am, and the hopeful sounds of compromise were in the air. Many thanked God for protecting the children who had needed oxygen during the night, and many thought the strike would be over by nightfall. But around 8 a.m., a contingent of about fifteen police- men arrived from the provincial town of Mouila. They immediately attacked the first of several barricades at the entrance to the town and with chain saws. Almost immediately, about thirty of Lébamba's townsmen massed behind the final barricade. Expecting the crowd to flee, the police stormed across the bridge with their clubs swinging. In the ensuing fight, one policeman was knocked unconscious, and several others were severely beaten before they retreated back across the bridge. The strikers swarmed after them and chased them into the woods on both sides of the road out of town! When they townspeople found the parked police van, they broke all its windows and turned it on its side. Then they poured kerosene on the bridge and tried to burn it. Fortunately, only part of the bridge burned and was not seriously damaged. The police withdrew to a safe distance, sent their wounded back to Mouila in another car, and waited for the governor.

When the governor arrived an hour later the strikers were in a foul mood. They made him wait at the bridge for several hours before they allowed him to cross alone on the partly burned bridge. The townspeople were still angry that the police had attacked them. Not surprisingly, the governor denied he had ordered them to use force. Nobody believed him, but because he remained cool, the crowd gradually calmed. Speaking softly but with authority, the governor insisted that before negotiations could begin all the barricades around the town had to be removed as a good faith gesture. After that, the demonstrators would have to restore the electricity to the town and to the other three towns in the province. This demand did not go well with the strikers and resulted in a stalemate. After several hours, the governor left, promising to get back in a day or two. He warned the strikers and town leaders that the federal government could decide at any moment to send in the army!

That night Serge told us that because of the fight at the bridge the young bucks wanted the strike to continue indefinitely. A cloud of gloom settled over us. We had food supplies for about another week. Thanks to the strikers, most if not all of the frozen food in Lébamba's stores had spoiled. Because the strikers had allowed the director of the hydroelectric plant to maintain the current to the hospital, the food in our freezers hadn't spoiled.

February 5, Friday. The next morning the town leaders and the strike organizers met and debated what to do. Cracks had started to form between the young men who had maintained the barricades and the older men who had given them the green light to set them up. The young men want to prolong the strike indefinitely and run a Malian family of shop keepers and truckers out of town. This was because the Malian storekeepers had refused to give the strikers diesel fuel and had insulted them. Unlike the Malians, they explained, Dr. Thompson and Pastor Serge had helped them and had treated them with respect. When I heard that I swallowed hard and thanked the Lord for His restraining grace!

In the end, a deal was struck: the young men could run the Malian merchants out of town, the electricity would be restored everywhere, and the barricades would come down. If the government acted on the town's demands, everything would remain peaceful. If not, the organizers would renew the strike.

Several hours later we heard the news that the strike was over. We were relieved that things would now return to normal, though we were saddened that the Malian merchants and their families had been forced to leave the town. It was the Malians who transported our medicines and construction supplies from Libreville in their trucks at a cost that we couldn't match. It was also the Malians who provided the majority of our fresh food. That night they closed their stores and fled to the next town. In less than a year most of them had quietly returned.

Keeping my mouth closed when I was angry was one of the wisest things I ever did. Sometime later, it occurred to me that God might have wanted more from me.

Jesus said to his disciples in Matthew 5:39-48,

"Do not resist an evil person. If someone strikes you on the right cheek, turn to him the other also... If someone forces you to go one mile, go with him two miles. Give to the one who asks you, and do not turn away from the one who wants to borrow from you... Love your enemies and pray for those who persecute you, that you may be sons of your Father in heaven. If you love those who love you, what reward will you get? Do not even pagans do that? Be perfect, therefore, as your heavenly Father is perfect."

The opportunity to love and forgive people who are nasty, ungrateful, and even evil, is a gift from God that we don't often appreciate. But it is critically important for God's servants who find themselves caught in the middle of conflict they did not start.

The Goat on the Roof

Ilobo's wife of forty-five years had worked as a cleaning woman at the hospital until dying of bone cancer two years before. He had loved her deeply and only now was beginning to smile again.

Following their mother's death, Ilobo's children had all moved to Libreville, Gabon's capital city. They had gone to great lengths to comfort their father and convince him to move to Libreville and live with them, but he steadfastly refused to leave his humble cement block house in Bongolo and move to the chaos of Libreville. As a concession, he agreed to visit them several times a year, and now he wanted to do something to thank them by bringing a goat to share with the family.

When he asked me if he could bring a goat along, I hesitated for almost a minute! In the end, friendship won over common sense. Perhaps I could tie the animal up on the roof where it could bleat and mess to its heart's content and not bother us below in the air-conditioned cabin. When I said yes, Ilobo's old face glowed with pleasure, and he readily accepted my one condition that someone from his house would tie the goat up on the roof rack when I came to pick him up in the morning.

The first hint of trouble appeared after I drove up to Ilobo's house in the dim light before sunrise. As I got out of my Landcruiser, one of his nephews was trying to tie the goat's feet together with a vine. It took less than a minute for the goat to free its legs from the vine and stand up, so someone provided a rope. This time, the young man succeeded in tying the goat's feet securely. For added measure, Ilobo's nephew stuffed the goat into an empty rice sack, leaving only it's head sticking out.

This must be the way to do it, I thought admiringly.

Another nephew dragged two, 100-pound sacks of manioc to my Toyota Landcruiser and loaded them on the roof rack next to the goat. I was not satisfied with the way the young man was tying the sacks on the roof, so I climbed up to help him. To make sure that the goat would not bounce out of the roof rack, I tied a second rope loosely around its neck and secured it to the railing.

Ilobo got in and I drove a few houses further to pick up Pastor Luke, the hospital's administrator. He brought out two more sacks of cassava which we added to the load already on the roof. The road was unpaved and rough, so I could only drive twenty or thirty miles an hour. The log bridges, blind curves and sudden mud holes kept me busy, and I soon forgot about the goat.

An hour into the trip, we heard a sudden thrashing and banging against a back window on the right side of the truck. To my surprise, the goat was hanging by its neck from the roof! Somehow it had squeezed itself through the 8-inch space between the rails that circled my roof rack. By the time I stopped the truck, and we got out of the car, the goat looked dead!

Over the years, I had personally contributed to the extermination from the hospital grounds of more than 100 of the creatures. I had to do it because every morning they did their best to spread droppings on every bench, sidewalk, or available floor. Since I had no animosity towards this particular goat, I climbed up onto the roof and gently squeezed the unconscious animal through the side rails and back onto the plywood floor of my roof rack. By squeezing its chest, I apparently revived it, and for the next few minutes it lay gasping like a fish out of water. As the goat recovered, I saw that it had made a complete hash of everything on the roof! Ropes, the sacks of manioc, the empty rice bag they had tied him in, and his choke rope were impossibly tangled and smeared with a sticky green slime, which turned out to be oozing from the goat.

It took me fifteen minutes to untie all the ropes, pile the sacks of manioc toward the front of the roof, lash the goat's feet together towards the back of the rack, and secure everything. When I was finished, green slime covered my hands, forearms, elbows, knees and shoes. I found a nearby puddle and washed the slime off as best as I could. As I climbed back into the driver's seat, Ilobo wisely chose to say nothing.

An hour later, we arrived in Mouila, the provincial capital, and the Peace Corps volunteer bid us goodbye. I needed to talk to the work inspector about an employee problem, so we drove to his office and parked the Landcruiser next to the building. Pastor Luke and I went inside and were warmly received. The meeting took longer than expected and would have gone on even longer had not one the work inspector's secretaries come running in to announce that the goat up on top of our truck appeared to be dying!

We emerged from the inspector's office to find four or five strangers doing their best to save our goat, as it had somehow worked itself over to the opposite side of the roof rack and in so doing, was strangling itself. Strands of gooey saliva ran from its blue tongue and down the windows of my Landcruiser. A man who had been waiting in the work inspector's office to file a claim against his employer was now tenderly loosening the rope around the goat's neck so it could breathe more easily. The employer had seated himself in the driver's seat of my Landcruiser and was shifting the gears into neutral so they could push my truck into the shade of a nearby tree! My mouth was already open in surprise, but the most astonishing display of mercy was one of the inspector's secretaries who was standing on her tip- toes trying to give the gasping animal a drink from a teacup, without getting green saliva on herself! Overall, it was the most astonishing animal rescue I had ever witnessed!

Embarrassed by our thoughtlessness, Pastor Luke, Ilobo and I thanked the inspector, thanked the goat's rescuers, promised to improve our treatment of the animal, and drove away quickly. As we bumped through town, I suggested to Ilobo that since his goat seemed determined to die, it might be best to leave it in Mouila with the local pastor, at least until he found a better way to transport it to Libreville.

"It's only meat," Ilobo replied, surprised at my concern. "If it dies, we'll eat it tonight when we get to Libreville." That sounded so heartless to my reawakened conscience that I hesitated. What was troubling me was the fact that we were killing Ilobo's goat by slow torture. And yet, if I untied its feet, I knew it would try to leap off the roof in an attempt to fly!

"Perhaps," I said hopefully, "once we got moving the wind will calm it." Just to be sure, I stopped outside of town and checked the goat again. It was laying on its side with its tongue hanging out but otherwise seemed to be recovering. For the next two hours, the challenges of simply staying on the poorly graded road made me forget the goat on the roof.

When we were about four hours from Libreville and rounding a curve, we saw a line of orange cones across the road indicating a police check. I slowed the car to a stop, and as I did the two officers sitting on chairs under a palm tree turned their heads toward us in slow motion. In perfect unison their mouths opened, and their right arms lifted into the air. As if choreographed, they pointed their index fingers towards the roof of my truck and in unison shouted, "Your goat is falling off!"

Sure enough, when we jerked around to see where they were pointing, we perceived the familiar blob of a strangling goat hanging from the roof rack. Once again flummoxed, I jumped out and looked up to see what had happened. The little Houdini had managed to squeeze its abdomen and torso through the eight-inch space between the top and bottom side rails of my roof rack. In Mouila I had removed the neck rope so it couldn't strangle itself, but the goat now hung by its feet! This time I was certain we had killed it.

Pastor Luke pushed from below while I pulled from above, and we again squeezed the goat back through the bars. Once again it was therapeutic enough to resuscitate the goat. As we stood there looking up at the animal's blue tongue, I felt trapped. If I didn't try to protect it for the last 80 miles of the trip to Libreville, Ilobo might decide to kill his goat on the spot! Fortunately for us, the police officers thought our technique of transporting goats was more amusing than criminal.

To the sound of their guffaws, I slunk back to my Landcruiser and drove on.

By then we were hungry, so after refueling in Lambaréné we drove to a favorite fast-food restaurant next to the river and ordered three egg omelets on a small loaf of French bread. Pastor Luke and I untied the goat and gently laid it down on the long grass beside the Landcruiser. For the first few minutes it appeared to be dead, looking up at the sky with one dull eye. Feeling sorry for it, I climbed down the riverbank and filled a tin can I found with water so it could drink. When it didn't respond, I poured some of the water on its nose. At that, the goat jumped to its feet, shook itself like a dog, and started chomping on the grass by the car as though it hadn't eaten in days! I tried to offer it water again, but it turned away in disgust, preferring the grass.

As we ate our sandwiches in the shade of a nearby tree, the goat got so frisky that Ilobo and I had to tackle it to tie it up again and get it back on the roof. This time we secured it so well that it couldn't get even close to the sides of the roof rack!

The trip between Lambaréné and Libreville is paved and usually takes around three hours. An hour outside of Libreville we were pounded by a heavy rainstorm. I hoped that it might clean up everything on the roof, but instead it turned the goat's prolific poop into a green film that drooled off the roof onto the sides and windows of the Landcruiser. The goat's ability to produce inexhaustible quantities of the green goo was amazing!

By the end of the trip and because of all the extra stops, our trip took twelve hours instead of ten. When we stopped at Pastor Luke's son's house, Ilobo got off with his goat. Once released, the goat wobbled over to a nearby tree, shook itself vigorously, and bleated once or twice. As I got back into the truck, I glanced at the goat one last time. It looked at me as though it wanted to say something! Later I learned that it played a key role in Ilobo's family celebration, though it was not exactly the guest of honor.

I've often thought about that goat and how we made it suffer up on my roof rack. A year or two later, I passed a minibus on the road carrying no less than four goats on its roof rack. To my astonishment, they were all standing together and happily facing into the wind, restrained with only a rope tied loosely around their necks and the roof rack! No matter how the minibus bounced and leaned as it raced around curves, the goats happily leaned into the turns! And suddenly it hit me: the goats were doing exactly what God made goats to do when they ride on bouncing roof racks or climb and jump on steep mountainsides: they are designed to stay on their *feet*! Even more surprising was to learn that this is mentioned in God's word! Psalms 104:18 states it clearly: "*High in the mountains live the wild goats, and the rocks form a refuge for the hyraxes.*"

If we're willing to read God's Word carefully, His wisdom is available to us! In Ethiopia, goats actually climb trees so they can eat the leaves! In Morocco and Western Algeria, goats climb 30 feet into Argan trees to eat their fruit! God *made* goats to be nimble on their feet, which is surely why Ilobo's goat traveled so miserably when we forced it to travel lying down. Maybe, just maybe the look I saw on the goat's face was a message to check out Psalm 104:18…!

Chapter Eight:

GOODNESS AND MERCY

A Narrow Escape

Though Gabon is filled with natural wonders, it is not one of the world's favorite tourist destinations. In recent decades, Muslim extremists in other African countries have become alarmed by the rapid growth of Christianity in Africa and have responded with hostage-taking and killings. Until now this has not happened in Gabon. Europeans and Americans come to Gabon primarily to make money, but Christians come to serve short-term at Bongolo Hospital as physicians and specialists, and as engineers and builders!

Since 1977, hundreds of Americans and Europeans have made the trip to the hospital. Most found their African experience enjoyable and well worth the trouble. But there are exceptions. One, whom I shall call Steve, faced a tragedy that challenged his faith and reminded us that our ability to live and work in Africa heavily depends on our Heavenly Father.

Steve came to Bongolo as a medical student, accompanied by his wife. Their French was quite limited, and though their lack of fluency limited Steve's ability to function independently at the hospital, it didn't hide his affection for the Gabonese people. After a stay of two months, their time in Gabon came to an end. A missionary nurse named Betty Keifer invited the couple to ride in her Toyota double cab pick-up truck to Libreville. The trip is 211 miles long, and in those days the first 125 miles from Bongolo were graded laterite and gravel. It usually took five to six hours of driving on dirt before reaching the paved part of the road, and by the time the three got to the paved section, Betty was tired and asked if Steve would be willing to drive the rest of the way. Steve kindly accepted.

By that time, they were driving due west, and it was late afternoon. As they drove, the sun was shining directly in their eyes. The road was mostly straight and smooth, and while most drivers drove that section of the road at 100 to 110 kilometers an hour, Steve drove between eight and ninety.

All of a sudden Steve saw a car parked 100 yards ahead of them on the left side of the road. A group of people stood around the rear of the car talking. As Steve approached on the right side of the road, he slowed to 40. At the moment Steve passed the parked car, a young woman darted into the road from his left. It happened so fast he could only slam on the brakes. But it was too late. The front of the pickup hit the woman squarely and threw her thirty feet.

In most countries in Africa, travelers who are involved in a serious accident like this one are advised *not to stop*. In Gabon, even the police advise foreign drivers who hit a pedestrian to continue without stopping until they get to the nearest police station and can report the incident. To ignore this advice is to risk death.

Of all the tribes in Gabon, the Fang tribe is most feared for its reputation of swift, lethal revenge. Steve could not know that he had just killed a Fang woman. Conditioned by a lifetime of Christian teaching and American law, he immediately pulled the car over to the side of the road and stopped. He and his wife and Betty, who was a nurse, rushed to the side of the woman to see if they could help. When they saw that she was dead, they gently carried her body off the road. The three of them were too stunned to think of their own safety.

The Africans who had witnessed the accident were stunned too, but they instantly descended on three foreigners in rage and began hitting them with their fists and slapping them. A large man kicked Betty from behind, and as Steve's wife tried to protect her dazed husband from the blows raining down on him, she deflected a punch to his face with her hand. Only later did she discover the blow had broken a bone. Several in the group ran to their houses to find machetes and spread the news.

The three Americans quickly realized that the people who had witnessed the accident were shocked and angered, but they had not yet comprehended that barring a miracle, they had only minutes to live. Instead of seeking refuge in the car, they tried to reason with the crowd. As precious seconds ticked by, one of the angered villagers reached into Betty's truck, removed the keys, and locked it so they couldn't take refuge in it.

At that moment, a miracle occurred that saved the three of them from death. The Chief of Police from Libreville just happened to be driving toward the accident from the other direction when he saw a crowd on the road swarming over three white foreigners. When he pulled his car to a stop, he saw the body of the victim and instantly understood what was happening. He was in uniform and driving an official car, and in a loud voice he began shouting at the crowd to move away from the foreigners. As the mob hesitated, he led the three to his car, ordered them inside, told them to roll up the windows, and locked the doors. His quick action saved them from certain death.

For the next thirty minutes the stunned trio sat in the stifling car while the policeman calmed the crowd and took statements from the witnesses. Some in the crowd came up to the car and screamed threats and insults at the three Americans, but when the policeman shouted at them, they stopped and moved away.

Eventually, the policeman retrieved the keys to Betty's car and gave them to her so the three of them could follow him five miles ahead to a police station. Once at the station, the policeman locked Steve in a room in the police barracks for his protection and allowed Betty to use the police phone to call the Mission director in Libreville, and he arrived at the police station an hour later. After introducing himself, he asked the police chief if he could stay with Steve while Steve's wife and Betty continued on to Libreville in her car. The police chief agreed, and Betty and Steve's wife continued on to the mission Guest House in Libreville. By this time, it was dark, and Clarence pointed out to the police chief that the victim's relatives lived only a few kilometers away. Unless guards were posted for the night outside the door and outside the room's window, Steve would not be safe from the family of the dead woman. The police chief agreed and allowed Steve and the Mission Director to drive to a recently built hotel in a town ten kilometers away. It was a terrible night for all of them.

As news of the accident spread, the missionaries in Bongolo and the Gabonese Christians in Libreville responded with a great outpouring of prayer on Steve's behalf. Steve and the mission

Field Director remained in the hotel for three days until the police investigation was completed and the paperwork was forwarded to Libreville. Only then were Steve and the Mission Director allowed to drive to Libreville.

It can take up to two months to get a judicial hearing in Gabon, but in less than two weeks, Steve's case came to trial. Mercifully, the judge ruled that since no crime had been committed, Steve could leave the country. The Mission was held responsible to reach a financial settlement with the family, but since the Mission was covered by liability insurance, the problem was turned over to the Mission's insurance company.

Steve and his wife may never know why God allowed that fatal accident on the road to Libreville, but nothing in the life of a Christian is unforeseen by our heavenly Father. When the three missionaries were completely helpless and in grave danger, God sent a policeman just minutes after the accident to deliver them from certain death.

Was it an accident that the chief of police arrived at the moment he did? I'm certain that it wasn't. The question we must ask is "Why would God allow young Steve and his wife to come close to a violent death on a Gabonese road, and then with perfect timing save them?" I can't think of a better example of God's providence.

King David wrote in Psalm 18:19-20, "*He led me to a place of safety; He rescued me because He delights in me. The Lord rewarded me for doing right; He restored me because of my innocence, for I have kept the ways of the Lord; I have not turned from my God to follow evil.* He wrote again about God's protection in Psalms 116:6-9.

Theologian Wayne Grudem writes about being thankful for all good things that happen: "If we genuinely believe that all good things are caused by God, then our hearts will indeed be full when we say, 'Bless the Lord, O my soul, and forget not all his benefits (Psalm 103:2) … We will 'give thanks in all circumstances'(I Thess 5:18). All things come to pass by God's wise providence. This means that we should adopt a much more 'personal' understanding of the universe and the events in it. The universe is not governed by impersonal fate or luck, but by a personal God. Nothing 'just happens,'—we should see God's hand in events throughout the day, causing all things to work together for good for those who love him. This confidence in God's wise providence certainly does not equal superstition, for it is not belief in impersonal or demonic control, nor is it control by a capricious deity concerned for meaningless ritual rather than obedience and faith. A deepened appreciation for the doctrine of providence will not make us more superstitious; it will make us trust in God more and obey him more fully."[8]

The book of Lamentations records Jeremiah's grief over the destruction of Jerusalem and its people (Lamentations 3:14-19):

"My own people laugh at me. All day long they sing their mocking songs. He has filled me with bitterness and given me a bitter cup of sorrow to drink. He has made me chew on gravel. He has rolled me in the dust. Peace has been stripped away, and I have forgotten what prosperity is. I cry out, 'My splendor is gone! Everything I had hoped for from the Lord is lost!' The thought of my suffering and homelessness is bitter beyond words."

But then in verses 20-26, Jeremiah reflects on all that has happened: *"I will never forget this awful time, as I grieve over my loss. Yet I still dare to hope when I remember this: The faithful love of the Lord never ends! His mercies never cease. Great is His faithfulness; His mercies begin afresh each morning. I say to myself, 'The Lord is my inheritance; therefore, I will hope in him! The Lord is good to those who depend on Him, to those who search for Him. So, it is good to wait quietly for salvation from the lord."'*

Preaching Wet

When Pastor Luke Mambela invited me to accompany him on Sunday to the four villages of Nzingui, Mbelenaletembet,

Yissinga and Nzoundou to preach, I accepted with pleasure. Earlier that year, Pastor Luke had been appointed the senior pastor of the Bongolo church, plus four of its daughter churches on back road.

He had retired from serving as the hospital administrator for 20 years, and I wanted to help him in any way I could. All four villages were situated on a road a logging company made several decades earlier through dense rain forest, and since then the government

8 *Systematic Theology: An Introduction to Biblical Doctrine*, Second Editon, Wayne Grudem, 2020, pp.464-5.

had taken it over. The road had many log bridges over streams and gullies, and every ten or fifteen years the bridges would collapse and need to be rebuilt. Since there were many pick-up truck taxis that ran up and down the roads, I knew the road would be passable.

As I prepared my sermon, I pictured myself standing in front of an attentive crowd of friendly Christians mixed with curious villagers. I would speak in French and Pastor Luke would translate my message into the Yinzebi language for the older folks.

The night before we left, a huge storm front moved in and dumped at least three inches of rain. I wasn't worried, since there were many storms like it during the rainy season. Besides, Becki and I had a two-year-old Nissan Patrol that had a powerful winch on the front bumper.

Becki and I picked up Pastor Luke at his house and left Bongolo at 6:30 a.m. There was a lot of mud, and the Patrol slid around a bit, but the deep treads on my tires and the Patrol's 4-wheel drive conquered every hill and hole we encountered. We were about five kilometers from the first village when I suddenly pulled up to an unfinished, thirty-foot log bridge over a deep stream. A government road crew had started rebuilding the bridge the week before, using forty-foot-long logs to span the stream 10 feet below.

The bridge-builders had begun nailing four-inch-thick boards crossways on top of the logs, starting on the far end of the bridge. But to reach the boards, I would have to drive for ten feet on top of slippery logs! To cross, I would have to drive the first ten feet on top of the parallel logs, then bump up onto the four-inch-thick boards nailed crossways.

Someone the day before the rains had come had shoveled dirt between the parallel logs to make it easier to cross, but the rain had washed much of it away and had turned the rest into mush.

Pastor Luke and Becki volunteered to walk to the far end of the bridge and direct me, so I put my SUV in low four-wheel drive and started out, watching their hand directions. My front wheels were apparently centered on the parallel logs because Pastor Luke held his hands straight up and down and motioned me forward. Becki was giving me the "c'mon on, c'mon, drive it!" sign, so I drove forward but moved so cautiously that when my front tires reached the six-inch thick boards, I didn't have enough momentum to bump up onto them. I would have to back up and try again with more speed.

I slowly backed up six feet, then stepped on the accelerator. This time I my front wheels almost made it, but my back wheels slid off the top of the logs and into the spaces between them. When I got out and looked under the car to see what happened, my heart sank. The front left wheel of my truck was just six inches from the edge of the bridge, my rear wheels had slipped off the logs and into the mush between the logs, and my differential was sitting up on a log between them. To move forward, I would have to get a jack under the axle, crank it up until the differential was free, then drive off without falling off the bridge!

Pastor Luke, Becki and I walked around the truck considering all this. At first, I thought I might be able to use the winch on the front bumper to pull the front end of the Nissan over to the center of the bridge and up onto the boards. If that worked, then maybe the winch could drag the back wheels out of the hole.

We all agreed that my idea might work, so I unwound fifty feet of cable from the winch and attached it to a tree at the far end of the bridge. When we were ready, I flipped the switch. Nothing happened! I couldn't believe it! The winch had never failed me!! I tried toggling the switch, shaking it and finally banging it with a rock, but the winch was dead. I finally gave up and went back to look at the rear axle and differential.

"Someone," I said to Pastor Luke, hoping he would volunteer, "will have to crawl under there, set the jack under the axle, and crank it up until the differential is no longer resting on the log."

I looked over at Pastor Luke to see if he was volunteering, but he was already looking for rocks to put under the tires. I looked down at my freshly ironed Dockers and my light cotton shirt and wondered what I had been thinking when I got dressed that morning!

Muttering to myself about the unfairness of it all, I got on all fours behind the truck and, gripping the heavy jack, gingerly crawled toward the axle.

The space was small, so small in fact that the only way I could get anywhere near the axle was to lie flat on my stomach. As I wriggled forward on mud, a blob of it slid between my skin and my belt.

As I advanced further, more mud slithered under my belt between the buttons of my shirt. By the time I got the jack into position I had mud in my mustache, my eyebrows, my ears, even my nose. When my neck muscles grew tired from holding my head out of the slime, I had to rest it on… mud! It occurred to me that the Lord could not have brought me down any lower from my high station as Bongolo Hospital's only surgeon!

It reminded me of how God humbled Joseph by allowing his jealous brothers throw him into a pit and then sell him into slavery. After he climbed to the top position in Potiphar's house, God humbled him again by sending him to prison after being falsely accused by Potiphar's wife.

I certainly didn't think of these great stories of the Bible as I struggled to place a jack under my SUV in six inches of mud. But I did briefly think, "Why are you doing this to me, Lord?" Perhaps it was God's way of reminding me that I was no less a sinner saved by grace than the villagers I would preach to later that day!

By the time I got the jack in place and cranked up enough to lift the differential up, Pastor Luke had collected more than 30 good rocks for me to put under the tires and was now almost as muddy as I was! Once they were in place under the rear tires, I crawled out from under my SUV.

Before making our final attempt to cross the bridge, Pastor Luke I went below the bridge, took off our shirts, pants, and shoes, clothes, and immersed ourselves in the stream. Our shirts would never look the same and my jeans were now brownish blue, but at least the mud was gone! We had no towels, so I climbed back into the truck dripping wet.

When all was ready, Pastor Luke suggested that we ask God to help us and to keep us from sliding off the bridge. We all knew that if the front wheels slipped just two inches to the left, our SUV would go over the side and down into the stream 10 feet below.

When we were ready, I started the motor, turned the front wheels to the right, and with my heart banging in both faith and fear, stepped on the accelerator and lunged the truck forward. The front wheels grabbed the boards, the rear wheels spun briefly, then grabbed and as we all cheered, our SUV surged up onto the bridge and over to the other side!

We arrived in the first village an hour late, and a crowd of about forty men, women, children, dogs, goats and curious chickens had gathered at the mudbrick church and were waiting patiently. If they found our appearance unusual, they gave no sign of it, singing, clapping in unison and welcoming us with wide smiles. Pastor Luke and I slogged to the front of the church, leaving wet and muddy footprints on the cement floor.

Fifteen minutes later, it was my turn to preach. In my stained, dripping clothes I shared with the villagers my testimony. Pastor Luke stood beside me in his matching outfit and as I preached in French and shared my testimony, he translated it into the tribal language.

That day, we preached four times in four different villages. Each time after sharing my testimony, I tried my best to explain why Jesus deserves our love. Had anyone else suffered and died for them? Had anyone else sent doctors and nurses with medicines and vaccinations to save their children from deadly diseases? Jesus did, and it was because of him that we were there for them.

Sometime later, I was again invited to preach at those same four villages. Confident that lightning wouldn't strike twice, I agreed to go. A cardiologist named Ron Johannsen was visiting the hospital then, and I invited him to go with me. Ron had come several times before to help out at the hospital, and over the years we had become close friends.

The evening before we were to leave, a storm front moved into the area and dumped three inches of rain in four hours, just like my previous trip with Pastor Luke! I should have wondered about the weather, but somehow it didn't register. Since Ron was the only person riding with me, I decided to take our small, four-wheel drive Suzuki Samurai instead of our big Nissan Patrol. We left Bongolo at 7 a.m. and were not surprised to find the road muddy and slippery. The little car spun and fishtailed repeatedly but never stopped moving forward. Several times we powered through deep, water-filled mudholes in four-wheel drive.

Then we came to a ten-foot-wide, flood-swollen stream. I had easily forded the same stream earlier in the week after a rainstorm, so and I was confident that it would not be a major problem. Slipping into four-wheel drive, I eased the Suzuki into the water. Suddenly the front bumper and headlights went underwater. As I gunned the motor we lurched and leaned thirty degrees to the left. Water flowed up over the hood, so I unsuccessfully tried to back out. By then water was pouring through the leaky door seals and rose to our laps. Our motor kept going, but we were firmly stuck. At that point, Ron grabbed his camera, and I grabbed my Bible and songbooks. We climbed out the passenger door that was still above water and pulled ourselves out of the stream and onto the road.

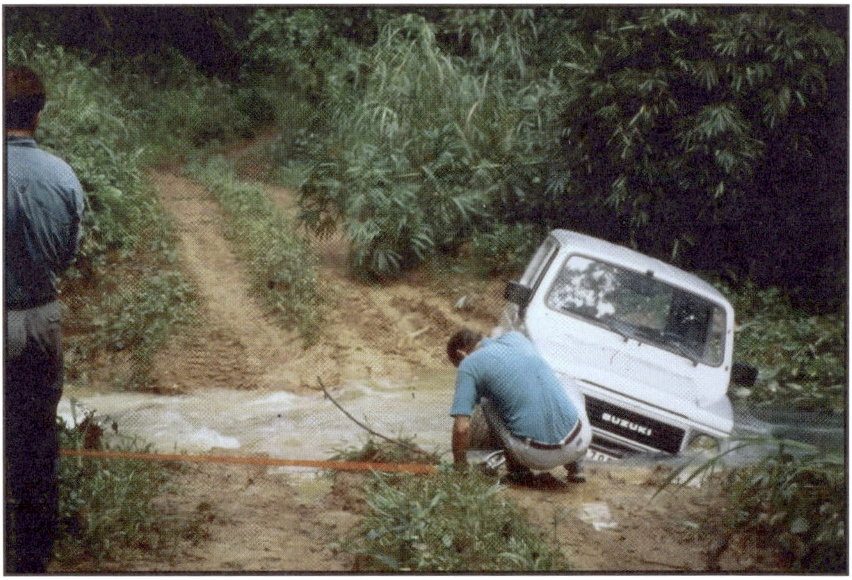

The author attaches the come-along strap to the Suzuki

As we stood on the bank and looked at our situation, we tried to figure out what to do next. I always carried a come-along in the Suzuki, so I waded to the back door and fished it out. We were surrounded by trees, but none of them were close to the stream. The cable on the come-along was at least twenty feet too short to reach the nearest tree. But fifteen feet from the Suzuki was a small clump of bamboo.

A mature bamboo stalk is as strong as cable and almost impossible to pull out by the roots, so I grabbed the nearest bamboo stalk and used my weight to pull the leafy end to the ground. Ron and I then hooked the come-along to the end of the bamboo. Ron waded in and hooked the other end of the come-along to a hook under the front bumper. The two of us took turns cranking the come- along until the car started to inch out of the hole. When the come-along wasn't strong enough to pull us any further, Ron suggested I try to drive the Suzuki out while he maintained pressure with the come-along. I waded into the stream and settled into the driver's seat. The water in the driver's seat was above my waist, but fortunately, the ignition key wasn't underwater. When I turned the key, the motor started on the third try, the exhaust bubbling up behind it like an outboard motor. After engaging 4-wheel drive I revved the motor, let out the clutch, and the feisty little car surged up onto dry land! Ron was doing some kind of victory dance, and I nearly ran him over!

An hour later, we arrived at the first scheduled service and were warmly welcomed by about 30 people. We walked to the front still wet and muddy and greeted the people warmly, explaining why we arrived wet and late. Most of the people had been to the hospital and knew me well, but when I introduced Ron as a visiting "heart doctor" they were thrilled! In each of the four churches that day, an elder translated for us as we gave our testimonies and I preached the message from God's word.

I don't really know how much or little God used our messages to strengthen and encourage the village Christians that day, but the lessons I took home was that: 1) God is willing to go to great lengths to keep his servants humble, and 2) God cares deeply about his children, especially those who live on a fraction of the incomes and blessings we require, and love Him anyway. Every time I visited Christians in the villages outside of Bongolo, I was deeply affected by their faith and courage.

How many of us would put money in our church offering plate if the only food we had to eat was what we grew ourselves? I saw our African Christians do this weekly. If we lived in a house we built out of mud bricks that we had to make ourselves, would we be thankful? Even if our completed house couldn't keep out cockroaches, spiders, rats and bats? For years I stood woodenly while African Christians danced with joy as they sang God's praises! If our monthly income amounted to $50 or $100, would I tithe? Would I share it with the needy? I saw my African friends give their money with joy, often dancing in a line to the front of a church with the offering place rested.

How great would our faith be If our only clean water was rain-water, and it didn't rain for a month? Would I sing God's praise on my five- mile walk home from my garden, while carrying 50 pounds of food on my back? If the nearest doctor was a four-hour drive away in an open pick-up truck and one stops in my village and has room for me, would I shout, "Praise you, Jesus!" If my children's only school had one teacher with a blackboard, the classroom had no desks, only benches, and the teacher could beat my kid with a stick if he falls asleep, would I count the school a blessing? How long would we call ourselves "Christians" if God allowed half of our children to die of malaria? Isaiah 61:1 is a prophecy about the Messiah's love for the poor, not the rich: "*The Spirit of the Sovereign Lord is upon me, for the Lord has anointed me to bring good news to the poor.*"

On God's Wings

In 1995, twenty-seven years after my parents died in Vietnam, I got a phone call from a retired missionary who had served in Vietnam until the end of the war in 1975. She asked me, "Have you and your brothers and sisters ever heard what happened to the B'nong people in Cambodia after your parents were killed?" Because in Africa we heard nothing about the B'nong people and Vietnam was still in the grip of a grim Communist government, we assumed the B'nong were still living in spiritual darkness. The story this retired missionary told us brought us to our knees.

In 1974, the North Vietnamese army moved into eastern Cambodia one last time. They came with tanks, troop carriers, long-range artillery, and an army twice as big as any previous army. Their invasion was the prelude to their final campaign to take over South Vietnam. As North Vietnam's army advanced towards Cambodia's eastern border, the soldiers ruthlessly burned the villages and the rice fields of the B'nong people, forcing them and other tribes living in eastern Cambodia to flee with whatever they could carry into Vietnam. There were no roads, just paths, so the refugees walked through the jungles on foot, carrying their children and whatever else they could bring on their backs. Within days they were out of food and water and were starving. Many of their children were sick from drinking foul water. Eventually, 100,000 Montagnard refugees fled into Vietnam's central highlands. The South Vietnamese government was overwhelmed by the crisis but managed to move most of them into former U.S. army bases. There the refugees found buildings to shelter in but no beds, blankets, water, food, or medicines.

Vietnamese and Montagnard Christians and the few American missionaries in the area realized what was happening and brought the desperate refugees food, clean water, blankets, medicines, and eventually, the gospel. When they heard the gospel, their leaders stood up and said, "Hey! We've heard this story before, in Cambodia, when Pastor Thompson and his wife came to our villages and told us about Jesus! Why aren't they here?"

With tears in their eyes, the Christians said to them, "The Thompsons came here to Banmethuot in 1968 to help our people on this side of the border. But 7 years ago, the Communists attacked Banmethuot and killed them! Their graves are over in Banmethout!"

When the B'nong heard the news, something broke in their hearts and they began to turn to Jesus; first a hundred, then a thousand, then 5,000! When the war was over and the Communist government allowed them to return to their lands in Cambodia, there were 7,000 B'nong Christians!

When Becki, my brothers and sisters and I heard the news, we wept, laughed, danced, and hugged each other! We immediately contacted the Vietnamese church leaders and began making plans to travel to Vietnam and if possible Banmethuot, to see mom and dad's grave. It was a grave we had only seen in photos. But when we applied for visas, we received a cold letter from the communist Vietnamese officials. They asked, "What crimes did your parents commit that resulted in their executions?" We were shocked and grieved by their harsh response, but there was nothing we could do.

Five years later, I received a letter from the Vietnamese Alliance church, encouraging us to apply again. We would later learn that this was through the efforts of Reg Reimer, one of the missionaries who was at my parents' grave for their funeral. This time we were granted visas and permission to travel to Banmethuot to see our parents' grave. In June of 2009, Becki, my siblings (Judith, Dale, Laurel and Tom) and I traveled to Vietnam. The plan was that Becki and I would fly out of Libreville, and we would all meet in Ho Chi Minh City before traveling together to Banmethuot.

Becki and I booked flights on Air Ethiopia out of Libreville, but because of a mechanical problem the flight was delayed for 24 hours. When we finally arrived in Addis Ababa, Air Ethiopia's flight to Saigon was ready to pull away from the gate. We sprinted to the nearest transfer counter in the terminal, only to learn that there were only enough empty seats for ten more passengers! Air Ethiopia would not have another flight to Ho Che Minh City until the following week!

By the time we got to the transfer counter, there were twenty people in front of us, all clamoring to get on! And we were at the very back of the line!

Convinced that it was hopeless, I sat down on a nearby stairwell, covered my face, and prayed, though with only a thimbleful of faith.

Becki, however, turned into a tiger and fought her way through the crowd to the counter, saying "Excuse me! Excuse me!" When she got there, she leaned over the counter said to the two harassed agents, "Do you see my husband sitting over there?" Their heads swiveled towards me and back to Becki. "He's been waiting to visit his mother and father's grave in Vietnam for more than 20 years, along with all his brothers and sisters! And now that we have permission to go, your airline messed up, and now you are making it impossible for him to be there with the rest of his family! Have pity on him! If we don't get there tomorrow, he will miss the ceremony and all of his family members!"

Both agents stopped what they were doing. Then one of them said something to the other one and they brought out two blank passes and wrote our names on them *by hand,* along with the flight number! Then they called their colleague at the gate with instructions to get us on the plane! While this was happening the crowd quieted down, obviously touched by our dilemma.

As soon as Becki and I got our tickets, we sprinted for the gate. In order to make room for us the attendants pulled a passenger off the plane who had thought he was going. As we ran up to the gate he was sitting forlornly on his suitcase. As we raced by him, I waved and thanked him!

Not surprisingly, the seats they gave us were far apart, but we didn't care! We were on God's wings! As we buckled our seatbelts the captain announced over the intercom that the "mechanical problem" that had delayed the flight had now been fixed! That was the first and only time I've been called a "mechanical problem!"

We landed in Ho Chi Minh City twelve hours later and caught up with my family members the next day in the city of Banmethuot. When we were finally able to visit our parents grave, we were shepherded by anxious Vietnamese security officials who were afraid we might make a scene. The mission houses had been razed, and a four-story hospital now occupied most of the property. On the back end there was a parking lot, and between the parking lot and a wall, we saw the grave.

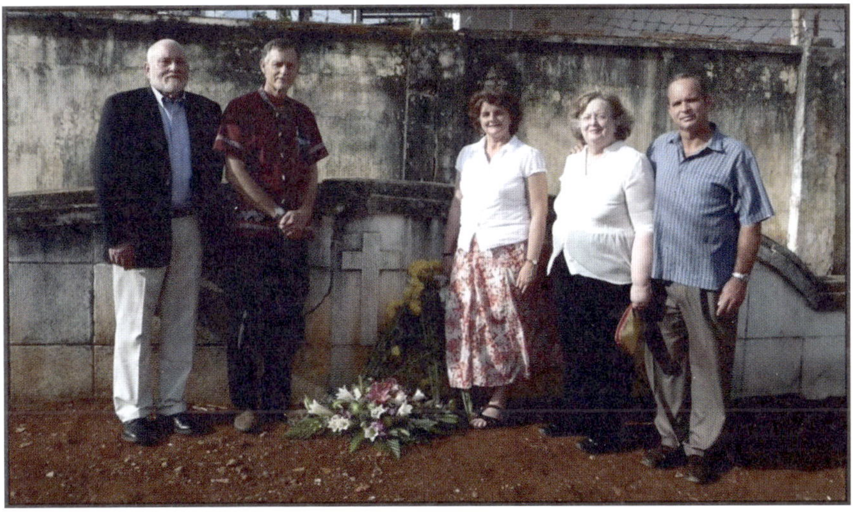

The Thompson children at their parents' grave in Banmethuot, Vietnam, 41 years after their parents' martyrdom. Left to right: Dale, the author, Laurel, Judy, and Tom.

Originally the grave had had headstones and two marble plaques on the ground inscribed with their names, the date of their deaths, and Jesus' words to His disciples in John 24:24 in English and Vietnamese: *"I tell you the truth, unless a kernel of wheat is planted in the soil and dies, it remains alone. But its death will produce many new kernels—a plentiful harvest of new lives."* The Communists took over the mission property and built a three-story hospital on it. Montagnard and Vietnamese church leaders requested permission to relocate the grave to church property, but the government refused. Since our visit in 2009, the grave continues to deteriorate. But the bones of the martyrs are still speaking!

The next day was Sunday, and the Montagnard Christians invited us to a "house church" that was outside of town in a coffee plantation. They drove the five of us in a minibus, and the drive over a rough gravel road that kept us bouncing took half an hour. When we finally arrived, we drove past an acre of coffee bushes, a large aluminum warehouse, and finally, a modest brick house. They sat us at a round table in the dining room and served us delicious coffee and pastries. We were perplexed because there were only about five people in the house drinking coffee with us, and we wondered when the service would begin. But as soon as we finished our coffee, they asked us to follow them out the door and over to the nearby warehouse. When we stepped inside, we were stunned to see more than 500 people sitting quietly on benches and facing away from us. Only then did we realize that the huge warehouse was the "house church" for the Montagnard Christians! As we walked to the front, many quietly waved and smiled at us. There were a few Americans there too, and they were smiling at our surprise.

The church service lasted an hour and a half and included three large choirs that took turns singing praises to Jesus in various languages. We were surprised again when the ushers opened large windows on both sides of the warehouse to let in light and air. Then they placed benches outside for the policemen who attended and gave them hymnals so they could sing with the congregation! The choirs and congregational singing lasted 45 minutes. Then the pastor invited each one of my brothers and sisters to say a few words. As we sat through what was clearly a memorial service for us and our parents, we couldn't keep the tears from filling our eyes and running down our cheeks.

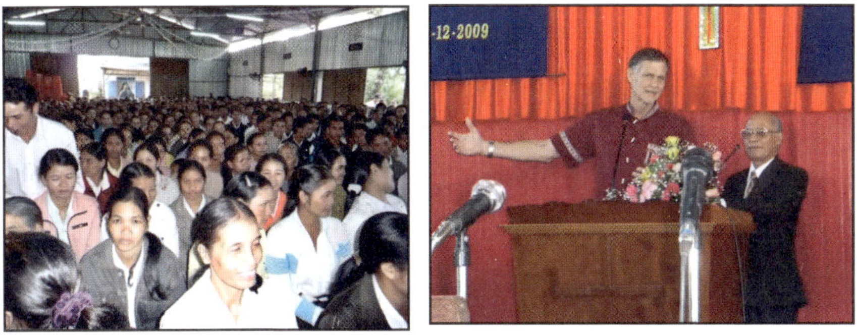

The "House Church" in the coffee warehouse.

I was the last to speak through a translator. I briefly told how God had comforted me and my siblings after the loss of our parents, and that we knew God was doing the same for them as they continued to trust and follow Jesus. Though we missed our parents, we knew they were in heaven, and that as they could see, God was still taking care of us and had made our faith in Jesus remain strong. I ended by briefly sharing how God sent Becki and me to Africa to share the gospel with the sick and the poor, and that we would be returning there after we left Vietnam. Finally, I gave them greetings from Becki's mother in America, who they all knew and loved.

When the war ended in late 1975, the Communist government allowed B'nong refugees to return to their homelands in Cambodia. By then, 7,000 of them had come to faith in Jesus and had burned their fetishes! But that was only the beginning. When the B'nong returned to their villages on Cambodia's side of the border, they took the gospel with them and led tens of thousands more of their relatives and friends to faith in Jesus! So many believed in Jesus that they lost count!

After we left Vietnam, Judy, Laurel, Dale, Becki and I flew to Phnom Penh and drove to Kratie. We stayed for a week and were able to visit all the houses where we had lived in Kratie.

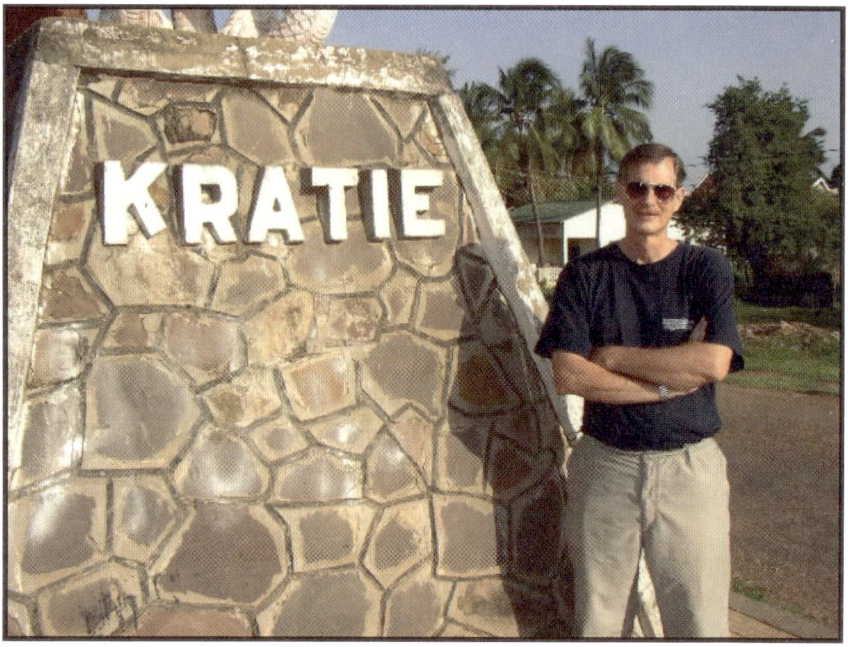

The author in 2009, at the entrance to the town of Kratie

At the time of our visit, our daughter Rachael was serving as a missionary in Cambodia, and she drove us into eastern lands of the B'nong. A Cambodian missionary to the B'nong guided us to a village where the Christians had built a church. As we stepped inside, we were astonished to see on the back wall the logo of the Christian & Missionary Alliance, the church our parents had served under. I turned to the pastor and asked him why they that logo was important to them. He asked the people to answer the question, and one of the elders said, "We have it up there because those were the people who loved us. They came to our villages and told us about Jesus, and some of them even died for us. We can never forget them!" That word alone made our trip unforgettable!

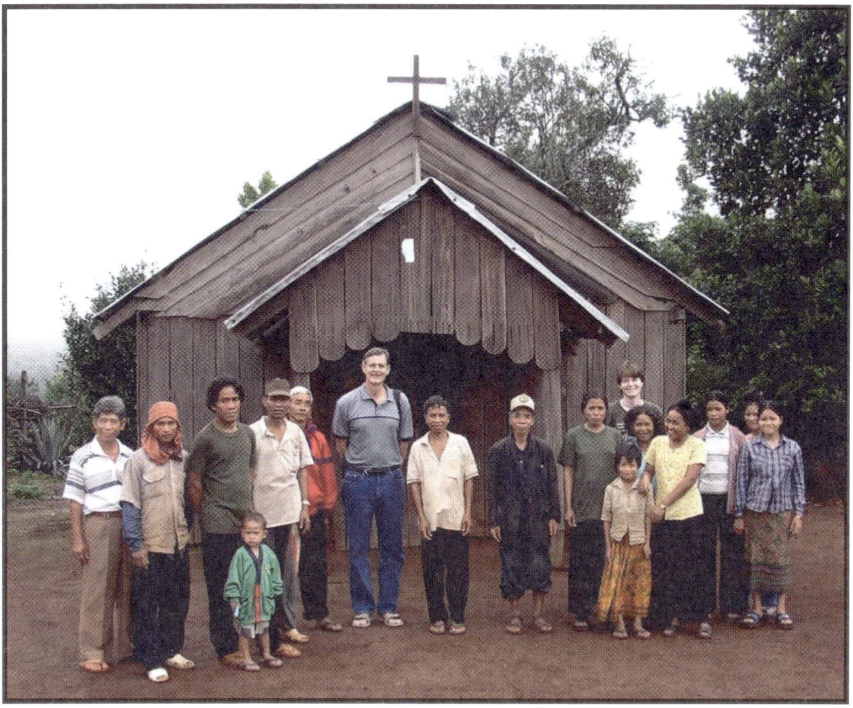

A B'nong church - 2009

In 2023, the B'nong Christians counted themselves in Cambodia and Vietnam. The number of those who declared themselves to be followers of Jesus Christ came to 107,000! God knew all along that it would take the blood of His saints—our parents were among a total of 10 missionaries who gave their lives over the years to win the B'nong, as well as hundreds of thousands of other Montagnards to faith in Jesus, a truly "plentiful harvest in new lives," (John 12:24).

Becki and I returned to our work in Gabon with renewed joy and faith, and with the promise of God in Isaiah 40:31 in our hearts: "*But those who trust in the Lord will find new strength. They will soar high on wings like eagles. They will run and not grow weary. They will walk and not faint.*"

Poisoned!

When our pediatrician Deborah Walker called me on the CB radio at 2 a.m. I was so groggy that it took me several minutes to understand what she was talking about. What I heard was something about a young woman who couldn't breathe, and that Deborah wanted permission to take her to our main operating room because it had bottled oxygen, which the woman desperately needed. Could I please come down and help?

It was dark and raining as I unlocked the garage doors. Why in the world would Dr. Walker need me come down to the hospital in the middle of the night for a case of asthma? I grumbled all the way down the hill, until I pulled my SUV to a stop in front of the surgery building and saw a crowd. I pushed through several anxious family members who were clustered outside the operating room doors and went inside.

When I entered the OR, I saw an unconscious young woman with blue lips, lying on her back on the operating table. Deborah had lowered the head of the OR table by six inches and was suctioning pink froth out of the young woman's mouth. Oxygen tubing with nasal prongs was already feeding oxygen into her nose, but her eyes were wide and desperate, and her chest was heaving violently from the effort to breathe. Every fifteen seconds she coughed out gobs of pink froth into an emesis basin that one of our nurses held next to her mouth. Dr. Walker was listening to the woman's chest with her stethoscope while a frightened nursing student took the patient's blood pressure and another student held the pulse oximeter monitor clip from falling off the woman's finger. The oxygen level recorded by the pulse oximeter was now in the high 80's, which was still low enough to precipitate cardiac arrest. The nurses rad managed to insert an IV in one arm, but only for medicines, since the woman clearly did not need more fluid. The burning question was, what would cause acute pulmonary edema in previously healthy young woman?

Dr. Walker quickly explained that when she first saw the young woman in the emergency room, she thought she was having an asthma attack. But when she started coughing up pink, frothy fluid, she rightly concluded that her patient was in acute congestive heart failure. Why would a perfectly healthy young woman suddenly develop congestive heart failure?

Just about then the oxygen monitor was alarming. I glanced at it and saw that the oxygen level was hovering again around eighty five percent. We had to dear her lungs more quickly and help her breathe, so I quickly slipped an endotracheal tube into her trachea, making it possible for us to suction deep into her lungs efficiently. This increased the oximeter reading to ninety percent, but we still didn't know what was causing our patient's heart failure.

I asked Dr. Walker if the young woman or her family had given any information about how the illness had started. All she knew was that the young woman's problem started a couple of hours ago, and suddenly. That sounded like poisoning, but when her symptoms had started, she had told her family that she hadn't eaten anything unusual. A family member had explained to Dr. Walker that our patient had never had a problem like this before. Her worsening condition made less and less sense.

Then Dr. Walker said, "Oh, her mother told me she's six weeks pregnant:' Deb added. A lightbulb went off in my head.

"Could she have taken something to abort her baby?" I asked. Dr. Walker said, "I already asked, and the family said no:'

Madeleine couldn't talk with an endotracheal tube in her throat, but we needed to find out if she was ready to tell us something. Putting my mouth next to her ear, I asked her if in the previous twenty-four hours had she swallowed something that a midwife in town gave her, or that a Nganga gave her. She shook her head. About then our chaplain, Boukila Simon, arrived Deb explained to him what was happening. He knelt next to her ear and after introducing himself, prayed that God would intervene to save her life and would give us wisdom on how to help her.

But then once again the young woman's oxygen saturation dropped to 85% again. Dr. Walker suggested to Pastor Simon that the young woman might be hiding something from us because her clinical picture didn't make sense. She couldn't talk, but as we continued to suction her trachea through the endotracheal tube, she was sometimes conscious enough to nod or shake her head. If there was something she could tell us that she was hiding from her family, we might be able to save her life. Otherwise, she could die. Pastor Simon knelt next to her and spoke urgently into her ear, explaining that unless God intervened, we couldn't save her. Was there anything more she could tell us? Barely conscious and as I continued suctioning her lungs, she apparently heard his question, only this time she did not shake her head "no."

Then he asked, "Did you take something to kill your baby?" After hesitating, she nodded. Just then her oxygen level dropped below 80% percent. At any moment she could arrest, and we might not be able to bring her back. Desperate, I asked everyone in the operating room to be quiet while I prayed one more time.

"Father," I cried out, my voice shaking with emotion, "please give this young woman another chance! If she doesn't know you Lord, and she dies now, it will be too late! We've done all we can, but it's not working! Please touch her and reverse the effect of the poisons she has put in her body! Please give her another chance!"

Medical grade oxygen monitors beep at different pitches with every heartbeat. The lower the oxygen level, the lower the beep, and vice versa. As I began my prayer, pleading for her life, the pitch of the monitor remained low, but ten seconds after I said "amen," the pitch began moving up! I turned and looked at the monitor, and as I watched, the oxygen level passed 80, then 85, then 90, and kept moving up, even though we weren't doing anything different!

Her oxygen level stayed in the 90's, and an hour later we extubated her and moved her to a hospital bed and gave her oxygen by mask. There was no doubt in any of our minds that God heard our prayers and intervened to save the young woman's life.

I wish I could report that she gave her heart to Jesus before she left the hospital, but she returned home knowing God had given her another chance to live. I still pray that someday she will repent of her sins and give her heart to Jesus.

God heals people today in response to prayers of faith. Some who doubt that might say this young woman recovered because of the medical measures we employed, that we breathed for her and suctioned her lungs so effectively that h er body's natural defenses won out over the poison she used. But Dr. Walker and I were there in that desperate moment, and we and the nurses who helped us saw exactly what happened!

There is a story in the Bible in Isaiah 38:15 that describes a Jewish king named Hezekiah. Hezekiah was a good and godly king, but one day he fell seriously ill. Isaiah the prophet wrote the story of what happened:

"This is what the LORD says: 'Put your house in order, because you are going to die; you will not recover.' Hezekiah turned his face to the wall and prayed to the LORD, 'Remember, O'LORD, how I have walked before you faithfully and with whole-hearted devotion and have done what is good in your eyes.' And Hezekiah wept bitterly. Then the word of the LORD came to Isaiah: 'Go and tell Hezekiah, This is what the LORD, the God of your father David, says: I have heard your prayer and seen your tears: I will add fifteen years to your life.'"

Then Isaiah said to the King's attendants, "Prepare a poultice of figs and apply it to the boil, and you will recover," (Isaiah 38:21). This was apparently done, and Hezekiah recovered.

So, what healed Hezekiah? God's power, or the figs? It's my medical opinion that God used both *natural* and *supernatural* means to heal the good king Hezekiah, and He still does it today!

A Boy Full of Cancer

In early 2000, a four-year-old boy came to our hospital with an intestinal obstruction. When he arrived, he was near death from vomiting and dehydration. Fortunately, with antibiotics and intravenous fluids we were able to reverse his state of shock and sepsis. I took him to the operating room fully expecting to find him full of worms. Instead, I found his abdomen was full of cancer.

The boy's intestinal obstruction had been caused by masses of tumors throughout his small intestine. They had migrated to his liver and spleen, and there were tumor implants throughout his abdominal cavity. With a sinking heart, I removed the portion of his intestine that was obstructed and sewed the two open ends back together. This would enable him to live and eventually resume eating after a few days, but it would not control the extensive cancer in his abdomen.

A biopsy of the tumor eventually revealed he had a highly invasive form of cancer that not very sensitive to chemotherapy or radiation.

When we finished the operation, I found the boy's mother waiting anxiously. She was a single mother, and the boy was her only child. As gently as I could, I explained to her what I had found and told her that only God could heal her boy. Her eyes grew round with horror, and she broke into loud cries, then fell to the ground at my feet, sobbing and beating her head against the cement floor, heartbroken.

I knelt down too but couldn't find words to say. Other patients came over and tried to comfort her, some of them crying with her. But she was so overcome that nothing we said comforted her.

The next day, when she was calmer and sitting next to her sleeping son, our chaplain came by to see her. As they talked, she suddenly asked, "Pastor, the doctor told me yesterday that only God could heal my child. What did he mean by that?"

Over the next thirty minutes the chaplain told her about Jesus and how He had healed people because He was God visiting earth as a man. The pastor told her the whole story of Jesus and asked her if she wanted to invite Him into her life.

"Yes," she said. After they prayed, the chaplain asked her if she believed that Jesus could heal her son.

"The doctor thinks He can!" she replied.

"Do you?" he asked.

After a moment, she said, "Yes!"

"Then let's pray and ask Him," the chaplain said. Placing a gentle hand on the sleeping boy, he prayed for his healing.

A week later we took the stitches out of the boy's abdominal incision. He was eating well, sitting up and walking around, but not demonstrably healed of his cancer. I could still feel a mass in his liver. Because the family lived some distance away, I gave the mother an appointment to come back in a month.

"Aren't you going to give me any medicine for my son?" she asked, disappointment evident in her eyes.

I told her no because he wasn't experiencing any pain and there was no medicine we could give him that would cure him. Then I added something I later regretted.

"In America or France, we could give your son some strong medicines to prolong his life, but they would not be able to cure him of the cancer."

The boy's mother sat up straighter.

"Could you give me a prescription so I could try to get them in Libreville?" she asked with renewed hope.

I tried to discourage her, telling her how expensive the chemotherapy drugs would be, that they would be hard to find, and that she would have to come back to the hospital with the medicines and the boy, because the treatment was complicated. Despite my explanation, she would not be deterred. In the end I wrote the prescription.

Four weeks later, the mother and her son missed their appointment. I thought he had probably succumbed to the cancer and died. But two weeks after that, they showed up. I was walking from the OR to my office when she approached me.

"I brought the medicines," she said. I recognized her immediately, but where was the boy? Puzzled, I took the bag and looked inside. Every medicine I had prescribed was there. It must have cost her over $500.

"Do you want to sell these?" I asked.

She looked confused. "No, they're for my son!" Just then a boy who looked at least six years old ran up to her.

"Where is he?" I asked, wondering who the boy was. She looked at me even more confused. "He's right here!" she said. Now it was my turn to look confused. The boy was at least an inch taller and pounds heavier than when I had last seen him. I pulled up his shirt and there was the scar of my operation running vertically down his abdomen. I motioned for them to follow me into the office.

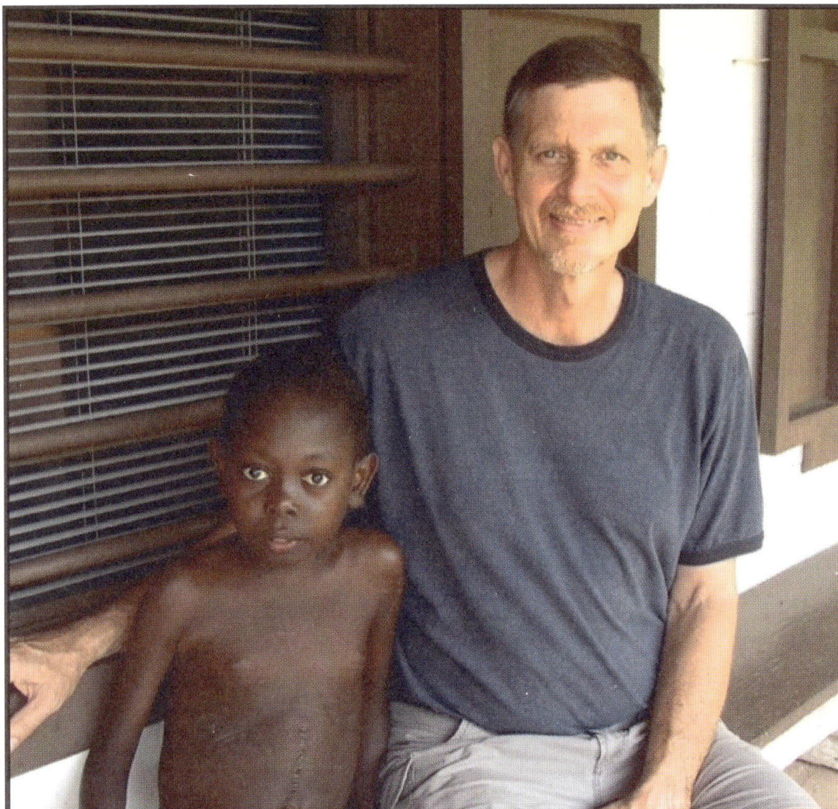

The boy healed from widespread intestinal cancer.

The boy hopped up onto the examining table and grinned at me. He was ticklish, and I had to calm him down so I could feel for his liver and spleen. The contrast from before when his liver was lumpy and enlarged, now it was smooth and normal in size. When I felt for his spleen, I could barely feel the tip of it. There were no lumps or bumps at all in his abdomen where previously there were massive tumors. Turning to the mother, I said, “Madam, God has healed your son!”

A huge smile spread across her face. “Will he still need the medicine?”

In one of the happiest moments of my medical career I said “No!”

What healed the boy? Was it my surgery, or was it God? It was both, of course. If I had not operated on him the day he first came, he would have died from the obstruction of his intestines. But if God had not then intervened and healed him in response to our prayers, he would also have died after the surgery. We followed him for years and his cancer never recurred.

God is the one who designed and made our world and everything in it, down to the smallest details. He created our immune systems and our bodies, and when we are ill, our bodies fight to heal themselves using natural, not supernatural means. God also has the knowledge and power to intervene in His creation and heal sicknesses. This is why the Bible tells us in Colossians 1:17, "in Him all things hold together," and why it says in Hebrews 1:3 that He is "sustaining all things by His powerful word."

There are, therefore, two streams through which God can bring healing to our bodies, and neither way precludes the other. He can bring healing through the natural, created responses of our bodies to disease or injury, and He can help us find healing by helping researchers discover new and effective medicines Finally, God can bring healing directly with His limitless and spiritual power!

This is no surprise to anyone who believes the Bible is true, because the Bible teaches that we live in a universe that is both physical and spiritual. There are physical beings in this world and there are powerful spiritual beings, both good and evil. We are much more than biological machines; we are a wonderful blend of both the physical and the spiritual. That blending remains mysterious to this day and continues to defy human attempts to fully understand it.

I have seen again and again that God willingly partners with His servants to bring healing when asked in faith. God *didn't ask*. The rule is simple: we have to ask for healing in faith. If it's God's will, the result will be healing. But if we don't believe enough to ask, we should not expect God to heal.

As a missionary physician and surgeon, it has been my delight to serve as one of God's junior partners. When I asked for His help, His mighty hand guided my scalpel too.

An Incurable Skin Infection

We first met Donald after a church service in Libreville. Becki and I had returned to Gabon the day before to begin another four-year term of service. We decided to attend a church in the capital city that in 18 years had grown from eight people to more than 3,000. As we worked our way through the crowd to where we had parked our car, a young woman rushed up to us and breathlessly asked, "Are you Dr. Thompson?" I didn't really want to hold a clinic in the church parking lot, but there was no way to deny it.

"Doctor," she said almost desperately, "my little boy has been in the Central Hospital here in Libreville for four months with a strange infection on his chest. The doctors have tried everything, but the infection just keeps getting worse and he is losing weight. My husband and I are afraid he's going to die from it!" Tears filled her eyes as she spoke, and I knew I couldn't refuse. I asked her what she wanted me to do.

"If you will wait, doctor, my husband and I will go get him from the hospital and bring him here." Becki and I agreed to wait, and thirty minutes later a taxi pulled into the church parking lot.

Donald's father stepped out of the taxi holding a thin, frightened, eight-year-old boy in his arms. After the introductions, I took a few moments to greet him and explain that I wanted to see his sore, not hurt him. Reluctantly, he pulled up his T-shirt and showed us a six-inch square bandage on the right side of his chest. He allowed me to lift the bandage, and I saw a baseball-sized hole with ragged, undetermined edges. I could see a bare rib at the base of the wound, and I recognized that he had what was called a "Buruli ulcer."

Buruli ulcers are named after the town in Africa called, "Buruli" where they were first described. They are caused by a bacteria named Mycobacterium Ulcerans, an evil cousin to tuberculosis that infects the skin in tropical climates instead of the lungs. Up until a few years ago, treatment with standard antibiotics did not alter the course of the disease. Untreated, the infection can go on for years and leave severe scarring, deformities and even death. I had seen Buruli ulcers before, but never one this large or deep, and never in a child.

I told Donald's mother and father that I thought we could help him, but the treatment would involve complete excision of all the infected tissue on his chest. After surgery, the wound would be four or five times larger than it was now. They would have to bring him to our hospital in Bongolo, and he would need to stay for several months. Both parents understood and agreed to bring him to Bongolo as soon as possible.

A week later, Donald and his mother showed up, and we admitted him to the surgery ward. The next day, I took him to the operating room and while his mother stood next to him and held his hand, we prayed that God would help us, heal Donald and give us wisdom. I also prayed that Donald would meet Jesus and invite Him into his heart during his stay. Once he was anesthetized his mother left the OR.

The bacteria that cause Buruli ulcers burrow under the skin and subcutaneous fat where there is minimal air. To expose the base of the wound to the air and to topical disinfectants, I had to remove all the infected tissue in the wound. Donald's infection had spread much farther than we expected, and we were forced to remove infected tissue over his entire chest. The disease had even reached into the base of his neck, down to his upper abdomen, and into his groin. Two hours later, at least a fourth of the skin on his body was gone, along with about a pint of blood that we had to replace with a transfusion. I was appalled at the extent of the wound we would have to eventually cover with skin grafts.

But first I covered the raw surfaces of his wound with dressings soaked in Betadine and changed them twice a day. Every time the nurses changed Donald's dressings, we could hear his screams all over the hospital. Even today that memory brings a lump to my throat and tears to my eyes.

Over the next four months, I prayed daily that God would give me the wisdom to save Donald's life. Our team performed a total of thirteen operations on him before we got control of the infection and could start covering his chest and abdomen with skin grafts. Several times he nearly died, and we transfused him six times. It took a total of five months in the hospital before his wounds were healed. Only God knows how he endured so much pain.

God also answered our prayers. As the skin grafts grew and the size of his open wound grew smaller, his pain diminished, his appetite increased, he gained weight, and he grew both physically and spiritually. Midway through his hospitalization he invited Jesus into his heart. All of our team and his parents rejoiced, knowing that no matter what happened to him, he would someday live forever with Jesus!

A year after his discharge, Donald's parents brought him back for follow-up. He had grown so much that at first, we didn't recognize him! When I checked his scars, I found no signs of recurrence and declared him entirely free of Buruli Ulcerans infection.

Twenty years later, Donald visited Bongolo Hospital to thank us for saving his life. He had grown into a strong teenager, and an even stronger faith in Jesus. When he showed us his scar, I was shocked! As his body had doubled, then tripled in size, the huge scar we had covered with skin grafts was reduced to a benign-looking scar ten abdomen.

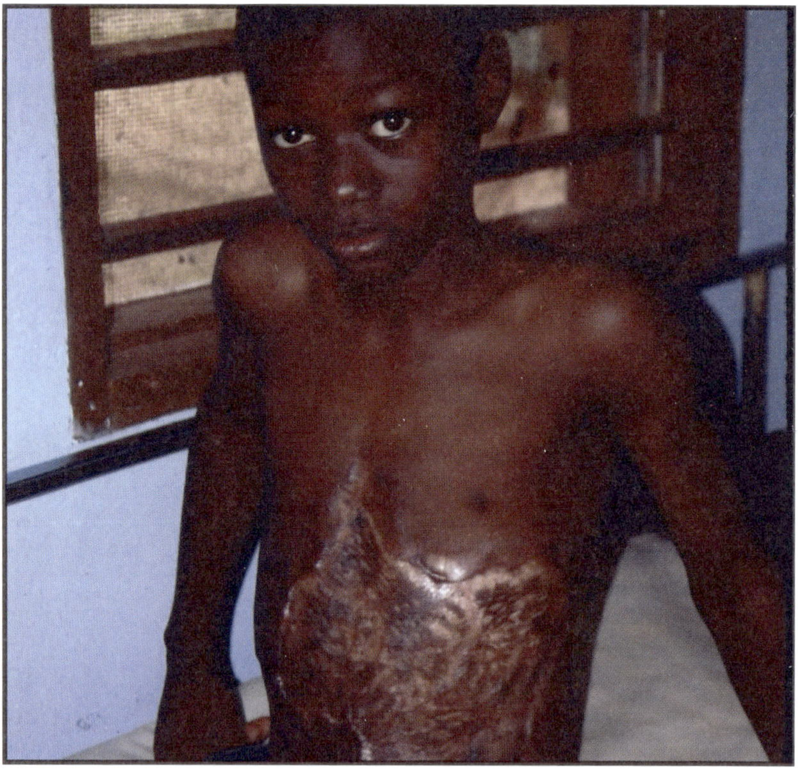

Donald, several years after his infection was surgically cleared and grafted.

Since those days, God in His mercy has led researchers to find an effective and affordable medical treatment for Buruli Ulcers that eliminates the need to surgically excise all infected tissues and cover the wounds with skin grafts.

What I can say about God's help for Donald as we were fighting for his life is what the psalmist wrote in Psalm 9:1-2– *"I will praise you, Lord, with all my heart; I will tell of all the marvelous things you have done. I will be filled with joy because of you! I will sing praises to your name, O Most High!"* In Deuteronomy 32:39 God sets the record straight: *"Look now; I myself am He! There is no other god but me! I am the one who kills and gives life; I am the one who wounds and heals; no one can be rescued from my powerful hand!"*

Saving Grace

The whole, heartbreaking tangle of events started simply enough: one day a seventeen-year-old pregnant girl wearing a torn, dirty dress wandered into Bongolo Hospital's outpatient clinic and asked for something to eat. She looked younger than seventeen and she informed the nurses in the maternity department that her name was Cornelia. She had walked 15 miles from Yishinga, a village of less than seventy souls in the dense forest west of Bongolo.

Cornelia may have been a seventeen-year-old physically, but her mind and emotions were that of a six-year-old. The demon gods still had a powerful grip in many of south Gabon's villages, including Yishinga. Cornelia's mother had five children and five husbands, and none of her husbands were supporting their children.

Cornelia was autistic, but by the time Cornelia was two her mother decided she was cursed. As Cornelia grew older her mother tried to control her using force and screaming at her. When Cornelia cried, she wasn't picked up and hugged, comforted, or loved, but was slapped, pinched, beaten, and shouted at until she obeyed. If she was fed, it was to stop her from crying. A more miserable child would be hard to find.

When Cornelia was in her teens a man in the village made sexual advances. Her mother and her older siblings laughed. When the man raped her, Cornelia was blamed. When she became pregnant, her family and neighbors shrugged. Cornelia's mother had five children by four different men, so how could she keep track of a crazy teenage girl if she disappeared from the village?

There was a s struggling Christian church in Yishinga that the early missionaries and pastors had established decades before. Once or twice a month, an itinerant pastor would come and lead a service, and he eventually helped the few Christians in village build a mud-brick chapel. Nevertheless, in most of the mudbrick and thatched homes the demon gods of Bwiti and Mwiri were worshipped, which meant that fear, threats, and hate were the most useful motivators for obedience, not kindness and love.

When Cornelia was six months pregnant, she left home and walked fifteen mi les through the forest to Bongolo Hospital. She was barefoot, unwashed, wore nothing but a ragged dress, and was famished. The nurses in the consultation area referred her to Maternity. The midwives immediately recognized that Cornelia was autistic and treated her kindly. They soon learned that she had left her family in Yishinga and had been mistreated.

With permission from the hospital director, they gave her food, cleaned her up, and evaluated her pregnancy. Since she was only six months along, they encouraged her to return to her village and her family until her next scheduled prenatal visit.

Cornelia had never experienced kindness from her family, so when the midwives told her to return home, she refused to leave. Instead, she found an empty bed in The Good Samaritan, a motel with twenty-five beds that the local church rented to outpatients who needed a place to stay. The cost was $ 2 a week, which she didn't have. Recognizing the complexity of her problems, the church let her stay anyway. For food, she stole or begged from others staying in the motel. This created such an uproar that she finally came to the attention of the hospital's pediatrician, Dr. Deborah Walker.

Dr. Walker gently and patiently drew from Cornelia her reasons for fleeing Yishinga and her family. When Cornelia's mother learned she was pregnant, she had locked Cornelia in a room for days at a time. Cornelia responded by attempting to set the house on fire. At that, her mother chased her away and told her to fend for herself. Someone in the village then told her that the people in Bongolo were kind and would help her, so she started walking. Whether that same person walked with her to Bongolo, or her heavenly father sent an angel to guide her, no one knows.

A week after Cornelia's first prenatal visit she had a grand mal seizure that lasted a full five minutes. She had suffered from seizures for years, but her family had never brought her to Bongolo for treatment. Out of compassion, Dr. Walker made the soon unpopular decision to give Cornelia a bed in the pediatric ward.

Once installed, Cornelia caused endless problems, stealing not only other patients' food, but also their belongings! The African ward nurses were kind-hearted, but they hadn't had any training on how to deal with autistic children. When simple kindness didn't work, they tried threats and anger. After a week, our African staff and many of the patients in the pediatric ward demanded that Dr. Walker discharge Cornelia and forcibly return her to her village.

We could all see that Cornelia had never experienced love and was severely incapacitated, but Dr. Walker couldn't bring herself to send the girl back to Yishinga, especially since it would probably end in tragedy. Her solution was to use her own money to buy daily meals for Cornelia, and she entreated our African staff to remember that Cornelia had the mind of a five or six-year-old child, not a teenager. She needed love more than discipline. Day after day Dr. Walker talked with Cornelia, gently but firmly explaining that Jesus loved her and wanted to become her father, but there were rules for staying in the hospital. When the ward nurses realized that Cornelia was responding, they did their best to follow Dr. Walker's lead. A sort of troubled truce was established.

Eventually, our African hospital administrator sent a request to Cornelia's mother to come and take care of her daughter, but Cornelia's mother never responded.

Cornelia's prenatal visits showed that her nutrition and general health had improved dramatically. With the regular medication prescribed by Dr. Walker, Cornelia's seizures became infrequent. Then one day she went into labor. Nobody slept that night in the maternity ward. Unable to comprehend the pain of her contractions, Cornelia fought the midwives, screaming at the top of her lungs until everyone was exhausted. In the middle of the night, she mercifully delivered a healthy baby girl!

The next day, Dr. Walker sent word to Cornelia's mother that her daughter had given birth to a normal, healthy child and that she needed to come and help care for her daughter and granddaughter. Once again, Cornelia's mother didn't respond. By this time, her daughter had lived at the hospital for more than four months.

When her baby was a month old and Cornelia seemed to be caring for her newborn under the supervision of the midwives reasonably well, our team decided the time had come to return both mother and baby to her family in Yishinga. One of our missionary nurses and midwife agreed to take them back to Yishinga.

When they arrived, they found Cornelia's mother and grandmother at home and encouraged them to see how much Cornelia had progressed. But neither of them was pleased to see the Cornelia. Arguing that they had too much work to do in their gardens just to provide food for the other members in their family, so they couldn't care for Cornelia and her baby. Carolyn refused to accept their excuses and told them it was time to shoulder their responsibilities for Cornelia and her baby. With that, she said goodbye to Cornelia and drove back to Bongolo. The hospital staff heaved a huge sigh of relief!

But three weeks later, Cornelia reappeared, holding a sickly two-month-old baby to her breast. Her baby was malnourished, covered with scabies, and was suffering from diarrhea from drinking river water. Dr. Walker hospitalized the two of them in the pediatric ward and once again, provided Cornelia with food.

To no one's surprise, Cornelia was not an attentive mother. Her mother and her grandmother's way of caring for children had taught Cornelia bad habits, such as pinching her baby when she cried, or slapping her in anger. Several times a day the hospital staff had to intervene to protect the little girl. At times, Cornelia would disappear for hours, leaving her baby on the bed for someone else to care for. Whenever this happened the nurses fed her baby and put the baby on their backs, carrying her around as they worked. Sometimes Cornelia would disappear for days. Not surprisingly, a bond began to grow between the nurses and Cornelia's little girl.

When Cornelia's baby was about five months old the nurses began calling her "Grace." Up until then she had had no name, since Cornelia couldn't make up her mind. The name "Grace" stuck, and as months passed Grace responded to the nurses' love and became more and more active and demanding for their attention. For her part, Cornelia was overwhelmed by Grace's needs and would periodically fly into a rage, screaming, weeping, and even hitting Grace before running away. Hours later she would return disheveled, dirty and contrite, and would sit quietly as the nurses or Dr. Walker scolded her, forgave her, and talked to her more about Jesus. Only when the nurses saw Cornelia was sorry and calm would they give Grace back to her.

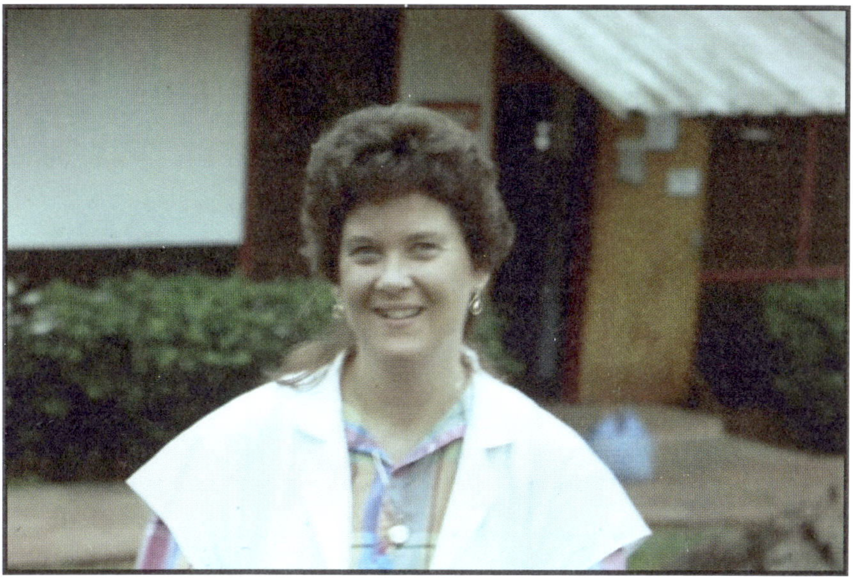

Dr. Deborah Walker

In addition to everything else Dr. Walker had to do, Dr. Walker and the hospital chaplain spent hours talking to Cornelia about how Jesus loved her and wanted to help her. Little by little their gentle and persistent explanations and assurances brought changes in Cornelia's behavior.

When Grace was six months old, Cornelia prayed a child's prayer with Dr. Walker, asking God to forgive her for her sin and inviting Jesus into her heart. She still had occasional rages and tantrums, but they occurred less and less frequently and didn't last as long.

One evening at the height of the rainy season, Cornelia went to the river to bathe, as was her custom, but never returned. The next morning, Dr. Walker went with Pastor Luke to the river to look for Cornelia. They found her sandals and clothes in a neat pile at the river's edge, but there was no sign of her. Suspecting that she might have drowned in the swift current, Pastor Luke sent word to her mother and grandmother that their daughter had disappeared. He then hired several men in canoes to search for her. Though they searched for miles downstream, the men found nothing. Two days later, a fisherman found her body. Our hospital maintenance men dug a grave and helped Pastor Luke and Dr. Walker wrap Cornelia's body in a blanket. We buried her after a simple service, and I wondered if her family was glad to be rid of her.

There are no orphanages in rural Gabon because up until recent times, there were no abandoned orphans. It is customary for the extended family to take in the children of deceased members and raise them as their own. So, when no one from Cornelia's family showed up to take Grace, the staff was conflicted. On the one hand Cornelia's mother had proven herself to be a careless and cruel mother, but in Gabon's culture and history, adoption was associated with child slavery. Several weeks passed while the nurses at the hospital continued to care for Grace, carrying her on their backs during the day and evening shifts, feeding and bathing her, and putting her to bed in the pediatric ward at night. Dr. Walker provided Grace with all the baby food and clothing she needed.

Several weeks later, Cornelia's mother finally appeared at the hospital with one of her own children, a thin, sickly, eight- month-old. She confronted Dr. Walker as she made rounds in the pediatric ward and told her that she had come to take her granddaughter home. The hospital staff responded to Cornelia's mother with a tidal wave of anger and indignation! Dr. Walker finally called the woman to her office to talk with her.

"Since your daughter Cornelia is no longer here to breast- feed baby Grace, how are you going to feed her?" she asked. "She can't eat solid food yet, and your own child is looking poorly nourished. You can't breast-feed your own child and Grace at the same time."

The woman shrugged and said, "I can't afford to buy her powdered milk."

Dr. Walker nodded and said, "Then perhaps Grace should stay here with us until she can eat solid food. That way, we'll know she's well nourished. We'll give you a place to stay so you can stay here near the hospital and take care of her."

Cornelia's mother shook her head and said, "I can't do that. I have to go back to my village to take care of my other children and keep up my gardens." After a long pause she said, "Since you're willing to take care of her, I'll leave Grace here with you for a while." The next day she returned to Yishinga.

Grace thrived on formula feedings and on the love and attention she got from the maternity and pediatric nursing staff. She filled out, reached her developmental markers ahead of schedule, and smiled and laughed easily. She was rapidly growing into a beautiful and delightful child. The only problem was that she had to be passed around with the nursing shifts like a sack of cassava! Added to that were the risks of living in the pediatric ward where there were all kinds of infectious diseases being treated.

Several months later, Grace's grandmother reappeared. By then, Grace was sitting up and crawling. Her grandmother saw how well she was doing and announced she was taking her home. When Dr. Walker heard the news, she sat down with her and again asked her how she could feed Grace while breast-feeding her own child– and caring for four other children, all without a husband's support. Even if she were to give Cornelia's grandmother formula and teach her how to mix it without boiled or filtered water, Grace's feedings would become hopelessly contaminated and result in chronic diarrhea.

Dr. Walker regularly saw children dying from diarrhea and malnutrition who were being cared for in rural villagers by their grandmothers. Many daughters from the villages went to the towns to attend high school, and many of them got pregnant and brought their babies back to the village for their mothers to raise.

To keep Grace healthy and happy, Dr. Walker invited Grace's grandmother to stay at the hospital and take care of Grace until she was old enough to eat regular food. Once again, Grace's grandmother angrily refused and returned to her village, leaving Grace in the nurse's care.

Grace's grandmother's threats led several of our African nurses to express concern that she might try to take Grace forcibly. Aware of this possibility, two of our missionary nurses named Terry Hotalen and

Karen Fitch volunteered to be Grace's foster parents until something acceptable could be worked out. They were deeply troubled that she was growing up in the hospital with haphazard adult supervision, not in a stable home. After praying for the Lord's guidance, the two women offered to take her to their home and care for her until something acceptable could be worked out for Grace's care.

The hospital administration, Dr. Walker, and the missionary team all agreed to Terry and Karen's plan. During the next six months, Grace settled into a safe and loving home and learned to walk, swim and speak words in both French and English. Several times a week, Terry brought Grace down to the hospital to visit with her numerous nurse-aunts and uncles, and on many days, she played with the other children her age on the mission compound. Grace soon blossomed into an inquisitive and affectionate child. But everyone knew the happy arrangement could not last forever.

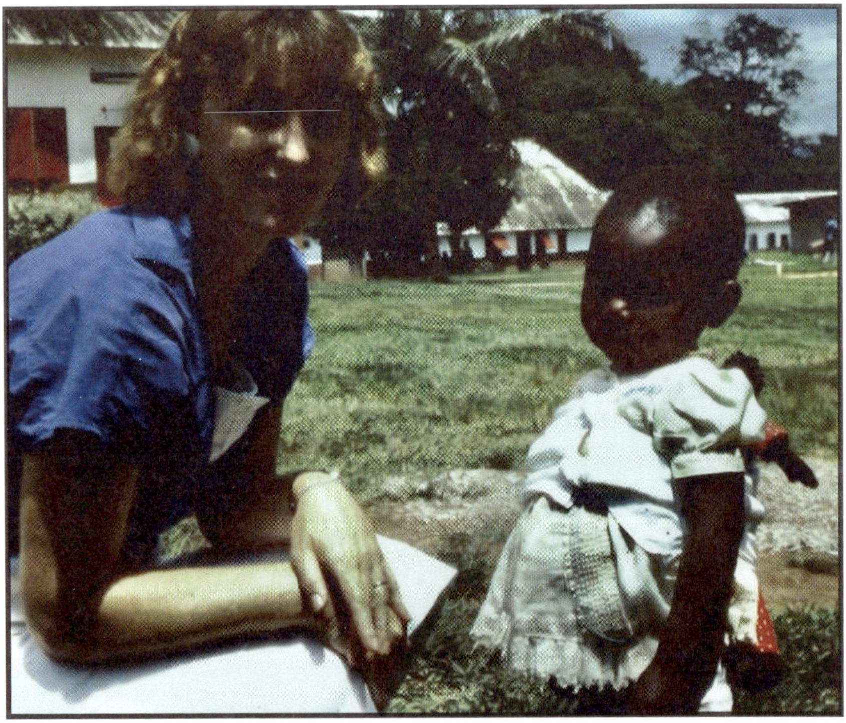

Nurse Terry, who for a year became Grace's foster parent

Gabonese tradition and law dictated that Grace's grandmother could not be indefinitely denied the right to take her grandchild home— even if she was incapable of caring for her, and this was the attitude of the local Gabonese authorities. It did not matter that her family had done nothing to help Cornelia give birth to Grace. Nor did it matter that returning Grace to her grandmother would relegate her to a life of poverty and perhaps even prostitution. As the conflict grew bitter, a wall of prayer rose to God from the hospital nurses and the missionary team on her behalf.

One day Grace's grandmother reappeared and came directly to Terry and Karen's door demanding that they hand Grace over immediately. When they refused and explained that the problem could not be settled that simply, the grandmother stood outside and screamed curses at them for several hours!

The next day, Pastor Luke called me over to his office for a meeting with him, Dr. Walker, and Grace's extended family, which had suddenly expanded to include one of Bongolo's three chiefs, a local congressman, a blind uncle we had never seen before, and an uncle who made a good living as a builder in town! Since Cornelia's first appearance, we had been told that the only family members in existence were Grace's grandmother and great- grandmother!

The irony of the family's sudden interest in Grace made it difficult for me to stay calm. The first to speak was the congressman. He thanked us for caring for Cornelia and went on to explain that since Grace's mother had had several lovers at the time he had known her, he could not be considered Grace's grandfather. "Since in Gabonese tradition children belong to the maternal side of the family," he continued, "I cannot be obliged to take responsibility for either Grace or her mother. Nevertheless, out of the goodness of my heart, I am offering to pay all of the expenses Cornelia and Grace have incurred up to now."

I could have told him then that I had in my pocket a complete and up-to-date accounting of those expenses totaling

$1,600, but since I doubted his sincerity, I kept quiet. The congressman finished his statement by emphasizing his unequivocal opposition to anyone outside of the family adopting Grace.

This ignited the blind uncle we had never seen before. He was a third or fourth cousin to Grace's grandmother, and to our surprise he launched into a passionate denunciation of our plans to sell Grace into slavery to recoup our losses! All of the other members of the family seemed to share this opinion except the congressman, who squirmed in discomfort. As the blind uncle's voice rose, Dr. Walker, Terry and I fought to keep our composure. Pastor Luke listened as though he were carved in stone.

When everyone from Grace's family had spoken, Pastor Luke calmly explained that the only thing the hospital wanted was for Grace to be raised with a mother and a father who loved her and would provide well for her needs. He asked, "Can't you find a Christian couple in your family or in the local church who could adopt Grace?"

To this, Grace's grandmother bitterly complained that Grace was hers by right and she would not accept that she be given to anyone else! This was more than Dr. Walker could handle, and trembling with suppressed anger, she left the room.

I leaned forward in my chair and, looking directly at Grace's grandmother said, "Since Cornelia was born and since Grace's birth you have never cared for either of these two children. As the medical director of this hospital, I will *never* agree to let you take Grace and raise her in Yishinga. If I did, I would be agreeing to child abuse!" There was an audible gasp from the blind uncle. Grace's grandmother stood and left the meeting in a rage.

Over the next forty-five minutes, those who remained in the meeting agreed that the best solution might be for our midwife, Julienne, and her husband, who was somehow related to Grace's family, to take Grace and raise her as their own child, since they were childless. Several weeks later, we were surprised to hear that in a separate meeting with Pastor Luke, Grace's grandmother had agreed to the arrangement! But the plan fell apart in less than two weeks. Julienne was suffering from a hernia and had to be scheduled for surgery the following week, so Terry agreed to keep Grace until Julienne recovered from her surgery.

The next day, the mayor from Lébamba and the chief of police stormed angrily into Pastor Luke's office.

Without even greeting him the mayor shouted, "Where is Dr.

Thompson? I demand to see him immediately!"

Pastor Luc stood and politely asked the mayor to sit down while he found me. But the mayor was too angry to sit. Instead, he stormed around outside the office while Pastor Luke went looking for me. He found me in the middle of an operation.

Concentrating on what I was doing, I told him I would come as soon as I finished, though it might take an hour. When pastor Luke explained this to the mayor, he threw up his hands and angrily ordered us to appear at his office the next morning at 8 a.m. sharp. He did not specifically state what he was angry about, but we surmised it had to do with Grace and my refusal to let her be taken back to Yishinga by her grandmother.

The next morning at 8 a.m., Pastor Luke, Terry Hotalen and I arrived at the mayor's office. We were surprised to find him sitting behind his desk in a suit and tie. In contrast to his demeanor the previous day, he was polite to the point of meekness. We chatted like old friends for about thirty minutes, until Grace's grandmother and a young woman she introduced as her younger sister, Veronica, entered the office, accompanied by the chief of police. After everyone was seated, the meeting got underway.

The mayor explained that Veronica was a close relative of Grace's grandmother and that she and her husband had agreed to take Grace and raise her as one of their own. They and their four other children lived in Franceville, 280 miles to the east. The couple had a comfortable home, and Veronica's husband earned a good income in a high paid government job. Veronica explained that she regularly attended the Alliance Church in Franceville and was a believer. She very much wanted to resolve the impasse over Grace's future by adopting her and raising her as one of her own children.

After Veronica finished talking, the mayor cleared his throat and explained that the reason he had come so suddenly to see us the day before was because the two women had come to his office and wept over the injustice of their situation, until he could bear it no longer. He hoped that by bringing us all together we could come up with a solution that would be both legal and would please everyone. Reassured by his conciliatory tone and by Veronica and her husband's evident maturity, we listened. The chief of police explained that if we agreed to the arrangement, he would write up a document that we could sign.

After a moment's silence, I asked what would keep Grace's grandmother from demanding that Veronica give Grace back to her the moment we drove away? Everyone shook their heads and vowed that such a thing would never happen. Though deeply skeptical, I gave my approval.

An hour later, the Chief of Police presented us with a document outlining the agreement. All of us signed our names to it.

To help Grace adjust to what would certainly be a painful separation and readjustment, Terry invited Veronica to come to her house to visit and play with Grace several hours a day. This seemed to go well, and after five days Veronica took Grace with her and left for Franceville. The separation was as traumatic for Terry as it was for Grace, but it seemed to be God's path to a good solution. Grace would now have a permanent home with a Christian mother and father who promised to love her and care for her as one of their own. Or so we thought.

A week later, a patient from a village on the road to Yishinga brought us the news that Grace and her aunt were both back in their village. It seemed unlikely, so we waited until we could confirm it. Two weeks later, an evangelistic team from the Bongolo church preached at the Yishinga church and saw that Grace was living with her grandmother. The villagers told them that Veronica had returned to Franceville without Grace! The news settled like a black cloud over the hospital and missionary staff. I was so troubled that the next day I went to see the mayor. Had he and the Chief of Police been in on the deception too? If I was ever going to trust the mayor again, I had to know.

When I told the mayor that Grace was back in the village with her grandmother, he seemed genuinely surprised. Before I left, he promised to send the police chief to investigate and report back. But five days later when Terry talked to the police chief, he said he knew nothing about it. I again took off from work at the hospital to see the mayor, but he was away. I didn't manage to see him until a week later.

This time, the mayor had more news. The Chief of Police had hitched a ride to Yishinga and had found Grace in the care of a nine-year-old girl. All the adults in the house had gone to the forest to work on their gardens, leaving the children by themselves for the day. He said Grace was dirty and unclothed but seemed to be in good health. He asked me if Terry was prepared to take Grace back on a moment's notice if he went and got her. I hadn't had time to ask her, but I told him I was sure she would accept to take care of Grace until Veronica could return.

The mayor had no car and asked if I could take him to Yishinga the following Sunday, but when I came to pick him up, he had left town, postponing again Grace's rescue. It was as if the demons of hell were playing games with us!

Days dragged into weeks as more delays, excuses and missed appointments continued. It gradually became clear that the mayor had no intention of rescuing Grace. The day after Christmas the mayor sent me a message, "My hands are tied and there is nothing I can do!"

Had the family threatened the mayor with sorcery? Had it become too politically messy? The mayor never explained, but Pastor Luke believed that Grace's grandmother had probably threatened to use sorcery against him if he interfered.

I was scheduled to leave in a few days on a month-long trip to the U.S. and Kenya. That morning as I prayed, I felt God directing me to go to Yishinga and confront Grace's grandmother. The next day, I drove Terry and the pastor of the Bongolo Church to Yishinga.

When we pulled into the village, a crowd of about thirty people quickly gathered. Many who came and greeted us were Christians or patients we had treated at the hospital. None of them expressed animosity, and several pointed out the grandmother's house and smiled knowingly as we walked towards it.

It was more a broken-down wooden shack than a house, worse than most of the houses in the village. It was built of thin, hand-hewn softwood boards nailed to a framework of vertical poles. The roof was covered by rusting roofing tins. Hearing a commotion, Grace's grandmother emerged from the house and greeted us with a scowl. After we explained that we had come to talk to her about Grace, she turned and motioned us brusquely inside. I had to duck to get under the five-foot high doorway, and once inside, my head was touching the rafters. The inside of the house was about six feet wide and maybe ten feet long, with a bedroom door on each side. The floor was packed earth, slanted and uneven. A wobbly table and chair were the only pieces of furniture. Someone brought two more chairs for us to sit on.

Within minutes, five or six distant relatives had crowded into the house. The only window, a two-foot square next to the door, was open, and two or three people leaned through it while others stood in the doorway. The room was stifling hot, and everyone seemed to be talking at once.

A minute later Grace's grandmother came out of one of the bedroom doors with Grace on her hip. She had awakened her from a nap, and the little girl was groggy. My heart sank when I saw how dirty and disheveled she was, and tears rolled down Terry cheeks. She had a large boil on her thigh, probably from an infected insect bite. When Grace saw Terry, she cried angrily and clung tightly to her grandmother. Terry softly talked to her and gently stroked her leg, and Grace looked at Terry and stopped crying.

In the midst of the crying and confusion, the pastor motioned for silence and explained why we had come. Then it was my turn, and I told Grace's grandmother that we were angry and upset that she had broken her promise and had taken Grace away from Veronica and had brought her back to Yishinga. She had lied to us, to the mayor, and to the chief of police. As I talked, a murmur of dissent spread around the room.

When I stopped, all heads turned to hear what Grace s grandmother would say. She shifted Grace to her other hip.

"I did not break my promise," she said defiantly. "The problem was Veronica's husband. He refused to take Grace, so I had no choice but to bring her back here!" We would later learn it was just another lie.

I looked at Terry, and she shook her head in disbelief.

About then, a middle-aged man smelling strongly of alcohol crowded into the room. Swaying slightly, he introduced himself as yet another one of Grace's multiplying uncles. How was it possible that she had become the cherished object of such a large and adoring family? In a long and rambling speech, he lent his support to the grandmother's lie. Then, to everyone's surprise, he concluded by saying that the missionaries should take care of Grace so there would be peace between the hospital and the village of Yishinga! A chorus of for and against noises arose from the crowd. Then Grace's grandmother motioned that she wanted to speak, and everyone quieted.

"You can talk all you want," she said as she hung tightly onto Grace, "but I'm never going to give up this child, either to you or anybody else!"

It was about 100 degrees in the airless room. I could feel the heat from the sun radiating through the roofing tins, and perspiration dripped off our faces and onto our clothes. Looking at Grace with obvious compassion, Terry spoke to the crowd for the first and last time.

"What you are doing to this little girl is wrong. You made a promise to us, to the mayor and to the Chief of Police that you would give Grace to Veronica and her husband, relatives of yours who have the means to take care of her, love her, teach her about God and give her a good education. Instead of keeping your promise, you deceived us." When she stopped, there was silence.

The pastor added a final word. "You can deceive men, but you cannot deceive God. He will have the last word in this matter. If you loved her more than you love yourself, you would give her to your sister and her husband to raise. You may get your way, but you are opposing God. If you insist on doing it your way and this child dies of neglect, you will be responsible for her death."

In the uneasy silence that followed, we pushed our way out the door. As Terry walked past Grace and her grandmother, her eyes followed Terry until she disappeared into the SUV and drove away.

One month later the Director of Social services in Lébamba came to the hospital to talk to us about Grace. It was the first I'd heard that Lébamba had such a person, and that he was only *now* aware of Grace's case! After introductions, he told us he had recently traveled to Yishinga to meet Grace and her grandmother and see how Grace was doing. He had quickly concluded that she was being badly cared for. The next day he drove 350 miles to Libreville to present her case to his superiors. They urged him to intervene and either place Grace with her aunt Veronica in Franceville or bring her to Libreville for adoption.

A week later, the governor abruptly and inexplicably replaced our mayor. When the Director of Social Services returned and recounted the entire convoluted story of Cornelia and Grace to the new mayor, he told the Director of Social Services to deal with the situation himself. The next day he came to Bongolo and explained the situation. Terry prayed that God would give him unusual courage and the boldness to do the right thing. When we opened our eyes, he thanked us with a look of amazement. Not until later did we realize what an impact that prayer would have on him.

Two weeks later, the Director of Social Services in Lébamba asked Pastor Luke, Terry and I to attend a meeting in his office with the mayor. It was a busy weekday morning, but since it was about the life of the precious little girl God had led us to save and protect, we canceled our appointments and drove to his office.

The Director was obviously nervous as Terry and I entered his office. The mayor, he explained, wasn't able to join us. Nevertheless, he wanted to report what he was trying to do. He had gone to Yishinga and on his own authority had ordered Grace's grandmother to bring Grace to Lebamba to meet with us. He had given her money for the trip and had fully expected her to come. He had also sent an official message to his counterpart in Franceville, ordering Veronica to travel back to Lebamba and explain her failure to take Grace with her to Franceville. We waited for two hours, but neither Grace's grandmother nor Veronica showed up.

For next month, there was no further news about Grace. Then, in April of 1998, the Director for Social Services again asked to see us. Veronica had come back to Yishinga and had reportedly taken Grace to Franceville without stopping in Lébamba to meet with him. He wondered if we would be willing to contact our missionaries in Franceville to check on Grace. We agreed to send them an e-mail and to ask them to be on the lookout for Veronica and Grace.

In May, we heard from Ray and Maureen Holcomb, who lived in Franceville. A woman holding a little girl had come up to them after church and introduced herself as Veronica. She had then introduced them to a little girl named Grace. The Holcombs invited Veronica and her daughter to their house for lunch and spent a pleasant afternoon with them. Grace appeared to be well cared for and happy. Her new mother explained that their family regularly attended one of the Alliance churches in Franceville.

Several years later, we received a report from the President of the Gabon Alliance Church that Grace was at an orphanage in a coastal town north of Libreville. The woman in charge of the orphanage was a member of local Alliance church and brought her children to church every Sunday. Grace was apparently one of the children living at the orphanage, and she was doing well. We were surprised but never found out why she had left her foster mother, Veronica. A decade later we heard that she was adopted by a Pastor and his wife who lived in Libreville and had other children. The pastor's last name was Nguémba, so from then on, she was known as "Grace Nguémba." After the pastor and his wife died, she continued to live with the Nguémba house with their surviving children.

Jesus said in Matthew 18:10, "*See that you do not look down on one of these little ones. For I tell you that their angels in heaven always see the face of my Father in heaven.*"

Like a mother eagle, God swooped down and lifted little Grace out of a life of squalor and hopelessness and gave her instead a life filled with love.

Chapter Nine:

A CLOUD THE SIZE OF A MAN'S HAND

By the early 1990's, I realized that my dream to serve God as a missionary surgeon was being fulfilled. Unfortunately, my capacity as a surgeon was nearing its limits. I was the only surgeon for roughly 200,000 people, which was not as bad as the numbers other missionary surgeons in Africa were facing. On average I was performing twenty to twenty-five operations a week, six or seven days a week. When I had to perform an emergency procedure above the diaphragm, I would put my patient to sleep with sodium pentothal, intubate him, and then turn him over to my best African nurse to keep him alive while I performed the operation. More times than I can recall I had to break scrub and take over to keep my patient alive— then rescrub and resume operating. I was on call for all emergencies 24/7, and ninety per cent of the time I was the only surgeon within 350 miles.

While I was grumbling about my long hours at Bongolo, Dr. Harold Adolph was serving 1,800 miles to the north at Galmi Hospital in Niger. He later wrote about a day when he operated for 12 hours on emergencies, finishing after dark. He was one of five formally trained surgeons in the entire country of Niger. In 1990 the population of Niger was 7.8 million, making Dr. Adolph the only surgeon for roughly 2 million people! He would later write, "It was a completely overwhelming situation, and I prayed more than I ever had in the past." I certainly did not have it as bad as Dr. Adolph.

Every four years, Becki and I returned to the U.S. with our kids and reconnected with our supporters in Alliance Churches and our families. During those years, a number of courageous surgeons stepped away from their mission hospitals or practices in the U.S. and stood in for me. The first one was Dr. Bob Greene, an orthopedist and general surgeon who served with his wife Elaine in Zaire (DRC) and Ethiopia for three or four decades. In addition to asking congregations to continue supporting us, we were blessed by the many who generously contributed to Bongolo Hospital's expansion. In 1989 and 1994, we shared with more than 30 churches Bongolo Hospital's urgent need for another missionary surgeon to join me. Of course, my wild stories of life and medical practice in Africa were perhaps not much of an inducement for young doctors and their families to uproot themselves, move to Africa, and work 100 to 120 hours a week on a missionary salary! Only God could make it happen, but God had some wonderful surprises in store!

Bongolo is a 4-hour drive from one of the most beautiful beaches in the world. We loved to take our kids on week-long or 10-day vacations twice a year and camp on the beach. We would often see chimpanzees, parrots, elephants, and other wildlife, and the fishing was fabulous! But when we arrived back in Bongolo, there were always patients with surgical emergencies waiting for my return, often for days. For some, I came back too late. There were other times when I operated half the night before coming home. I began to pray and ask God daily to call another surgeon or two to come help!

Back in 1978, Becki and six other missionary nurses started a three-year nursing school and began training nurses for our hospital. One of the nurses was Moukoumbi Etienne, who excelled in his classes. After he graduated, I added him to our surgical team. First, I trained him to circulate and assist in the operating room. He was bright, conscientious, and a quick learner, so I began teaching him surgical skills and minor surgical procedures. He did so well that over the next year I taught him how to give spinal anesthesia, perform C-sections, repair inguinal hernias, and perform simple urological procedures.

The next year, I taught Etienne to operate on strangulated hernias that required bowel resection and anastomosis (sewing to cut ends together). This provided a mostly successful solution for the trips to the capital city that periodically I had to make, as well as week-long vacation times. But Etienne did not have the training to improvise, and we all knew that in a culture that justified vengeance, a mistake that caused a patient irreparable harm or death would result in severe consequences, including death threats. While this provided a temporary bridge, it was not a long-term solution for the hospital.

By 1994, I had been asking God for surgical help for four years! God had answered many other prayers, so I couldn't understand why he didn't answer this one! He had provided wonderfully for a new surgery ward, a two-story HIV/AIDS building, an expansion of the maternity ward, and later for a new ophthalmology building. So why wouldn't he answer my prayer for another surgeon or two?

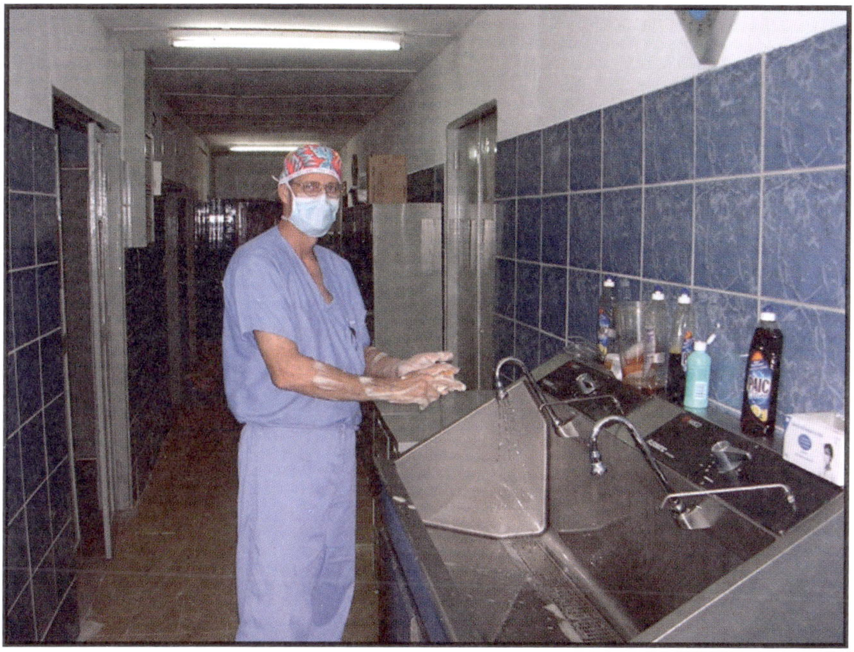

"*You* train them David!"

One early morning as I was again praying pleading for help, God spoke just four words: *"You train them, David."*

Surprised, I smiled and said to myself, "Wow, now that was a random thought!"

Almost immediately, the Lord said it again, "*You train them, David!*" Aghast, I said, "Lord, how in the world could I do that? I'm working as hard as I can already, the government would never approve, and who would apply to learn surgery *here*?" My complaints sounded a bit like Moses, and that's when I knew in my heart that God was serious.

A few months later, Becki and I received an invitation from the Christian Medical and Dental Association to attend a Conference in Kenya for medical missionaries. We had been wondering how we could maintain our medical credentials, and this sounded like a good solution. We signed up for the conference and a few months later, flew to Nairobi. The conference was scheduled to take place at a retreat center called Brackenhurst. It turned out to be a beautiful and restful conference center. Not only were there lectures for the major medical specialties, like internal medicine, general surgery, pediatrics, and more, there were lectures for nurses too!

Halfway through the conference, several missionary surgeons from hospitals in Kenya called for surgeons attending the conference to meet in the late afternoon. Only six of us showed up, and to my surprise, the topic was the growing shortage of missionary surgeons! Several noted that as missionary surgeons reached their seventies and retired, younger surgeons were not volunteering to take their places. Since the 1960's, hundreds of mission hospitals across Africa had closed for lack of surgeons! Even gloomier was the realization that multiple informal efforts to train African surgeons in mission hospitals "on the job" were neither recognized by African governments nor producing the broadly qualified surgeons Africa needed.

The most troubling observation that came out of our meeting was that nobody had a workable plan to solve the problem! All but two of were working alone, were overworked, and were discouraged. I was the youngest surgeon there, but for some reason, young, Christian American surgeons weren't responding to a call to "burn out for Jesus in Africa!" Towards the end of the meeting, I brought up the idea of starting residency programs in our hospitals, though I didn't share that God had said to me earlier that year, "You train them, David!" The consensus was that a training program could only happen if some of us left our hospitals and joined one or two of the big hospitals in Kenya, some of which already had two surgeons on staff. Notably, nobody at the meeting volunteered.

Over the next two years I prayed for a clear vision of how we could move forward. Little by little, God gave me an idea. If for five years I used the same curriculum that I was taught as a surgery resident, the same textbooks, the same way of teaching in the operating room, weekly reading assignments and quizzes, and we required our residents to take an annual examination before advancing to the next level, it might be possible to train surgeons! Of course, we would also have to include a discipleship program for our residents, but that was not our biggest challenge. I had no idea where to start.

In January 1996, I wrote a letter to the Christian Medical and Dental Society (now the Christian Medical and Dental Associations) asking for their help to pull together the various mission hospitals in Africa and help us establish a program to train and disciple African surgeons. I thought that in time, such a project could become one of the most effective and prestigious training programs in Africa.

A few months later, Becki and I flew to Kenya to attend our second CMDA— Continuing Medical Education Conference for medical missionaries at the Brackenhurst Retreat Center. This time we recognized many from the previous conference and made many new friends. On the second day of the conference, I asked all of the missionary surgeons and lecturers to meet with me after lunch to hear a proposal for surgical education. About five other surgeons showed up. At that meeting I shared the vision God had given me to join with other missionary surgeons and mission hospitals and begin training and discipling Christian African surgeons at our hospitals. From the moment I began talking, there was intense interest.

The next day, about ten surgeons and the CMDA-CME Coordinator, Gerald Swim, attended our meeting. Others who attended included several surgical lecturers, most notably Dr. Bruce MacFadyen from the Medical College of Georgia, Dr. Adrian Park, missionary surgeon Harold Adolph, Dick Bransford from Kijabe Hospital, Bob Greene from the DRC, and Dr. Bob Foster from the Evangelical Hospital of Lubango, in Angola. On February 14, 1996, as the conference drew to an end, ten or eleven of us agreed to establish the Pan- African College of Christian Surgeons (PACCS), which shortly after we amended to the Pan-African Academy of Christian Surgeons (PAA-CS). After signing our names to a simple charter, we asked God for His guidance, for His provision for the needed finances, and for applicants. We had no money, no mandate from any government to proceed, no curriculum, and no applicants. Nevertheless, our doctors in all of the mission hospitals we represented. Gerald Swim would be the secretary of the organization and would represent us to the CMDA, along with Dr. MacFadyen, a former president. We also agreed that I would serve as a "PAACS Coordinator."

Some who were present were concerned that African governments would oppose us, but I argued that because most African governments were not training surgeons for the needs of their people, they might instead be grateful that mission hospitals were doing it. All of us could see that no matter how many missionary surgeons we recruited, there would never be enough to fill the widening gap between Africa's burgeoning population and surgical needs. Recruiting more expatriates would only increase Africa's dependency on foreign surgeons and would not build competency within the African healthcare sector.

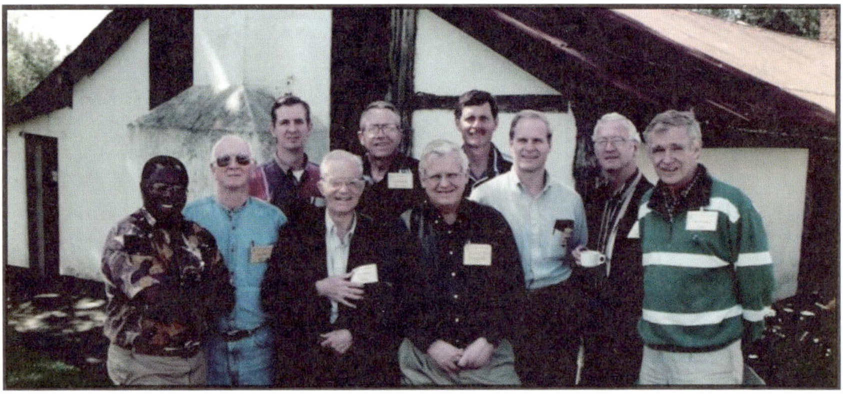

The twelve missionary surgeons who signed the PAACS charter that day included Dr. Harold Adolph, from Galmi Hospital in Niger; Dr. John Fletcher, from Good Shepherd Hospital in Tshikiaji, Zaire; Dr. Dick Bransford, from Kijabe Hospital, Kenya; Dr. Bob Wesche, Tenwek Hospital, Kenya; Dr. Robert Greene, from Virunga Hospital, Zaire; Dr. Bob Foster, from Evangelical Hospital of Lubango, Angola; Dr. David Fort, from Baptist Medical Centre in Gambaju, Ghana; Dr. Henri Obiang, from Dongola Hospital, Cameroun; Dr. Stan Tople (from Zaire?); Dr. Susan Smith, Mr. Gerald Swim, the CMDA Representative for the conference, and myself.

None of us could have known that our step of faith would be like "the cloud about the size of a man's hand rising from the sea" that Elijah's servant initially saw as Elijah began praying for rain. As Elijah continued to pray, the cloud grew into a mighty thunderstorm that ended years of drought and famine in Israel, drenching the land with blessing! (1 Kings 18:44).

Though initially we didn't have funding to either support our residents financially or build housing for them, there was so much excitement among Christian surgeons and missions- minded churches that within a year, we received enough money to build and furnish the apartments we needed and financially support our residents in Bongolo.

Several months after the meetings at Brackenhurst that led to the establishment of PAACS, I received a letter from a Dr. Paulo Baltazar, an Angolan doctor who was working with Dr. Stephen Foster at the "Centreo Evangélico de Medicina do Lubango" (CEML). Dr. Foster had attended some of the discussions that led to PAACS and encouraged Dr. Baltazar to apply. Surprised and excited by God's answer to my prayers for an applicant, I quickly created an application form and mailed it back for Dr. Baltazar to fill out, along with a request for a letter of recommendation from Dr. Bob Foster, who knew him well. A few weeks later I received Dr. Baltazar's completed application and recommendation letter. After consulting with our "PAACS Advisory Group," in August of 1996, we accepted Dr. Baltazar to be our first general surgery PAACS resident!

Midway through the year, I received a second application, this time from Madagascar. The applicant had the longest name I had ever seen: Rasamimanana Sahalanirina Harison! He was working at a Lutheran Hospital in the capital of Madagascar and had learned surgery "on the job" while working for several years with missionary surgeons. We accepted him to start in August of 1997. In August of 1998, I added another applicant to our program. By 2001 we had three more Christian residents, bringing our total to five residents.

During those first years of our residency program, I was the only long-term faculty surgeon. Soon after we started, however, God began calling American surgeons to come for weeks at a time and help train my residents with weekly academic lectures and operate with them. They also gave weekly academic lectures and developed quizzes over the residents' weekly reading assignments. In addition to academic lectures and hands on training in the operating room, I also asked our visiting surgeons to lead some of our weekly Bible studies. Our goal from the beginning was to develop a two-track curriculum that included both academic and spiritual teaching. I also taught our residents to pray with their patients and share the gospel with them. A constant reminder of the two roads every person must choose between was a painting that a visitor painted on the waiting room wall.

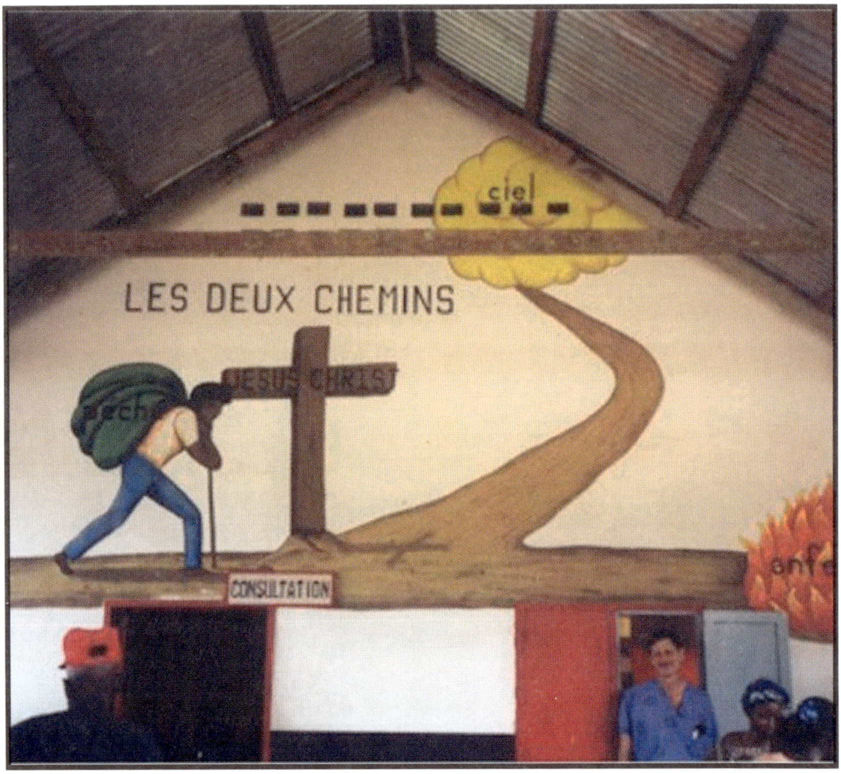

From the beginning, our goal was to train excellent African surgeons who would unashamedly share the gospel with their patients. By the fourth year of our surgical training program in Bongolo, my residents were completing their weekly reading assignments in their Ameri- can surgical textbooks, taking emergency calls at night, performing increasingly complex operations, and passing the toughest annual examination I could devise. If they passed the exam, they advanced to the next level of training. If they failed, they repeated the year.

Two years after we started training our residents at Bongolo Hospital, Becki, my two residents and I attended the bi-annual CMDA meeting in Kenya. During the 10-day conference a number of American Academic Surgeons joined our board and strongly encouraged us. These included Canadian pediatric surgeon Dan Poenaru, a Canadian pediatric surgeon, Dr. Adrian Park, a surgical program director in Baltimore, and Dr. Bruce Steffes, a remarkably gifted teacher and general and vascular surgeon from North Carolina.

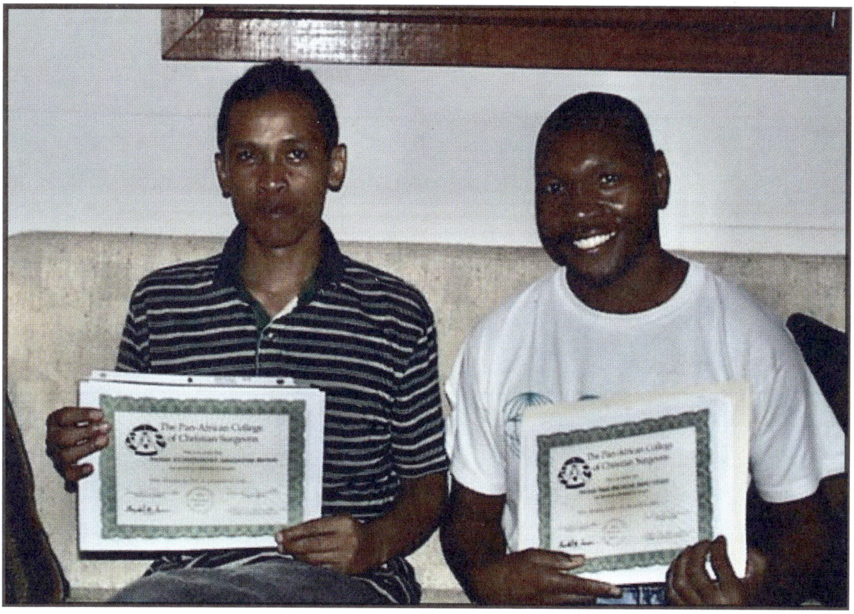

The first two PAACS graduates

In 2002, Dr. Harison and Dr. Baltazar passed their 5th year examinations and graduated. Dr. Harison and his family returned to serve at a Lutheran Hospital in Madagascar, where at the time of this writing, he still serves as a surgeon. Because Dr. Baltazar had to learn two languages (French and English) he had to spend an additional year in Kenya learning English and graduated the same year as Dr. Harison. Dr. Baltazar returned to the CEML mission hospital in Angola where he is still serving.

By the time Drs. Harison and Baltazar graduated, five residents were in training with PAACS at Bongolo Hospital. The residents were a tremendous help, but as the PAACS Coordinator I needed to respond to requests to visit mission hospitals in Cameroun, Niger, and Ethiopia that wanted to open training programs under PAACS.

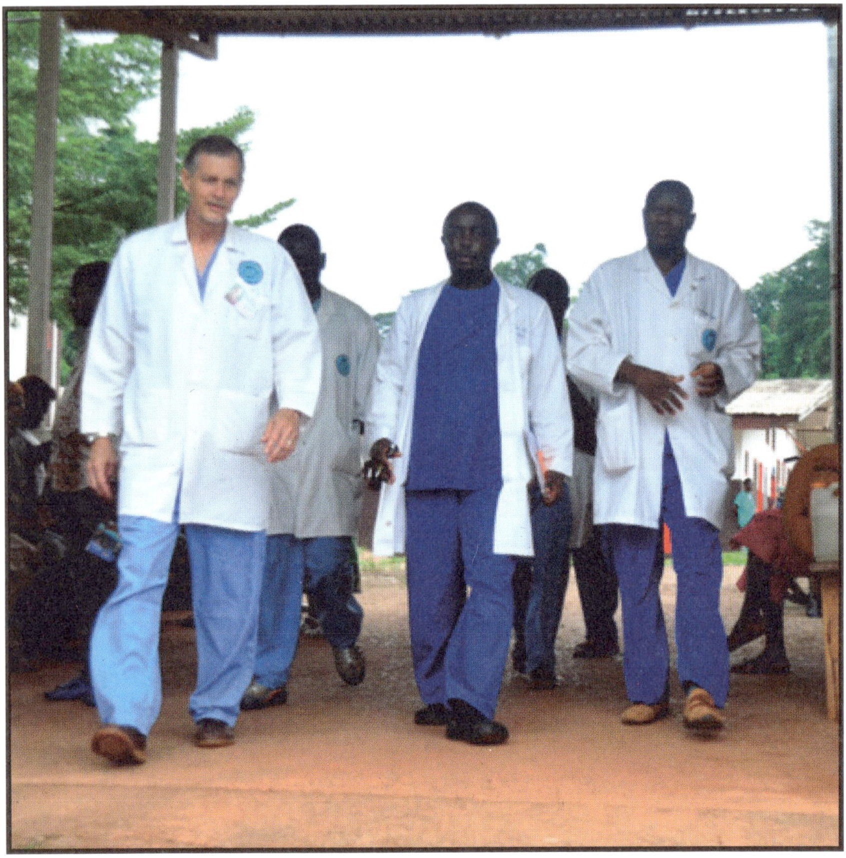

Dr. Thompson with his residents.

By 2005, the challenges of training my residents in Bongolo and at the same time helping start new PAACS programs at other Christian hospitals in Africa became overwhelming. In February, Dr. Bruce MacFadyen and I asked Dr. Bruce Steffes to take on the role of CEO of PAACS. We had no funds to provide him with a salary, no clear job description, and no funds to cover his travel expenses between Africa and his home in North Carolina! A month later he graciously accepted the challenge. Over the next eleven years under Dr. Steffes' leadership, PAACS grew from two training sites to nine, from nine surgery residents to 76, from three graduates to 59, and from 12 board members to 20! In 2013, PAACS was finally able to begin paying Dr. Steffes a modest salary and cover his travel expenses.

That same year a young surgeon named Keir Thelander joined our team in Bongolo, giving us two faculty surgeons.

In 2017, Dr. Steffes stepped down as the PAACS CE. Susan Koshy took over as the PAACS CEO, and Dr. Keir Thelander became the Executive Vice President of PAACS.

Today the surgical specialties open to Christian African residents through PAACS include pediatric surgery, orthopedics, pediatric orthopedics, neurosurgery, head and neck surgery, obstetrics and gynecology, anesthesia, plastic surgery, and cardiothoracic surgery. Two additional specialties in urology and surgical endoscopy will soon be added.

Because of God's foresight and blessing and the extraordinary leadership God has provided over the years, PAACS continues to open new training programs at Christian hospitals in Africa. PAACS has also been recognized by two of Africa's colleges of surgery, the West African College of Surgery (WACS) and the College of Surgeons of East, Central, and Southern Africa (COSECSA). PAACS has also received strong academic support from Loma Linda University in California, which granted PAACS the right to include its logo on PAACS diplomas. Every two to three years, members of Loma Linda's surgical faculty visit the PAACS training programs to review them and make recommendations for improving its academic training.

Another encouraging development has been the rapid increase of PAACS faculty surgeons. When I started in 1996, I was the only faculty member! Today more than 70 Christian faculty surgeons are training PAACS residents, one third of whom are PAACS graduates. The rest are career missionaries.

As of 2025, PAACS was financially supporting 190 residents —both men and women– in 28 surgical training programs at 18 mission hospitals, and at an annual cost of $5 million. At the time of this writing, more than 180 PAACS-trained surgeons have graduated and are serving the poor in 25 African countries. Were all the events that came together to create PAACS simply a result of the hard work and sacrifices of good people? The answer is no! The Master Architect of this remarkable ministry is God. Every day that I was privileged to train and disciple my African residents, I got to watch God's transforming work in their hearts, see their families grow in faith and the knowledge of God's Word, and rejoice with them as they shared the gospel with their patients! Like me, our PAACS residents came to believe and live by the words the Apostle Paul wrote in Ephesians 2:10: "*For we are God's masterpiece. He has created us anew in Christ Jesus, so we can do the good things He planned for us long ago.*" They learn in weekly Bible studies and through the struggles of life what God means when He says through the Apostle Paul in 2 Corinthians 2:9-10, "*My power works best in weakness. So now I am glad to boast about my weaknesses, so that the power of Christ can work through me. That's why I take pleasure in my weaknesses, and in the insults, hardships, persecutions, and troubles that I suffer for Christ. For when I am weak, then I am strong.*"

Conclusion:

CRUSHING THE CURSE

The curse of Bongolo Falls came from demons, God's rebellious and twisted angels. But it was only a small portion of Satan's ancient, worldwide, and destructive work. The Bible tells us that before Satan rebelled against God, Satan was one God's most beautiful and powerful angels in creation. When he revolted, he took with him a third of the angels that to this day serve in his rebellious army. Though Satan's fallen angels deceptively claim to be God's servants, their goal is to enslave the human race and disrupt God's merciful and gracious plans for the world.

In 1933 when Don Fairley and Joseph Nicholson arrived in the village of Makombo, the tribes of south Gabon believed that their demon gods Bwiti and Mwiri were their friends and protectors. The Fairleys didn't know that they were some of the world's most impoverished and miserable people. They didn't know that Satan's demons had deceived the village people into believing that there were no natural deaths, and that their neighbors and even their relatives were the cause of their sorrows through secret sorcery. Husbands did not marry their wives for love, but for sexual pleasure, to have women to grow their food, and to give them children. That only a quarter of their children would survive to adulthood seemed inevitable. Only the Ngangas could know which enemy had caused a family member to die, and they learned who the guilty were by consulting their treacherous spirit Gods, Bwiti and Mwiri. Worse yet, the punishment for the accused wasn't banishment, shaming, or whipping. The punishment for those accused of murder by sorcery was death! The result were constant executions of falsely accused villagers which only weakened the tribes. The people's worst fears, miseries, and sorrows were the works of the very demon gods they worshipped.

The contrast between the rule of the demon gods and the rule of Jesus was almost too great measure. That Jesus would die for their sins was at first incomprehensible. To become a child of God, they only had to turn from worshipping the demon gods, destroy their fetishes and idols, and believe in a Godman named Jesus who died on a cross for their sins and forever afterwards called those who believed in Him His children!

The contrast was too huge to comprehend and burst into the darkness of their lives like an explosion of light. Even Ngangas who repented and believed in Jesus were freed from the curse of their demon gods! Men and women who had worn fetishes around their necks since childhood to protect themselves from evil now burned their fetishes publicly, were baptized, and became exuberant followers of Jesus! In the place of misery and unending sorrow, there was now peace and joy!

Within a decade, young men who loved Jesus and were discipled and walked to distant villages to preach God's Word. When the missionaries opened a Bible school in Bongolo, some became evangelists and pastors. The result was that within two decades, the gospel of Jesus was being proclaimed to many of the tribes in the south! With every advance of the church of Jesus, the blessings of God grew greater, and the curse of the demon gods grew weaker. Within five decades there were Alliance churches in every province in Gabon, led by capable and spirit-filled Gabonese pastors.

But it wasn't just the spiritual war that was won. Where fetishes failed to protect the people from leopards, prayer chased them away! Where villagers once hated their neighbors, Christians from all the tribes learned to love each other! Where once they trembled as they approached Bongolo Falls, now they laughed at the idea that human souls lived under it and rejoiced that God sent His servants from the other side of the world to turn water to light! Where once disease, accidents, and childbirth ended the lives of thousands, excellent and affordable healthcare was available at Bongolo's Hospital.

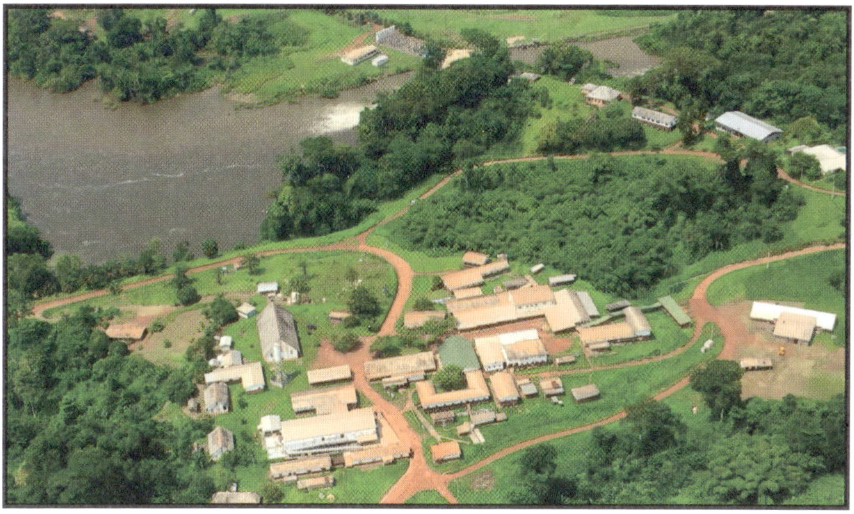

Bongolo Hospital in 2020

In three decades, Bongolo Hospital grew from two small buildings to twenty-five, and continues to grow to expand its services. Twenty years after Becki and I arrived in Bongolo, dam builders from Canada harnessed the river and the falls, installing huge turbines that today produce electricity for Lebamba and three other southern towns. Because the government built the dam on Bongolo's land, Bongolo receives electricity from the dam at no cost! Then in 1997, Gabon, Canada, and the United States provided the money to build a bridge across the Louetsi River.

Sixty years before all these events happened, Bwiti, Mwiri and their Ngangas ruled a kingdom of fear and misery. But when Jesus came, the Gospel of Jesus brought life, forgiveness, blessing, and light to a dying and sin-cursed land.

Becki and I still marvel that God turned us away from Asia where we wanted to go, and instead sent us to Gabon, a country we had never heard of. It wasn't in Africa that I saw a seriously injured man die and wondered where his soul would awaken; it was in Asia. But that vision would take us to Africa.

Once more I return to Ephesians 2:10 where the Apostle Paul wrote, "*He [God] has created us anew in Christ Jesus, so we can do the good things He planned for us long ago!*"

From the moment Don Fairley and Harold Pierson took ownership of the Bongolo property in. 1936 and brought the gospel to people in darkness, the curse of Bongolo Falls began to die. By the time our medical team arrived in 1977, it was a fading legend. In its place, God went on to create a lasting blessing— a hospital that has ministered to hundreds of thousands of sick and suffering Africans, has led more than 20,000 to faith in Jesus, and that continues to this day to proclaim the Good News of Jesus to all who come.

The hospital was a great and wonderful blessing, but God wasn't finished! More than 60 years after the Fairleys and the Piersons set foot in Bongolo and began proclaiming the Good News of Jesus to Gabon's southern tribes, God chose little Bongolo Hospital to host the first surgical training program of the Pan-African Academy of Christian Surgeons. Since 1996, Bongolo Hospital has graduated 23 African surgeons who today are serving the sick and proclaiming the gospel of Jesus in Guinea, Mali, the Democratic Republic of Congo, Angola, Zimbabwe, Madagascar and Cameroun, and continues to train more! But God's vision was greater than that.

As more and more training programs opened up at Christian hospitals in Africa, God sent thousands of short-term surgeons and specialists to help and support the new training programs. He also raised up hundreds of Christ proclaiming surgeons from the United States, Europe, and Australia to come with their families and serve in PAACS training programs for *decades*! At the time of this writing, PAACS has opened training programs in 22 Christian hospitals in Africa, and the number continues to climb. To date, God's servants in PAACS have trained and discipled more than 180 gospel-witnessing surgeons. Two of our graduates have died (one from Ebola and the other from cancer, but the rest are serving the poor in 25 African countries). At the time of this writing, 190 more future surgeon-evangelists are being trained and discipled by PAACS. I am asking God to enable PAACS to graduate and send out a thousand Christian surgeons by the end of this decade. Only God could carry out such a marvelous plan, and in His grace and wisdom he chose to start PAACS in the humblest of places: Bongolo!

As a missionary physician, my goal in life was to love God with all my heart, obey Jesus in every situation, serve my patients to the best of my ability with compassion and love, and proclaim the Good News of Jesus Christ to all of our patients. It never even occurred to me that God might use me to be a small part of crushing the curse of Bongolo Falls and turning it instead into a growing blessing for Africa.

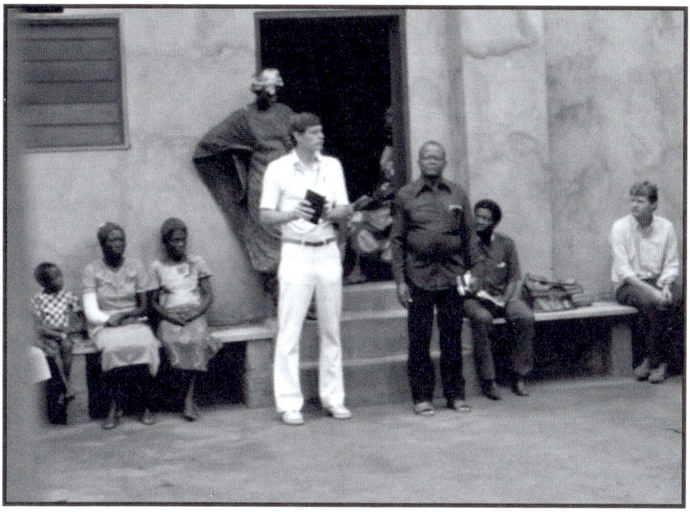

Psalms 66:16-20 states my closing thoughts:

"Come and listen, all you who fear God, and I will tell you what He did for me. For I cried out to Him for help, praising Him as I spoke. If I had not confessed the sin in my heart, the Lord would not have listened. But God did listen! He paid attention to my prayer. Praise God, who did not ignore my prayer or withdraw His unfailing love!"

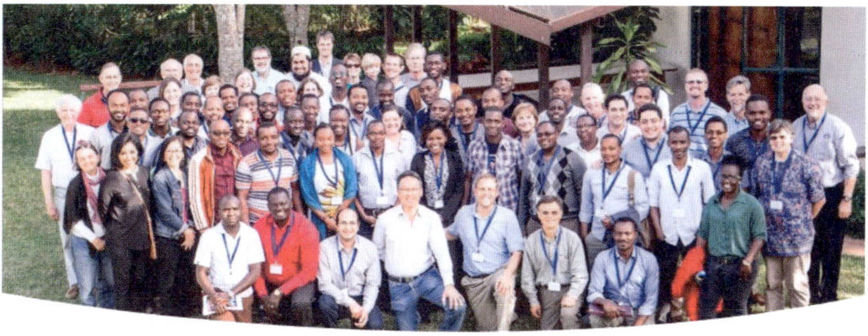

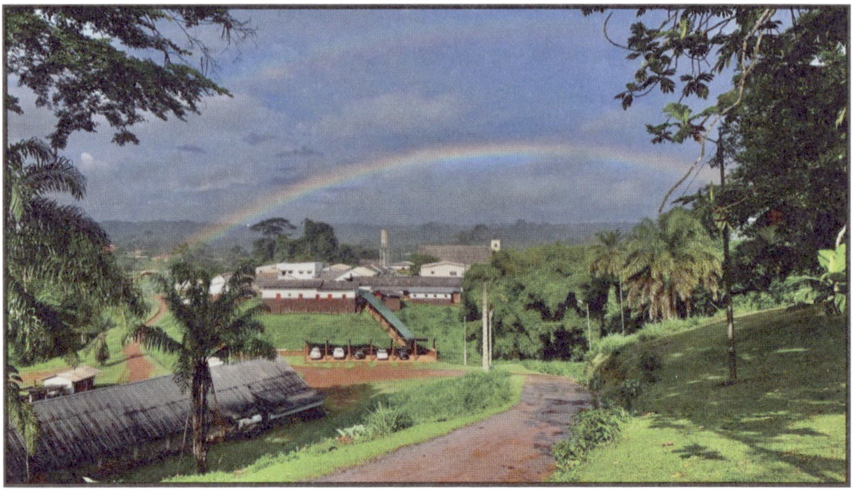

The End

REFERENCES

1. Chambers, Oswald. *My Utmost for His Highest,* Barbour Books, 1963, https://a.co/d/5FcWYiu, Accessed 23 October, 2025.

2. Fairley, Donald. *Hunting Pygmy Hunters,* Fundamental Truth Publishers, 1929.

3. Grudem, Wayne. *Systemic Theology: An Introduction to Biblical Doctrine,* Second Edition, 2020, pp.464-5.

4. *New Living Translation Bible,* Tyndale Publishers.

5. Pan-African Academy of Christian Surgeons, https://paacs.net/.

6. Payne, Karl I. M.D. *Spiritual Warfare: Christians, Demonization, and Deliverance,* Republic Book Publishers, 2020, p.129, https://www.worldofbooks.com/products/spiritual-warfare-book-karl-i-payne-, Accessed 24 October, 2025.

7. Reimer, Reg. *On the Cruel Edges of the World:* A memoir of carrying help and hope into dark places in dangerous times, 2024, https://a.co/d/dGvRNQ3, Accessed 17 October, (Amazon).

8. Taylor, William, Antonia van der Meer and Reg Reimer. *Sorrow & Blood: Christian Mission in Contexts of Suffering, Persecution, and Martyrdom (Globalization of Mission),* 2012, https://a.co/d/1u63N1w, Accessed 17 October, 2025(Amazon).

9. Thompson, David M.D. *Beyond the Mist, The Story of Donald and Dorothy Fairley (The Jaffray Collection of Missionary Portraits),* Moody Publishers, 2002, https://a.co/d/2B1XsPF, Accessed 17 October, 2025(Amazon).

ABOUT THE AUTHOR

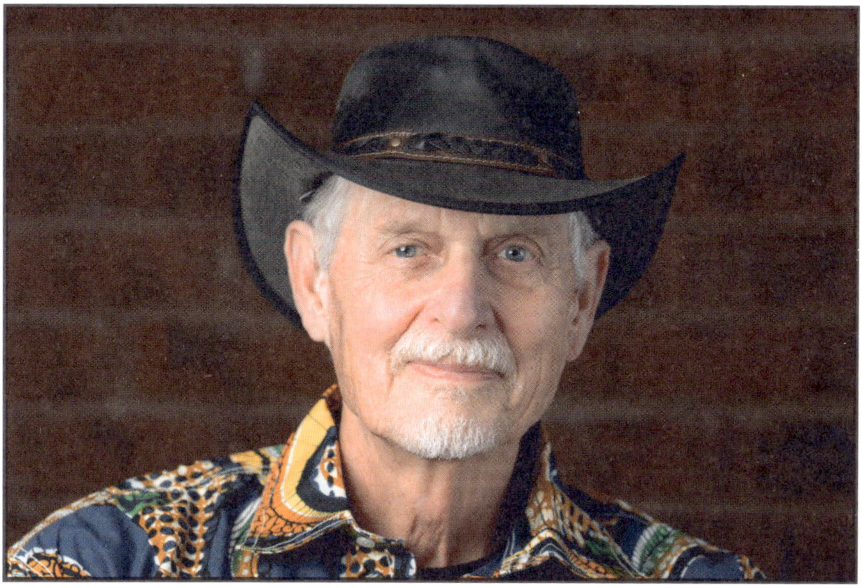

Dr. David Thompson is a retired Alliance missionary surgeon who, with his wife Rebecca, served under the Christian & Missionary Alliance at Bongolo Hospital, in the country of Gabon, for 35 years, and at Harpur Memorial Hospital in Egypt for 5 years, retiring in 2018.

David grew up in Cambodia, the son of missionary parents Ed and Ruth Thompson, both of whom were martyred in Banmethuot, Vietnam, in 1968. David and his wife Becki married in 1971 and have three children and six grandchildren. He is currently retired and living in Redding, California. He is currently 77 years old.

Dr. Thompson led the Alliance team in Gabon that built Bongolo Hospital. Since the hospital's inception, more than 20,000 patients have come to faith in Jesus and many churches have been planted in the region, several of which the Thompsons personally started.

In 1996, Dr. Thompson helped establish the Pan-African Academy of Christian Surgeons (www.paacs.net), and in 1997 started the first PAACS program to train African doctors to be surgeons at Bongolo Hospital. Between 2013 and 2018, Dr. Thompson and his wife Rebecca moved to Egypt to open a new PAACS training program and a nursing school, both of which are still thriving. The Thompsons left Egypt in December 2017, after turning their work over to other IW's.[1]

Since retiring from fulltime missionary service in 2018, Dr. Thompson has remained active on the PAACS Board of Directors and on the Bongolo Hospital board. He has made several trips to Gabon and this year served as the Interim Medical Director of Bongolo Hospital during the month of June. He also serves on the board of Bongolo Friends and of Partners in Evangelism (PIEI) Grace Hospital, a new hospital in Isiro, northeast DRC that one of the surgeons he trained is heading up.[2]

Here in Redding, Dr. Thompson is a part-time volunteer, be-friending and serving Redding's homeless community by providing primary medical care in homeless camps as needed, sharing the gospel with those willing to engage, and working with other volunteers from Redding's churches to develop resources that will help the homeless overcome addictions and rebuild their lives.

Dr. Thompson has authored five books describing his years of overseas experience: *On Call, The Hand on My Scalpel, Beyond the Mist, Christian Mercy, and Training God's Surgeons for Africa.* His latest book, *The Curse of Bongolo Falls,* is a revised compilation of *On Call* and *The Hand on My Scalpel. The Curse of Bongolo Falls* has been revised to give readers an exciting, chronological look at Thompson's time in Gabon, Africa. New content has been added to reflect the years that have passed and the stories that have transpired since the original two books were published.

When asked why he became a writer, Thompson explained that the incredible, miraculous and true stories that he witnessed were not his, but that they belonged to God. Therefore, the stories must be told.

1 IW's: an abbreviation for International Workers.

2 Isiro is a city in northeast Congo that grew up during the endless civil war in that region as refugees fled their villages. Today it has half a million people.